SURGERY IN INFANCY AND CHILDHOOD

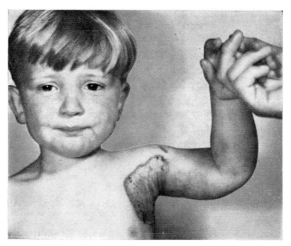

Wringer injury.   Child's arm was drawn into the wringer of
an automatic washing machine (see Chap. III).

Surgery in Infancy and Childhood

A HANDBOOK FOR MEDICAL STUDENTS AND GENERAL PRACTITIONERS

BY

MATTHEW WHITE

M.A., M.B., Ch.B., F.R.F.P.S.(Glas.), F.R.C.S.(Edin.)

Consulting Surgeon, Royal Hospital for Sick Children, Glasgow.
Lately, Barclay Lecturer in Orthopædics and Surgery in relation
to Infancy and Childhood, University of Glasgow. Consulting
Surgeon, East Park Home for Infirm Children.

AND

WALLACE M. DENNISON

M.D., F.R.F.P.S.(Glas.), F.R.C.S.(Edin.), F.I.C.S.

Barclay Lecturer in Surgery in relation to Infancy and Childhood,
University of Glasgow. Surgeon, Royal Hospital for Sick Children,
Glasgow. Pædiatric Surgeon, Royal Maternity and Women's
Hospital and Stobhill General Hospital, Glasgow.

E. & S. LIVINGSTONE LTD.

EDINBURGH AND LONDON

1958

Printed in Great Britain

THIS BOOK IS DEDICATED TO

THE NURSING STAFF

ROYAL HOSPITAL FOR SICK CHILDREN

GLASGOW

PREFACE

THIS book is designed to introduce to the senior student some of the surgical problems encountered in infancy and childhood. It is not a book of reference for the pædiatric surgeon; it does not presume to be complete and in many ways it is unbalanced. We hope that some of the information within these pages will help to refresh the memories of our colleagues in general practice. The teaching is based on our experience in the Royal Hospital for Sick Children, Glasgow.

For approximately a quarter of a century the final-year medical student in the Glasgow Medical School has been required to attend a ten-week course on the problems of Surgery in Infancy and Childhood. In the Final Examination a compulsory question on Pædiatric Surgery is included in the written paper and clinical and *viva voce* examinations are also held. Much of the teaching is carried out at the bedside and in the out-patient department, but in the time available it is impossible to cover the subject adequately. The clinical teaching has therefore been supplemented by systematic lectures, tutorials and clinical-pathological demonstrations. This book is based on these lectures and demonstrations; we hope that it may replace many of the lectures and allow more time for bedside teaching.

Pædiatric surgeons and anæsthetists work in close collaboration with their medical colleagues, and we take this opportunity to thank Professor Stanley Graham, Dr J. H. Hutchison and their staffs for their co-operation. We are fortunate in our colleagues in the Departments of Pathology, Biochemistry and Radiology, whose specialised advice has greatly aided many of the recent advances in pædiatrics. It is a great pleasure to thank Dr A. M. MacDonald, Dr H. Ellis C. Wilson and Dr S. P. Rawson. Dr W. Auld, who guides us in the field of anæsthesia, wrote the section on Anæsthesia and Operative Care. The photographs, line drawings and X-ray reproductions are from the teaching library in the Department of Medical Illustration. They were prepared by Mr J. L. A. Evatt, and we thank him for his enthusiastic co-operation. Most of our own diagrams have been redrawn and greatly improved by Mr R. W. Matthews of Messrs E. & S. Livingstone. Mr J. J. Mason Brown, Mr J. F. R. Bentley and Dr Gavin Arneil read the original manuscript and made many valuable suggestions. We thank also Mr J. P. Fleming and Dr R. A. Shanks for their help in proof-reading.

The book could never have been completed without the secretarial assistance of Mrs J. Glover; she has cheerfully typed and retyped it many times. We thank her for all the help she has given us. We are grateful to the Editors of the following journals who have allowed us to reproduce illustrations which we have previously published: *Archives of Diseases in Childhood, Glasgow Medical Journal, Journal of Bone and Joint Surgery, Lancet* and *Surgo.* Finally, we thank Mr Charles Macmillan of Messrs E. & S. Livingstone for his patience and enthusiasm and for his guidance in the realms of the publisher's art.

MATTHEW WHITE.
WALLACE M. DENNISON.

GLASGOW, *April* 1958.

CONTENTS

ix

CHAPTER I

Surgery in Infancy and Childhood

PÆDIATRIC surgery is not a special branch of surgery but is the whole of surgery applied to a special age group. Between birth and puberty children suffer from many of the diseases which affect older individuals but they are also subject to developmental anomalies and to types of infection seldom encountered in later life. Many of the problems which arise in this age group cannot be dealt with in a small handbook but in this chapter we present some of the differences between children and adults, so that the reader may appreciate how the effects of disease and trauma are modified in the actively growing child.

The unborn child is designed to undertake what may very well be a traumatising journey. There is a protective mechanism which persists for several days after birth and should the infant suffer from some remediable developmental anomaly, he is usually well nourished, is fully supplied with blood and as a rule is a good risk for even major surgery during the first week of life. The protective mechanism is soon lost and from the end of the first week until the age of 3 months the infant is not such a good surgical risk and only essential surgery is carried out during this period.

In the growing child all the vital processes are extremely active. Along with intensive functional activity there must be corresponding structural changes and there is a continuous process of adaptation of structure to function. Not only has nature to make good the effects of ordinary wear and tear as in the adult, she has at the same time to undertake a constant series of replacements. Should the body structure of the child be damaged either by injury or disease, a process of repair sets in at once and the normal structure is restored with remarkable speed and exactness. The most obvious example is the repair of bone. A birth fracture is firmly united in fourteen to twenty-one days and a birth fracture of the femur which has been allowed to unite, literally at right angles with gross over-lapping, will in six to nine months be difficult to distinguish radiographically from the normal femur. Knowledge of this process of repair does not excuse careless obstetrics leading to birth fractures nor does it relieve the clinician of the responsibility for treating adequately such fractures when they do occur.

Children can recover quickly and completely from the immediate effects of even severe injuries which in the adult might prove fatal. Injuries which in the adult would require physiotherapy and rehabilitation and would lead to permanent disability may leave little or no trace and physiotherapy is rarely necessary. There is evidence that wounds of the liver, kidney and lung heal readily and with minimal scar tissue and organs such as the appendix can recover in a remarkable fashion from severe inflammation.

In recent years the reaction of the growing child to infection has presented a somewhat confusing picture. Few surgical infections are allowed to progress without the exhibition of some chemotherapeutic agent. We do not understand the mechanism whereby immunity to infection is developed, but it does seem clear that the defence is slowly built up during infancy and childhood. The newborn infant is bacteriologically sterile and one of his early problems is to select the organisms with which he intends to live in symbiosis and to repulse all the others. The passive immunity that he obtains from transplacental passage of maternal gamma globulins with antibody properties is transient and is followed by active immunity derived from repeated exposure to sublethal infections. The effect of the antibiotic group of drugs has been dramatic and life-saving through control of blood-stream infection. Before their introduction infection in infancy and childhood carried a very high mortality from septicæmia. For example, the mortality from acute hæmatogenous osteitis until about 1940 was over 30 per cent.; it is now less than 2 per cent. (Fig. 1). The indirect effect of the antibiotics upon the reaction of the tissues at the local focus and upon the develop-ment of immunity has yet to be assessed. The response of the fixed tissue cells at the local focus seems to have become slower and less violent. In many patients formation of a local abscess tends to be delayed and, indeed, in many cases aborted; in others the response resembles that of a chronic type of infection so that a pyogenic cervical adenitis may simulate tuberculosis. We have yet to learn what effect such changes may have upon the development of immunity during childhood. A further complication has arisen—particularly in hospital practice—in the appearance of strains of organisms resistant to one or more of the antibiotic drugs commonly in use. It is to be hoped that the human organism will prove equally efficient in acquiring resistance to these bacteria in turn.

Apart from the general reaction of the growing child to trauma and infection there are certain aspects of the growth process that give rise to surgical problems. Growth, like all living processes, is periodic in character. The normal growth curve of the human individual shows a steep ascending curve up to puberty, when it gradually flattens out and then remains more or less horizontal until the slight drop of old age occurs. When examined in greater detail the curve shows certain well-marked and distinctive periods of accelerated growth followed by longer intervals of slower growth. The first period

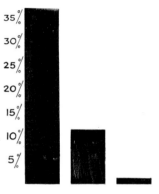

GROUP I   GROUP II   GROUP III

Fig. 1

Mortality from acute hæmatogenous osteitis during three five-year periods. Group I, before introduction of chemotherapy; Group II, treated with sulphathiazole; Group III, treated with penicillin.

of rapid growth is that of infancy, the second commences about 5 years of age when the child goes to school, and the third is that of puberty. Each of these periods of accelerated growth is accompanied by well-marked and characteristic anatomical, physiological and psychological changes. They are periods of instability during which disturbances of structure and function and indeed of health generally are apt to occur and they are periods when the so-called postural defects are commonly met with. The infant learning to walk is often a source of anxiety to the young parents. They fear he has " flat feet " because the everted heel and valgus posture of the normal child resembles the flat foot of the adult and the arch is obscured by the normal pad of fat in the infant foot. Or it may be that the infant turns in his toes and visions of a hen-toed, bow-legged child arise to worry the parents. This hen-toed gait is physiological rather than pathological and is soon abandoned as the child grows. No permanent deformity results as long as the child is given adequate periods of rest. One of the most interesting examples of this periodicity in growth is that afforded by congenital torticollis. Of a series of 180 children with this deformity 130 were aged from 5 to 12 years. Almost invariably it was not the parents who first noticed the wry neck, but, significantly, the school teacher or the school medical officer. The parents admit the presence of the deformity once their attention has been drawn to it but are emphatic in declaring it to be of recent origin. The explanation of this apparent lack of observation is that about the age of 5 a period of accelerated growth is normal. The neck and spine in particular grow rapidly and the shoulders " fall away " from the head. The shortened neck muscles and fascia, which have been present since intra-uterine life, are obscured by the normal short neck of the baby and young child and the deformity is revealed only when at school age the neck lengthens (Chap. XX). Another complaint common at this age is knock knee. This is a postural defect having no relation to rickets and common in young children " on their feet from morning till night." It is self-curing with adequate rest and avoidance of fatigue.

The most obvious and well-known period of rapid growth is that of puberty. It occurs earlier and more noticeably in the female and is associated with much more profound physio-logical and psychological changes. The faulty posture of this age group is well known—rounded shoulders, head thrust forward, slouching gait, knock knees and flat feet ; and the anxious mother complains that her child is always tired. Yet all the defects may be physiological in origin and due essentially to lack of muscle tone associated with this period of rapid growth. It is as though nature had arranged for a general slackening of muscle tone and joint ligaments to allow for the rapid lengthening of the bony skeleton. If, during this period, continued strain is permitted postural defects will follow. Adequate and frequent rest is the cure, although appropriate postural exercises will be of value. Our forebears were well aware of the postural defects of puberty, and classes in " deportment " were the forerunners of the postural exercises in the modern physiotherapy department. Not infrequently, there appears to be some loss of moral tone. Indeed in all these periods of postural strain there is often an associated psychological strain not unconnected with the anxiety of the parents—an element in the clinical picture that is often overlooked.

The endocrine glands present a most confused and variegated picture of growth activity. Each gland seems to have its own specific period of growth, reaching maturity and exerting its maximum influence at varying periods and in varying degrees. They seem to act as pace-makers, regulating and controlling the onset, rate of growth and senescence of every system in the body. When their growth is interfered with the various permutations and combinations of endocrine disturbance are endless.

Within the skeletal system itself there are many examples of inequality of the growth process. A physiological example is that of the well-known change in the body proportions from infancy onwards. The infant has relatively short limbs in comparison with the trunk but about the second dentition the arms and legs grow rapidly, the tibia and fibula faster than the femur, the forearm faster than the arm, and the changing proportions present a problem to the mother in adapting the clothes.

From time to time local inequalities of growth occur and may present surgical problems of peculiar difficulty. Developmental aplasia or hyperplasia of a limb or part of a limb is not infrequent and is usually beyond surgical aid. The short limb following anterior poliomyelitis is well known and in some cases the operation of leg lengthening may be called for to reduce the amount of shortening. Perhaps the most intractable inequality is that caused by damage to the epiphyseal cartilage, whether traumatic or inflammatory. The resultant inequality of growth is very difficult to control by any means, operative or instrumental, and may indeed call for amputation. By way of contrast, lengthening of one limb is by no means uncommon. It is usually caused by a local increase in the blood supply whether developmental, traumatic or inflammatory in origin (Chap. V). Hypertrophy of one limb does occur without apparent cause but the presence of multiple angiomata or of an arteriovenous shunt of developmental origin is always accompanied by an overgrowth of the affected limb. Fracture of a long bone, especially if allowed to unite with angulation or overlap, may be followed by a degree of temporary

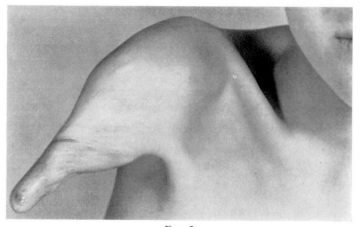

Fig. 2

" Conical stump " in boy of 11 years, following traumatic amputation six years previously.

lengthening more than sufficient to offset the overlap and even to the extent of requiring a temporary raising for the shoe of the sound leg.

It is evident then that in dealing with infants and children the surgeon must constantly bear in mind the fact that he is dealing with a rapidly growing organism and all his methods of treatment must allow for that fact. Not the least important result of growth is that a pair of shoes, a spinal brace or a leg caliper, specially and carefully made, may be too small in a few months' time. In an amputation stump the bone grows faster than the soft tissues and may require to be shortened on one or more occasions, lest it ulcerate through the soft tissues of the stump—the so-called conical stump (Fig. 2).

DEVELOPMENTAL ANOMALIES [1]

Parents whose child is born with some defect are always concerned to know the cause. Two questions are always put to their doctor : " Is the defect due to any fault in the father or mother ? " and secondly, " Will a second child be likely to have a similar or any other defect ? " Unfortunately a satisfying answer to either question is not always possible. It is now generally accepted that the genes are the particles responsible for the transmission of inherited characters. Any alteration in the genetic make-up of the germ cell may thus be represented in the offspring in the form of anatomical, physiological or biochemical defects. Spontaneous alteration in the structure or position of the genes is known to occur but we are largely ignorant of the cause of such mutations and the resulting defects are in the nature of an " occupational risk " for normal parents. In some cases the mutant gene is not lethal and may be transmitted to the offspring. Many such defects are thus familial in their incidence. Parents with a family history of such defects must accept a greater risk of producing a defective child and the increased risk applies to subsequent children. So many factors are involved that the laws of simple Mendelian inheritance cannot be applied and the risk cannot be expressed in figures. Where parents have one defective child the risk of a further child being also defective has been stated to be about twenty-four times greater than that amongst the population in general, when all types of defects are considered. Though in the past the mutation rate in any community has remained remarkably constant whether the resulting defect is lethal in the pre-reproductive age or not, there is increasing evidence that exposure of the gonads, at any age, to radioactive material is followed by an increase in the incidence of mutation.

Apart from defects of genetic origin there are other factors that influence the development of the embryo to such an extent as to cause actual defects. It is known, for example, that maternal rubella or vaccinia in the early months of pregnancy may cause such anomalies as congenital cataract, deaf mutism,

---

[1] The term congenital, so frequently used in relation to defects, should be employed only in its simple derivative sense of being present when the child is born and not with any ætiological connotation.

cardiac abnormalities and microcephaly. In the lower animals, vitamin deficiency has been shown to result in defects among the offspring but this has not been demonstrated in the human subject.

It has been suggested that intra-uterine pressure or adhesions have been the cause of anatomical defect in the offspring but the evidence is far from convincing and it seems likely that disturbances of growth and development are essentially genetic in origin.

MALIGNANT DISEASE IN CHILDHOOD

Malignant disease plays a large part in the mortality of childhood and more children die from neoplasm than are killed by motor vehicles in traffic accidents. The tumours which come within the province of the pædiatric surgeon are discussed briefly in appropriate chapters, but for the convenience of the student a survey of the present position is given at this point.

Leukæmia is the most common form of malignant disease in childhood. The disease is not often seen in the surgical wards of a children's hospital but patients with leukæmia present in the surgical out-patient department with palpable lymph nodes, enlargement of liver or spleen or with vague pains in the limbs. *Tumours of the central nervous system* are not uncommon. Most are astrocytomas or medulloblastomas and they are generally subtentorial. Vomiting is one of the early symptoms and unexplained persistent or recurrent vomiting in a child should always suggest the possibility of brain tumour. *Tumours of the sympathetic nervous system* are the highly malignant neuroblastomas and the more benign ganglioneuromas. Most arise from the adrenal glands but tumours may originate from any part of the sympathetic chain. *Nephroblastoma* (*Wilms' tumour*) of the kidney is the most common malignant tumour dealt with by the pædiatric surgeon. It is usually encountered in the first two years of life and presents with painless abdominal swelling. *Sarcoma* may present as a painless swelling anywhere in the body. Lymphosarcoma and reticulosarcoma may be difficult to differentiate from one another and some children diagnosed as suffering from lymphosarcoma may develop the blood picture of leukæmia.   True bone sarcomata are uncommon.   *Teratomata* are most commonly seen in the sacrococcygeal region but they occasionally present in the testis.   Other malignant tumours seen in childhood are the *rhabdomyosarcoma* of bladder or vagina and *primary tumours of the liver* and the *salivary glands.*

Few surgeons have extensive experience of malignant tumours in children.   From our own experience, we have been impressed by the number of apparent " cures " following early surgery and we feel that every solid tumour in an infant or child should be investigated at the earliest possible moment.

CHAPTER II

Pre-operative Care, Anæsthesia and Post-operative Care

WHILE many advances in surgery are due to the availability of blood, plasma and plasma substitutes, to chemotherapy, to the great advances in anæsthetic techniques and to detailed attention to pre-operative and post-operative care, another factor applies in the advances in pædiatric surgery. A staff which devotes the major part of its time to pædiatrics learns to understand the child himself. The nurse is a very important member of the surgical team and, particularly in the surgical problems of the newborn, it is skilled nursing more than any other factor which influences the sick infant's prospects of survival.

PRE-OPERATIVE CARE

Infants and small children cannot be prepared mentally for admission to hospital nor can they understand the significance of the procedures that are carried out on their persons. We do not yet know what permanent psychological trauma is inflicted on an infant or young child by separation from the home and parents and it is fashionable to stress the mental upset which follows admission to hospital. In the older child, the parents and family doctor should attempt to explain to the child that he is going to hospital to have his pain taken away, that the parents will be coming to see him every day and that he will soon be home again. Children vary in their adaptation to hospital life. Some proclaim their immediate displeasure in a loud voice, others merely take a reluctant interest in all that goes on around them. Most children settle down quickly but they should, as far as possible, be allowed to do so in their own time. They are, by nature friendly and co-operative ; they look to the hospital staff for that friendship and they must not be let down. We must never say that a procedure such as a pre-operative injection of atropine will not hurt, because we know quite well that it will. If we do, the child will distrust everything we say. There *are* some spoiled and badly brought up children but usually if a child is completely unco-operative, he or she is ill or scared or both, and much patience may be required before the patient's confidence is gained and anxiety dispelled.

Feeding.—An infant should never be starved before operation and unless there is some obstruction the stomach is empty two hours after a feed. The last feed four hours before operation should be replaced by glucose water. The older child should be allowed the normal evening meal the night before operation. If the patient has been seriously ill and is dehydrated and starved, any time available before operation is devoted to at least partial correction of the fluid loss by administration of parenteral fluid. Minor degrees of electrolytic imbalance will be restored when the underlying surgical lesion is corrected. Routine use of enemata is quite unnecessary and only when a surgical attack is planned on the colon, rectum or anus is there any necessity for pre-operative irrigation of the bowel.

Intravenous Fluid.—The renal function of the neonate differs from that of the adult in that there is inability to excrete excessive sodium load. This continues until the child is 3 months old, when there is some improvement, but it may be three years before adult efficiency is reached. Fluid requirements must therefore be carefully assessed since excess readily produces œdema and death. In the early months of life, normal saline should never be given and hypotonic saline only is administered. One-quarter normal saline or glucose saline and the plasma substitutes all have their place.

Blood.—If a long or extensive operation is to be performed, the patient's blood is typed and matched beforehand. If the hæmoglobin is below 10 g. per 100 ml., no surgical procedure is carried out until the anæmia has been treated by transfusion of whole blood.

In older children, blood and intravenous fluids can usually be given through a needle inserted percutaneously into a vein in the cubital fossa.   In all babies and most infants fluid and blood can be given into a scalp vein (Fig. 3) or into a vein on the back of the hand.   If the infusion is to be continued

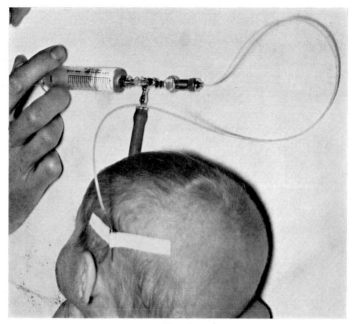

Fig. 3
Transfusion into scalp vein of infant.

throughout the operation it may be advisable to cut down on the saphenous vein at the medial malleolus and to insert a metal cannula or fine polythene tubing.

Sedation.—In young infants pre-operative sedation is rarely necessary and only atropine is given.   Over the age of 2 years a child should never be taken to the operating theatre unless he is asleep or at least drowsy and unafraid.   A satisfactory pre-operative sedative for children has yet to be found but the barbiturates, morphine and pethidine all have their place. Average doses are tabulated in the section on Anæsthesia (p. 17).

Vitamin K (Synkavit, 1 mg.) is administered pre-operatively to all newborn infants since they usually have a bleeding tendency due to transient hypoprothrombinæmia.

OPERATIVE CARE AND ANÆSTHESIA

The response of infants and young children to anæsthesia and surgery presents problems which cannot be solved by regarding the patients as small adults. Pædiatric patients differ from adults in many ways which are of importance to the anæsthetist. Their physiology and anatomy are different, their response to pain, illness and surgical stimulation is different; so, too, is their power of recovery. These factors vary also in the several age groups into which the patients can be divided. A knowledge of these differences is essential for the anæsthetist, and consideration of them and of the nature and duration of the proposed surgical procedure determines the choice of anæsthetic.

OPERATIVE CARE

Respiration.—In infancy respirations are shallow and rapid. The thoracic muscles are weak and in the supine position the abdominal viscera press upon the diaphragm and embarrass respiration. Surgery and anæsthesia stimulate respiration, and the respiratory rate may be thus increased from 40 to 100 breaths per minute. If allowed to continue this will produce exhaustion and shock. The tidal air and dead space so closely approximate each other that only a few cubic centimetres are available for respiratory interchange and a condition of marginal anoxia exists. Atelectasis is a common condition at birth and varies from partial to complete, but a considerable degree of atelectasis is compatible with adequate oxygenation.

The oxygen requirement of children is greater than that of the adult, and infants and young children cannot tolerate anoxia. The anæsthetic, therefore, must be so designed that full oxygenation will be maintained throughout.

Blood Loss.—The blood volume of the newborn infant is given as 100 ml. per kg. body weight, so that the normal full-time infant may be expected to have 350 to 400 ml. of blood. This may be diminished by 100 ml. if the umbilical cord is cut too soon. It is essential that the circulating blood volume be maintained and blood loss must be accurately estimated during operation by weighing swabs, and blood is replaced as it is lost.

Temperature Control.—The temperature regulating mechanism of the neonate is inefficient and the infant's temperature tends to vary with that of its environment and should be carefully watched, especially after operation. During operative

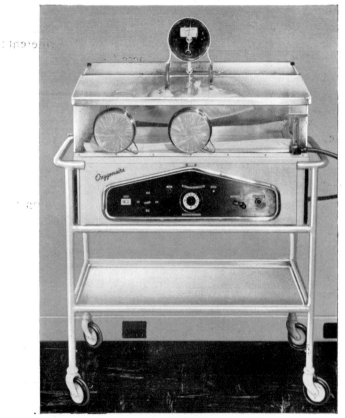

FIG. 4
Modern Oxygenaire incubator.

procedures the temperature falls: 2° or 3° F. in a short operation such as a pyloromyotomy for pyloric stenosis; 10° F. in a longer procedure such as repair of œsophageal atresia. Incubators are now available which allow accurate control and the temperature should be brought up to normal levels within three hours (Fig. 4).

Nervous System.—The nervous system is not fully developed at birth. Pain sensibility, though present, is not well developed and it may be six weeks before the pain sense in the skin shows normal adult levels. Because of this increased pain tolerance of sensory nerves, anæsthesia may be maintained at lighter levels and with less toxic drugs than in older patients.

ANÆSTHESIA

The choice of anæsthetic agent depends largely upon the skill of the anæsthetist. For those who have no special experience in pædiatric work ether is the safest agent. Ether anæsthesia, whether given by the open mask or by one of the machines, can provide adequate anæsthesia with safety. It has disadvantages however. Ether is a tissue poison and it stimulates respiration and circulation. It has been shown that in the infant a condition of shock develops after forty-five to fifty minutes of its use, and if surgery of such duration is contemplated special skill is called for. At present the anæsthetic of choice in such circumstances is nitrous oxide-oxygen, using Flaxedil to obtain muscular relaxation, and in this way no toxic drug is administered. If the operation is likely to be prolonged the respiratory muscles are paralysed and the infant is relieved of the muscular effort involved in rapid respiration, this effort being undertaken by the anæsthetist. Such a technique should be used only by those having special skill. If the operator is gentle in his manipulations and if blood loss is made good as it occurs, major surgical procedures of three or four hours' duration can be performed without exhaustion or shock to the patient.

In his choice of anæsthetic the anæsthetist divides children into four age groups: (1) *Birth to seven days*; (2) *seven days to three months*; (3) *three months to five years*; (4) *five years onwards.*

Group 1: *Birth to Seven Days.*—The newborn child is fit and well, is well nourished, has a good airway, is fully supplied with blood and there is no infection or major biochemical upset. Should such a child suffer from some remediable defect, he is a good risk for major surgery. If more than forty-five minutes is required for operation, ether and other toxic substances should be avoided if possible; blood loss is measured and replaced as it occurs. The neonate must be handled gently, for although a good risk he has little reserve of strength and, if allowed to become upset, especially by anoxia or over-stimulation, collapse may occur and never be fully overcome. Most surgical conditions at this age affect the alimentary tract and are obstructive in type, and chemical changes and fluid imbalance develop rapidly. These infants recover quickly when the obstruction has been relieved, and if the surgeon wishes to operate the anæsthetist must be prepared to anæsthetise the patient who appears to be a poor risk.

Group 2 : *Seven Days to Three Months.*—This group has a decreased anæsthetic and surgical tolerance and only essential surgery should be attempted. The need for surgery in the neonate is usually recognised, however, before the child is seven days old. The most frequent operations performed on the child between the ages of 7 days and 3 months are pyloromyotomy and circumcision, both of which, fortunately, are of short duration. Many people favour local anæsthesia for pyloromyotomy although satisfactory results can be obtained using general anæsthesia.

Group 3 : *Three Months to Five Years.*—Generally speaking these children are good risks. Their condition will, of course, vary with the illness necessitating operation. At this age the effect of ether anæsthesia of forty-five to fifty minutes is to produce a condition akin to shock. If no special anæsthetic skill is available there should, however, be no hesitation in using ether, keeping the depth of anæsthesia as light as is compatible with the nature of the surgical stimulation.

Group 4 : *Five Years Onwards.*—These patients should be treated more or less as adults.

PREMEDICATION

Atropine.—Atropine is essential at all ages and for all anæsthetics. An adequate dose should be given, as even a small amount of mucus can cause obstruction. The required dose in the average child is shown in Table I and this should be given thirty minutes before operation.

TABLE I

Dosage of Atropine at Different Ages

Age Group	Atropine Dosage
1 day to 2 months	$\frac{1}{300}$ gr.
3 months to 5 months	$\frac{1}{250}$ gr.
6 months to 1 year	$\frac{1}{200}$ gr.
2 years to 4 years	$\frac{1}{150}$ gr.
5 years onwards	$\frac{1}{100}$ gr.

Sedation.—Co-operation cannot be expected from a child and sedation is desirable over the age of 2 years. The ideal sedative for a child has not yet been found, but any of the following drugs may be used in the dosage indicated (Table II); they are given one hour before operation. The dose is modified if the patient is in poor condition.

TABLE II

Dose of Pre-operative Sedatives

Age	Morphine (by subcutaneous injection)	Pethidine (by subcutaneous injection)	Nembutal
2 to 3 years	$\frac{1}{60}$ gr. (1 mg.)	20 mg.	
3 to 5 years	$\frac{1}{48}$ gr. (1·25 mg.)	25 mg.	$\frac{1}{2}$ gr. (32 mg.)
5 to 8 years	$\frac{1}{36}$ gr. (1·85 mg.)	40 mg.	per stone
8 to 10 years	$\frac{1}{24}$ gr. (2·5 mg.)	45 mg.	(6·4 kg.) body
10 to 12 years	$\frac{1}{12}$ gr. (5 mg.)	50 mg.	weight given
12 to 14 years	$\frac{1}{6}$ gr. (10 mg.)	50 mg.	by mouth

When nembutal is used it occasionally causes stimulation and makes post-operative management difficult. This is readily controlled by the hypodermic administration of papaveratum, 2 per cent., in a dosage of 1 minim (0·06 ml.) per year of age.

INDUCTION

Induction of anæsthesia should be carried out carefully. Poor induction produces mucus secretion and causes trouble which may last for the duration of the operation. A small quantity of mucus will obstruct the narrow air passages of the infant and cause anoxia with all its attendant troubles. In children, relatively large amounts of ether are required for

2

induction but only small quantities for maintenance. When ether is being used as the principal anæsthetic agent, the depth of anæsthesia should vary with the nature of the surgical manipulations, there being periods when light anæsthesia will suffice. Change in the depth of anæsthesia can show suddenly and without warning, especially at the extremes of light and deep. Constant vigilance is necessary to protect the patient from the harmful effects of surgical stimulation on the one hand and anæsthetic shock on the other. The responses of a child are exaggerated and shock develops quickly after the first signs are apparent.

The major difficulties during induction of anæsthesia are breath holding, vomiting and mucus secretion.

Breath holding is most commonly due to sudden increase in the concentration of ether vapour. It may be prevented by gradual but constant increase in ether vapour strength during induction. If it does occur, the administration should be interrupted, the lips rubbed with a swab and a breath or two of air allowed when breathing resumes.

The dangers associated with vomitus and excess mucus in the respiratory passages cannot be exaggerated and every effort should be made to prevent such an occurrence. The routine case, having been prepared as previously described, will have an empty stomach. Most emergencies, however, must be considered to have material in the stomach. This is especially so in patients with intestinal obstruction and injury and a stomach tube is passed in such patients before anæsthesia is commenced. The introduction of the tube will frequently initiate vomiting and thus eject from the stomach material which would be too large to be removed by the tube. Some emergencies may be allowed to wait for a few hours but it must never be assumed that vomiting, the passing of a stomach tube or the lapse of time do in fact empty the stomach and the inexperienced anæsthetist should induce anæsthesia by inhalation methods. Using such methods, the laryngeal reflexes are present when vomiting is most likely during induction and laryngeal spasm is least likely to be prolonged. If a tube was not introduced while the patient was conscious, it should be passed immediately unconsciousness occurs, that is, while the laryngeal reflexes are present and the trachea protected against any regurgitation which may result. The tube is secured in position by adhesive strapping and remains until the cough reflex has returned. If vomiting or regurgitation occurs during anæsthesia the patient is turned on the side, head down, and the mouth and nose cleared with suction or a swab and the anæsthetic then resumed. Excessive secretion of mucus should be prevented by adequate dosage of atropine and smooth induction, but if secretion pours out and causes obstruction the upper respiratory passages are cleared by suction or swabbing and the anæsthetic again resumed.

The success of surgical procedures is now properly regarded as the result of team work. The part the anæsthetist plays is not the least important, for he has in his charge the well-being of the patient during the operation. His knowledge of physiology will assist him in this. Thereafter he has to provide satisfactory anæsthesia, and this will be obtained if the primary rules are observed : *good induction, a clear airway, full oxygenation, a depth of anæsthesia proportional to the degree of surgical stimulation and replacement of blood loss as it occurs.*

POST-OPERATIVE CARE

Sedatives are administered as required and the patients are kept under close observation until consciousness returns. Complications, such as aspiration of vomitus, happen with dramatic suddenness and constant nursing care is necessary. The small and sick infant is very liable to hypostatic pneumonia and he should be turned in his cot every few hours ; older children are encouraged to move around in bed as much as possible. In the whole field of nursing care there is no more exacting or responsible task than that of nursing the sick infant and the surgical nursing of the neonate requires the highest degree of nursing skill.

Except after major intra-abdominal procedures, oral feeding should usually be resumed six to eight hours after operation. Infants are given glucose water and resume the pre-operative feeding regime within twelve hours ; children are given clear fluids to drink, then light diet, and within twenty-four hours should be taking normal diet. Gavage or tube feeding is necessary in premature babies and may be required in weakly full-term infants. It may also be required in patients with anorexia following extensive burns or scalds. Patients in the surgical wards receive supplementary vitamins.

Few infants and children require intravenous fluid following surgical procedures and any fluid loss is rapidly made up when the patient begins to drink a few hours after operation. But severe fluid deficiency in ill children must be dealt with promptly and adequately by intravenous therapy. It must be remembered, however, that in babies and infants the danger of fluid retention may be almost as great as that of fluid deficiency. The immature kidneys of the young have only a limited capacity for excreting excess fluid and following surgery and anæsthesia there may be a temporary depression of renal function. Although intravenous fluid therapy is important in saving life, many small children have died of over-hydration. In the neonate, intravenous potassium is rarely required but if gastric suction is continued for more than three days, hypo-kalæmia is prevented by infusing Darrow's solution.[1] In all age groups, parenteral replacement of potassium must be made with great caution. The common intravenous fluids used are quarter-normal and half-normal saline or glucose-saline, blood plasma and the plasma substitutes.

All premature babies and all neonates who have been subjected to major surgery should be nursed in an incubator (Fig. 4). The temperature is kept constant, hypothermia is quickly corrected, oxygen is administered and the atmosphere is maintained at a high degree of humidity. In premature babies, administration of oxygen is very carefully controlled because of the risk of inducing retrolental fibroplasia in a high oxygen atmosphere. The incubator has small apertures for intravenous and suction tubes. The place of the oxygen tent in older children and the use of post-operative antibiotics will be considered in appropriate chapters. Sedation has been discussed on page 17. Papaveratum B.P. is given post-operatively when nembutal has been used as a pre-operative sedative; aspirin, morphine derivatives and pethidine are all given to relieve pain and no routine can be laid down.

[1] *Darrow's Solution.*—Potassium chloride, sodium chloride and sodium lactate.

CHAPTER III

Trauma

BIRTH INJURIES

ANTENATAL supervision and improved obstetrics have greatly reduced the dangers to the fœtus during delivery but birth injury still ranks as an important cause of stillbirth and neonatal death. Many avoidable birth injuries still occur and no structure of the body is entirely immune. Only the common types of injury will be considered here.

Superficial Structures.

Caput succedaneum consists of an œdematous swelling, often associated with ecchymosis, which occurs over the presenting part of the fœtus. It is most commonly seen over the parietal region in vertex deliveries but it may occur over any presenting part. In breech presentations the scrotum, labia or buttocks may be severely œdematous and markedly discoloured. The swelling usually subsides within a few days but the staining following ecchymosis may take some time to disappear. In *cephalhæmatoma* the hæmorrhage is between the periosteum and the skull, usually in the parietal region. The hæmatoma is limited to the area of the affected bone

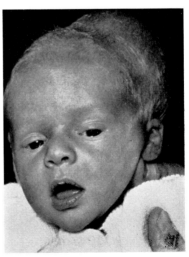

FIG. 5
Cephalhæmatoma.

by the attachment of the periosteum at the suture lines (Fig. 5). It usually appears on the second day after birth and may persist for many weeks, but invariably it disappears. The marginal blood clot (and later, calcification) may give the impression of a ring of bone with a central depression and the condition is often mistaken for a depressed fracture. Aspiration is seldom indicated, but should the hæmatoma become infected the infected blood clot is evacuated through a small incision. *Bruising and ecchymoses* are not uncommon but require no treatment. *Abrasions and lacerations* may be caused by slipping of the forceps and are treated with 1 per cent. gentian violet. Slightly blanched ridges are seen in different areas of the body and have been termed *fat necrosis*. The pathology of these lesions is not understood but they are probably due to pressure and usually disappear spontaneously within a year.

Muscle.

The so-called *sternomastoid tumour* appears in the lower third of the sternomastoid a few weeks after birth. For a few weeks it is tender to the touch but the tenderness goes and the swelling disappears spontaneously within three months. It is probably due to damage to a muscle, already the seat of developmental hypoplasia, and sternomastoid tumour may be followed later by torticollis (Chap. XX).

Injury to the Abdomen.

In assisted deliveries there may be damage to the *liver*, *spleen* or *bowel* and similar injuries may be caused by mismanaged artificial respiration. There is sudden collapse and evidence of an intraperitoneal catastrophe. Only prompt laparotomy can save life.

Fractures.

Fractures of the *clavicle, humerus* and *femur* are usually recognised by pseudo-paralysis. There may be obvious deformity and crepitus. Healing takes place rapidly with gross callus formation (Fig. 6) and even with inadequate correction of angulation these fractures show no permanent deformity. The parents should be warned that a hard mass of callus (like a plumber's joint) will be felt, but this will disappear within a month or two. An infant with a fracture is more comfortable and is more easily handled if the painful part is gently immobilised. After separating skin surfaces with white lint, the arm is bound to the chest in fractures of the clavicle or shaft of the humerus and the thigh is bound to the abdomen in fractures of the femoral shaft. Immobilisation is discontinued after ten or twelve days. Fractures of the *skull*

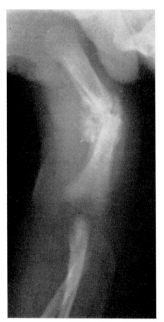

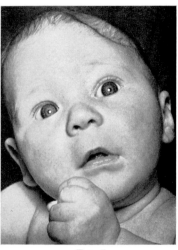

Fig. 6
Birth fracture of humerus with angulation and callus formation.

Fig. 7
Birth fracture of skull—
" pond fracture."

are uncommon. They are usually stellate, but depressed fractures may be caused by pressure on the sacral promontory (Fig. 7). The depression usually disappears spontaneously and operative elevation is seldom required.

Extracranial Nerves.

Facial paralysis is usually due to pressure of the forceps blades on the facial nerve, but supranuclear paralysis may be due to cerebral trauma. Movements of the affected side of the face are diminished and the mouth is drawn to the uninjured side when the infant cries. The eye on the affected side may remain partly open. There is no interference with sucking and normal function is usually restored within two or three weeks.

Permanent paralysis is very rare. The *brachial plexus* may be damaged by stretching or lateral flexion of the neck, usually in a breech delivery (Chap. XXIV). The fifth and sixth cervical nerves or their roots are most commonly damaged (*Erb-Duchenne paralysis*), but the injury may be more extensive with paralysis of the whole arm. (The authors have never seen *Klumpke palsy*

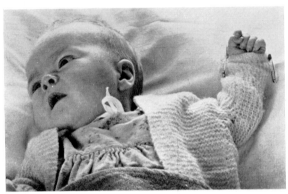

FIG. 8

First-aid treatment of Erb's palsy; sleeve pinned to pillow.

from damage to the eighth cervical and first thoracic nerves.) In Erb's palsy the arm hangs limply at the side, internally rotated with the fingers flexed. As a first-aid measure the sleeve is pinned to the pillow to keep the shoulder abducted and the elbow flexed (Fig. 8). Most cases recover within ten days. *Radial nerve palsy* is rare and the drop-wrist recovers completely after immobilisation in a cock-up splint.

Intracranial Injuries.

Intracranial damage is the most serious form of birth trauma. Extensive lacerations and gross cerebral damage cause death during or shortly after delivery. There may be no more than œdema or congestion of the skull contents and the signs of cerebral irritation and shock may disappear within two or three days. Even without actual trauma, the venous congestion present in *asphyxia neonatorum* favours cerebral bleeding and the importance of asphyxia is impossible to exaggerate. Non-fatal injuries may result in such permanent disabilities as *cerebral palsy, hydrocephalus* and *mental defect.* If the falx cerebri or tentorium cerebelli are torn there is a grave risk of fatal hæmorrhage from one of the veins or sinuses. Hæmorrhage may also be subarachnoid, intraventricular or into the brain substance.

Clinical Features.—Clinical evidence of intracranial damage manifests itself in many ways. The condition is frequently overlooked but it should be suspected when the infant appears shocked, is difficult to resuscitate and fails to cry normally. Twitching or convulsions may occur. In the fatal case the condition deteriorates, with signs of depression of the respiratory and other vital centres, and life ebbs away in a few hours. Most cases, however, gradually improve and signs of irritation appear some twelve hours after birth. The infant becomes restless and there is a shrill high-pitched cry. There may be twitching movements, nystagmus and convulsions and there may be stiffness of the limbs and neck. Vomiting may occur.

Treatment.—The infant is kept warm and if necessary nursed in oxygen. Handling is reduced to a minimum and sedatives (usually chloral hydrate) given if the infant is restless.

Late Effects.—HYDROCEPHALUS from birth hæmorrhage is usually progressive but occasionally there are spontaneous remissions. Normal intelligence is compatible with gross hydrocephalus but the mental development varies greatly in different cases. The principles of treatment are considered in Chapter XVIII.

CHRONIC SUBDURAL HÆMATOMA.—The hæmatoma may lie over one hemisphere but is often bilateral. The infant fails to thrive and there is bulging of the anterior fontanelle. The cerebrospinal fluid obtained by lumbar puncture is xanthochromic and the diagnosis is confirmed by aspiration of blood, serosanguinous fluid or xanthochromic fluid through a needle inserted through the lateral angle of the anterior fontanelle. The hæmatoma may resolve after repeated aspiration but operation may be required. The hæmatoma is evacuated and its lining membrane removed to allow the brain to expand.

CEREBRAL PALSY.—Asphyxia in the newborn and intracranial birth injury are the most important causes of the symptoms in the group of cases classed under the title of cerebral palsy. Spastic patients probably represent almost half the total and the handling of this group is considered in Chapter XXIV.

Successful delivery is no assurance that the newborn baby is no longer exposed to the risks of trauma. Burns due to

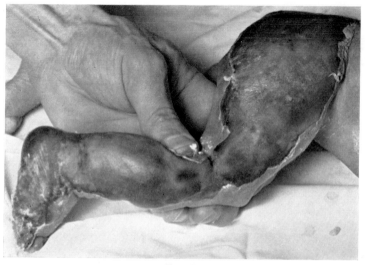

FIG. 9

Dermal necrosis in infant aged 6 days, caused by bursting of hot-water bottle in cot. After resuscitation and early skin grafting, made an excellent recovery.

lapses in nursing techniques in the use of hot-water bottles, electric blankets and strong antiseptics occur too frequently, not only in the home but also in nursing homes and hospitals. Figure 9 shows dermal necrosis in a 6-day-old baby caused by the bursting of a hot-water bottle in the cot.

WOUNDS

Children are subject to the same forms of trauma as are sustained by the adult and the principles of treatment are also the same. Two types of wound, particularly common in childhood, should always be regarded as potentially serious. These are *spike wounds* and the so-called *wringer injuries*.

Spike Wounds.

Children quite regularly impale themselves on spiked railings and penetrating wounds are sustained to the buttocks, perineum and, less commonly, the chest or abdomen. There may be early evidence of visceral injury indicating the need for urgent surgical intervention but very often the wound of entry is insignificant and the child appears well. Such wounds should be regarded with grave suspicion and should be carefully examined. Quite apart from the fact that signs of visceral damage may not be evident for some time, penetration may be deep and foreign material can be carried a long way into the body.

Penicillin and antitetanic serum (or tetanus toxoid) are administered and the wound carefully examined under general anæsthesia. The outer portion of the wound is excised and the depths examined as thoroughly as possible and any foreign material removed. Radiography may reveal an unexpected lesion in the thoracic or peritoneal cavity.

Foreign Bodies in the Soft Tissues.—It is not uncommon for large foreign bodies to become embedded in a child's tissues through a very small wound of entry. After a fall from a tree or wooden fence, large portions of wood may be buried and remain unsuspected for a lengthy period. Radio-opaque foreign bodies such as air-gun pellets, needles, etc., present the same problems in localisation as in the adult.

Wringer Injuries.

Although this title is applied to the crush injury sustained when a child's hand and arm are drawn into the wringer of an automatic washing machine, the same pathology may be encountered in a " run-over " accident. In the typical lesion there is little laceration and no avulsion of skin. The limb is swollen and there may be abrasions and ecchymosis but on initial examination the injury appears to be a minor one (*Frontispiece*). The serious element of the injury is the progressive tissue destruction which is hidden beneath the skin surface. A sleeve of skin is separated from the underlying fascia, sheering off the blood supply. Within twenty-four to forty-eight hours skin which was apparently viable changes colour and if left untreated becomes black and necrotic.

Destruction of muscle is rarely marked in children and the underlying bones usually escape injury.

Treatment.—When there is a history of this type of sheering injury the prognosis should be guarded for at least forty-eight hours. The limb is X-rayed and any fracture reduced. After thorough cleansing under general anæsthesia any large hæmatoma is evacuated and lacerations loosely sutured. A pressure bandage is applied over a tulle gras dressing. The fingers (or toes) are left exposed so that circulation can be carefully watched. The limb is elevated and the dressing taken down at intervals to determine the progress of the condition. If in spite of treatment the integument should slough, the raw area is allowed to granulate and then covered with a split-skin graft. Penicillin is given from the time of admission to hospital.

TETANUS

Tetanus neonatorum is now a rare disease in this country. Infection occurs through the umbilicus. Mild cases may respond to antitetanic serum but the mortality is generally very high.

Tetanus in Childhood.—Although tetanus in adults is most likely to follow contamination in deep punctured wounds, the few cases we have seen in childhood have been associated with quite superficial wounds which have scabbed over early. As in the adult, the longer the incubation period the better is the prognosis. In three of our patients in whom the incubation period was under ten days the outcome was fatal. The symptoms are the same as in adult life, trismus, muscular rigidity and reflex spasm. The spasms become generalised, the back arches and breathing is arrested during the spasm.

Diagnosis.—The trismus must be differentiated from the jaw stiffness associated with local infection of the mouth, jaws and fauces. In the early stages tetanus may simulate poliomyelitis or meningitis.

Prophylaxis.—1,500 units of antitetanic serum should be given to all children with contaminated wounds. Intradermal tests of sensitivity to the serum are valueless and a small subcutaneous test dose should be given before all but the first inoculation.

Treatment.—A massive dose (200,000 units) of antitoxin is injected intravenously as soon as possible. As with the ordinary prophylactic dose, the risk of anaphylaxis should be borne in mind and 1 in 1,000 adrenaline should always be at hand. Any local treatment to the wound is delayed for at least an hour after the injection of antitoxin. Under general anæsthesia the wound is opened widely, any foreign or necrotic material removed and the wound flooded with hydrogen peroxide. A long-acting preparation of penicillin is injected intramuscularly. The child is nursed in silence in a darkened room. The spasms can be abolished by the use of one of the relaxants but respiration must be continued through an endotracheal tube using an anæsthetic machine or by manual compression of a bag. Bronchial secretions are aspirated and nutrition maintained partly by intravenous glucose saline and partly by a gastric drip through a catheter passed through the nose into the stomach. Following the success of routine tracheotomy and positive pressure respiration in bulbar poliomyelitis, some workers recommend routine tracheotomy in tetanus. A relaxant is administered and the paralysed and anæsthetised patient is treated in the same way as one with bulbar poliomyelitis.

The quantity, timing and route of administration of A.T.S. vary in different centres and bear no relation to the final outcome of the disease. Severe anaphylactic reaction and even death following A.T.S. is not uncommon. The intradermal test for sensitivity is unreliable and should be replaced by the subcutaneous trial dose method. The patient is given subcutaneously 0·2 ml. of a 1 in 10 dilution of serum and is watched for half an hour ; if no reaction occurs, 0·2 ml. of undiluted serum is given. If there is still no reaction after a further half-hour, the full dose for prophylaxis or treatment is then given intramuscularly. (Once a patient has received an injection of any horse-serum antitoxin he should be promptly immunised against diphtheria and tetanus with the appropriate toxoid.) Many infants are immunised against whooping cough and diphtheria and it is now practicable to administer a triple prophylactic at the third or fourth month. Three doses of 1 ml. of the combined diphtheria-pertussis-tetanus are given at intervals of four weeks and a reinforcing dose is given before the child goes to school.

HÆMOPHILIA

In this disease there is an inherited tendency to bleed from minor injuries, associated with a prolonged coagulation time. Hæmophilia occurs almost exclusively among males but is transmitted by females. The sons of hæmophiliacs do not develop the disease nor do they transmit it; the daughters are the carriers. The disease is determined by a rare sex-linked recessive gene. In our experience there is rarely a family history of the disease. As hæmophilia results in severe disability few of the patients survive to adult life to have children. There is presumably a steady loss of the abnormal gene in each generation, the loss being offset by new spontaneous mutations.

Although bleeding time is normal, coagulation time is prolonged and there is a deficiency of anti-hæmophilic globulin (A.H.G.). In a few otherwise identical cases the A.H.G. is present in normal amounts but there is a deficiency of the plasma thromboplastin component (P.T.C. or Christmas factor). This rarer *Christmas disease* is clinically indistinguishable from classical hæmophilia.

Clinical Features.—Hæmophilia is never manifest at birth and significant hæmorrhage is seldom seen before the age of 2 years. The eruption or extraction of a tooth or some minor scratch or cut draws attention to the disease. Although not alarming in severity the hæmorrhage continues in spite of all efforts to arrest it and it may lead to profound anæmia and collapse. After minor bumps, hæmatomata may occur in any part of the body and may be very extensive (Fig. 10). Retroperitoneal hæmatoma can be particularly alarming but fortunately secondary infection is very rare. Hæmarthrosis is one of the most frequent manifestations and the knee joint is most commonly affected. The same joints are repeatedly affected; movement is restricted and arthritic changes are almost inevitable. Hæmorrhages may occur from mucous membranes following minor trauma but spontaneous hæmorrhage is rare.

The tendency to bleed varies from time to time in each patient. Every children's hospital has its regular " customers " and it is usually possible to tell from the child's expression on admission whether or not the episode is going to be a severe one. An anxious expression should warn the hospital staff that the patient is probably in a bleeding phase. The prognosis must always be guarded. All the activities of childhood are fraught with danger and the frequency of serious episodes varies with the measure of protection which the patient can receive. The patient may die or become a complete cripple before puberty. In those who survive beyond this period the hæmorrhagic episodes decrease in frequency and sometimes in severity.

Treatment.—There is no cure for hæmophilia. Sometimes bleeding from cuts or tooth sockets ceases with simple pressure and hæmatomata and hæmarthroses may absorb with simple rest in bed. Sooner or later blood transfusion is required in every case, either to replace blood lost or to control

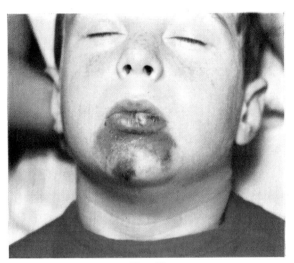

FIG. 10

Hæmophilia. A minor injury led to extensive bruising of the mouth, chin and tissues of the neck and severe dyspnœa and dysphagia.

bleeding. Repeated transfusion, preferably of fresh blood or fresh plasma, may be necessary. Active concentrates of *anti-hæmophilic globulin* are now available and are given to arrest bleeding or to raise the level of A.H.G. in the circulating blood before any surgical procedure is carried out.

Epistaxis is usually controlled by packing the anterior nares. Bleeding tooth sockets should be lightly packed, the pack being held in place by a small dental splint. Each time a hæmophilic patient is admitted to hospital for whatever reason, his mouth should be examined by the dental consultant. Good conservative dentistry may prevent bleeding from the gums, cheek and tongue.

The Ministry of Health has issued a booklet on hæmophilia for the guidance of patients and their relatives. It discusses the management of the disease, protective measures, social services available to hæmophiliacs and suitable hobbies and leisure activities. Copies are available free of charge to any general practitioner at the local clinic or laboratory which acts as a reference centre for hæmophilia.

PSEUDOHÆMOPHILIA

There is a group of conditions distinguished from hæmophilia by their occurrence in both sexes, by a normal clotting time and by a marked prolongation of bleeding time. The symptoms are variable in intensity but hæmorrhage rarely endangers life and the disability is less severe than true hæmophilia.

Affected children bruise readily, there is excessive bleeding from minor cuts or following tooth extraction and epistaxis is common. Blood transfusion may be indicated for anæmia but there is no specific treatment. Local pressure may arrest hæmorrhage.

Among the uncommon conditions which might be confused with hæmophilia are *hæmorrhagic telangiectasia* and the *Ehlers-Danlos syndrome*.

HÆMORRHAGIC TELANGIECTASIA

In this condition there may be repeated and profuse epistaxis; more rarely there may be hæmatemesis or melæna. Small telangiectatic lesions are present on the lips, tongue and fauces and there may be similar lesions in the nose or in the skin. Both sexes are affected.

In general, spontaneous oozing from mucous membranes and the occurrence of petechiæ or ecchymosis in the skin suggest the group of hæmorrhagic purpuras.

EHLERS-DANLOS SYNDROME

There is hyperextensibility of the joints and the fingers can be bent backwards to an abnormal degree and the elbows can be hyperextended. The skin is elastic and can be pulled out as in the " elastic skin man " in the circus sideshow. The skin is excessively fragile and tears readily and the scar tissue stretches until there are pouches of skin over the knees and

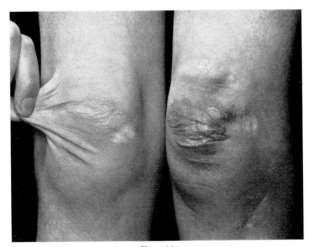

FIG. 11
Ehlers-Danlos syndrome—scarring and elastic skin of knees.

elbows (Fig. 11). There may be troublesome hæmorrhage from wounds and operation sites. The syndrome is inherited as a simple dominant and is probably due to a fault in the formation of collagen.

BURNS AND SCALDS

It is customary to describe the lesions due to dry heat as " burns " and those due to moist heat as " scalds." There is, however, no essential difference in the two lesions save that in scalds the lesions are usually more superficial and dermal necrosis is less common. In infants and young children, scalds are more common than burns and are usually caused by hot water, soup or tea. Burns are sustained by clothes catching fire or by the child clutching hot coals or the bar of an electric fire.

Most domestic burns and scalds are preventable and in

many homes the most elementary precautions against accident are neglected. All open fires should be adequately protected by fireguards and guards are now available for all types of gas and electric fires. The common fabrics used for clothing should be graded in terms of inflammability. Flannelette and winceyette are commonly used for children's nightwear and present a serious hazard in the home. Expensive materials like natural silk and wool do not catch fire or burn easily, but artificial silks (rayon), lacquered nets and loosely woven fabrics are highly inflammable. Cotton and rayon can now be rendered relatively flame-resistant by chemical processes such as treatment with salts of antimony and titanium.

The diverse mechanism of scalds presents a serious problem to all parents and it is the duty of the family doctor to point out the hazards which exist in the home. The main agents responsible for scalds in the home are: (1) Pulling cups, jugs and teapots off the table; (2) knocking pans and kettles off the hob or kitchen stove; (3) falling into a bucket or bath of hot water; (4) collision with another child or an adult carrying a utensil full of hot fluid. A disturbing factor is the number of young children who are scalded late at night and in these cases there is usually evidence of overcrowding in the home.

The prevention of accidents in the home is an exercise in social medicine in its widest sense. It is part of the duty of the family doctor to instruct his patients, particularly those with a young family, in the prevention of household accidents. Having acquired some knowledge of first-aid himself, the doctor should take every opportunity of imparting this knowledge to the parents.

CLINICAL FEATURES

It is difficult to assess the severity of a burn in a young child. There is a striking lack of anxiety after the initial fright has passed and the child appears to suffer little pain—the only complaint being of thirst. Primary shock is uncommon and there is usually a marked contrast between the child and the frightened parents.

Secondary (oligæmic) shock, however, soon develops due to loss of fluid both externally and into the tissues, unless hæmoconcentration is prevented. In spite of copious *oral fluids* the patient may shiver and complain of cold. At this time the pulse-rate may increase and the nose and extremities feel cold. Restlessness develops and the colour becomes poor and there may be slight cyanosis. There may be vomiting at this stage and there are alternating periods of drowsiness and restlessness. Only then is there any marked fall in blood-pressure. If a hæmatocrit reading is made at this stage it will indicate hæmoconcentration. Air hunger and loss of consciousness follow quickly unless the disturbance in fluid balance is corrected by the intravenous administration of fluids.

If a scald involves the chin, neck and chest, the lips and mouth should be examined for evidence of damage. Children may attempt to drink from the spout of a kettle and hot water or steam may be inhaled or swallowed and œdema of the glottis may occur. Lung lesions may follow inhalation of hot air and smoke in burning accidents. Chest complications are common in burns and scalds involving the chest wall.

TREATMENT

The small superficial lesions which occur in the home usually heal well, whatever method of treatment is adopted. One of the most satisfactory applications is an antihistamine cream, which relieves pain and prevents œdema. If there is superficial destruction of the epidermis, dibromopropamidine cream with 2 per cent. promethazine (Phenergan cream, May & Baker) can be applied without preliminary cleansing, bandaged in place, and left for four or five days. In small superficial lesions of the face, dusting with a good talcum powder expedites clotting of the surface plasma exudate and no bandage is required. If the burn is more than trivial, a clean dry dressing should be applied and the child sent to hospital. Greasy dressings may interfere with subsequent treatment. If the lesion is extensive and the patient's home far from hospital, intravenous or subcutaneous fluid should be given and the drip continued during transport.

In Hospital.—If the burn or scald involves 10 per cent. or more of the body surface, intravenous fluid will probably be required. Sedatives are administered as required and blood is taken to assess hæmoconcentration. Repeated hæmoglobin estimations give a rough guide to the extent of hæmo-concentration but more accuracy is obtained from hæmatocrit readings. Urinary output must be carefully observed and fluid intake and output charts are kept. The intravenous fluid of choice may be blood, plasma, plasma substitutes or glucose saline and the requirements in childhood are finally assessed on clinical judgment. Anoxia may be relieved by nursing the child in an oxygen tent.

Local Treatment.—There are many methods of local treatment of the burned area but their success finally depends on the co-operation and enthusiasm of the nursing staff. The local treatment should vary with the site of the lesion and the nursing problems arising therefrom. In the absence of dermal necrosis most scalds and burns heal uneventfully in fourteen to twenty-one days.

In a surgical unit of the Royal Hospital for Sick Children, Glasgow, burns and scalds have been nursed in a small *Burns Unit* since 1937. Until tannic acid became unfashionable in 1940, the lesions were gently cleansed under sedation or light general anæsthesia and the surface coagulated with a solution of tannic acid or silver nitrate or one of the antiseptic dyes. " Open " methods of treatment were then adopted and bland dressings, pressure dressings, Stannard envelopes, Bunyan bags, local sulphonamides and local penicillin were all tried and in the hands of the enthusiast gave reasonably satisfactory results. During this time there were great advances in the general treatment of the burned patient and inevitably this led to improved results in the local lesion irrespective of the method of local treatment adopted. The " exposure method " of treatment was then rediscovered and was used as a routine procedure for two years, at first with penicillin powder ; later without any antibiotic or antiseptic. To avoid the need for cleansing the burned area in the severely burned child dibromopropamidine was introduced and in the form of Brulidine and Phenergan cream (M. & B.), was used for almost three years. Although an ideal first-aid dressing dibromopropamidine was found to delay healing and, in deep lesions, was used only during the first ten days of treatment. During 1955 Hibitane (bis-*p*-chlorophenyldiguanidohexane (I.C.I.)) became available and the early results following application of a 0·25 per cent. solution were so satisfactory that this preparation has for the present supplanted previous forms of treatment. Anatomical regions present their own nursing problems. Lesions of the chin and anterior aspect of the neck must be nursed with the head extended; burns of the buttocks and perineum are nursed with the patient lying prone or with the legs slung from a gallows splint; lesions involving the front and back of the body present exceedingly difficult nursing problems. It may be difficult to assess the depth of the lesion in children. Dermal necrosis may occur in what at first appears to be a superficial scald, and burns which initially appear to be deep epithelialise in a remarkable fashion.

It is usually possible to assess the extent of dermal necrosis within a few days of admission and the surgeon must start to plan what skin coverage will be required and the site of the donor areas. Local treatment should be directed towards obtaining a clean granulating surface suitable for grafting in eighteen to twenty-one days. In extensive burns temporary cover may be obtained by the use of homografts, from a skin " bank " or with skin taken from parents or relatives. In children, homografts may give temporary cover for three or four weeks. The patient's own donor areas can be used over and over again at intervals of a week or ten days.

General Treatment.—In addition to replacement fluids, requirement fluids to make up loss from kidneys, gut, skin and lungs must also be given. Even with extensive lesions, fluid balance is usually restored within forty-eight hours. If there is more than 15 per cent. loss of skin, the clinical picture tends to follow a similar pattern in all patients without prophylactic treatment. About four days after the injury there is a rise in urinary urea with a fall in blood hæmoglobin and plasma proteins. Excess protein catabolism leads to depression of hæmoglobin synthesis. The main source of loss is the burned area. The burned surface will not heal until the hæmoglobin is over 60 per cent.; the anæmia will persist until the burn heals. This condition is associated with anorexia and the circle is difficult to break.

Blood transfusion during the period of fluid imbalance may prevent the onset of marked anæmia. If anæmia does occur it is treated with repeated small blood transfusions. Intravenous

3

protein hydrolysates have on the whole been rather disappointing and we have depended on the early administration of a high protein diet. Dry skimmed milk (100 gm.) in 200 ml. water gives 34 gm. protein and 52 gm. carbohydrate (*i.e.*, more protein than a quart of milk and only one-fifth the volume). The patient is given frequent milk shakes made from this mixture and the colour and flavour are varied throughout the day. Collagen fibres do not form in absence of vitamin C and proliferating mesodermal cells do not mature. All patients are therefore given massive doses of vitamin C.

Infection is prevented by isolation, aseptic and antiseptic precautions and the administration of antibiotics as required. Antibiotics should not be used locally. Applied to the burned area they tend to delay healing, they encourage the growth of resistant strains of bacteria and they may lead to drug sensitisation. Deformity is prevented by early grafting and suitable splinting.

CHAPTER IV

Infection

SEPSIS IN THE NEWBORN

AFTER the first week of life infection is the most important single cause of neonatal death, pneumonia and gastro-enteritis being of outstanding importance. It is perhaps not generally recognised that either pneumonia or gastro-enteritis may be the presenting signs of septicæmia; and if treatment is delayed or inadequate, pyæmic lesions may form in any organ. Although the infant may be born with congenital immunity to certain organisms to which the mother is immune, the capacity for antibody formation during the neonatal period is generally very poor. Before the introduction of antibiotics the prognosis in septicæmia of the newborn was poor and few babies lived long enough to show evidence of bone infection (p. 43).

The fœtus is usually bacteriologically sterile until the membranes rupture, although there is evidence to show that intrauterine infection may be more common than is generally appreciated. After rupture of the membranes the fœtus may inhale or swallow infected liquor amnii or may encounter virulent organisms in the vagina. After delivery there are many possible sources of infection, particularly the skin and upper respiratory tract of the mother and attendants. Before there is evidence of severe infection, paronychia, skin pustules or infection of the cord stump may be observed. Minor staphylococcal infections appear in 10 to 15 per cent. of infants born in maternity units and the incidence of such infection is increasing. In hospital such apparently minor lesions must be treated seriously by the obstetrician or the pædiatrician because major infections rarely develop until the mother and child have gone home.

SITES OF INFECTION

Skin.—Skin infections may present as *pustules*, *infected vesicles* or *dermatitis* with or without exfoliation. Infected areas should be covered to prevent spread to other parts and the appropriate antibiotic administered.

Nail Folds.—Paronychia is not uncommon and is favoured by finger sucking. There is redness and swelling of the nail fold and a bead of pus may appear. The condition usually responds quickly to local application of 1 per cent. gentian violet ; further spread may be prevented by cotton mittens. If the infection becomes more severe the condition should be treated by the oral administration of one of the wide-spectrum antibiotics such as tetracycline in one of its proprietary forms.

Eyes.—Conjunctivitis and purulent ophthalmia are common. The eyes are irrigated frequently with saline or antibiotic drops and ung. hydrarg. ox. flav. is smeared on the lids.

Subcutaneous Tissues.—Abscesses may be found in any situation and infection may occur at pressure points such as the back of the head and heels. One must always suspect underlying bone infection in cases with cellulitis or abscess formation. A cephalhæmatoma may become infected and although infection may subside with simple aspiration a small incision may be necessary to evacuate the infected blood clot.

Parotitis.—The infection may be unilateral or bilateral. The causal organism can be cultured from the bead of pus expressed from the duct by gentle pressure over the gland. Incision should be avoided if possible, because of the risk of fistula formation.

Breasts.—True *mastitis* follows acute infection of physiologically engorged breasts (Fig. 12). This may be due to lack of cleanliness, attempts to express the so-called " witch's milk " or abrasion of the areola from resuscitation of the infant by rubbing the chest with a rough towel. As soon as there is fluctuation the abscess must be incised to prevent a spreading infection of the chest wall (Fig. 13).

Umbilicus.—Periomphalitis may be followed by umbilical abscess. There may be only redness or moisture of the cord stump but this may spread to the abdominal wall and there is always the risk of thrombosis of the umbilical vein. Treatment is by antibiotics and surgical drainage when indicated.

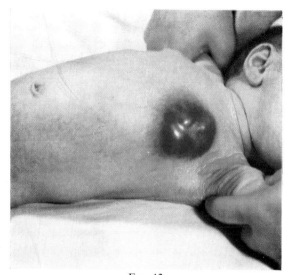

FIG. 12
Mastitis neonatorum.

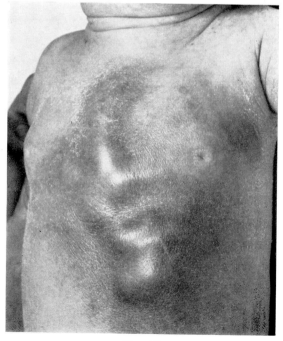

FIG. 13
Cellulitis of chest wall in newborn.

Respiratory, alimentary and urinary infections are considered fully in medical textbooks but it should be remembered that any of them may be the first manifestation of a septicæmia.

Peritonitis.

Meconium Peritonitis.—If an abnormal communication should occur between the bowel and the peritoneal cavity

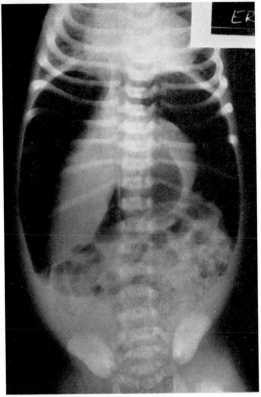

FIG. 14

Pneumoperitoneum following perforation proximal to jejuno-ileal atresia.

during the last few months of intra-uterine life, a non-bacterial foreign body and chemical peritonitis will follow. Meconium peritonitis usually follows antenatal intestinal obstruction with perforation of the gut proximal to the obstruction (see Chap. IX).

If the perforation is still present after birth, the sterile chemical peritonitis will become infected and secondary pyogenic peritonitis will develop. There is usually evidence of shock, the respirations are grunting in type, there may be cyanosis and there is often œdema of the flanks and scrotum. There may be absence of liver dullness due to pneumoperitoneum (Fig. 14). Treatment is by laparotomy and relief of the intestinal obstruction (Chap. IX). Resection and anastomoses may be required.

Primary Peritonitis.—Primary peritonitis may occur in the neonatal period as a manifestation of septicæmia or from infection of the umbilical stump. The infection is usually streptococcal. The early clinical features are vomiting and diarrhœa with pyrexia and a diagnosis of gastro-enteritis is usually made. The infant is listless and toxic and there is doughy swelling of the abdomen.

A wide-spectrum antibiotic (tetracycline) is injected pre-operatively. If no perforation is found at laparotomy, pus is evacuated by sucker and the wound closed without drainage. Antibiotic therapy is continued after operation and the infant is nursed in an incubator or oxygen tent.

Hæmatogenous Osteitis in the Newborn.

As a result of the successful treatment of septicæmia in the newborn, more small infants are living long enough to show clinical evidence of hæmatogenous osteitis. The organism is commonly a coagulase-positive staphylococcus and in the Royal Hospital for Sick Children, Glasgow, the staphylococcus is resistant to penicillin in over 80 per cent. Acute hæmatogenous osteitis is discussed fully in Chapter V, but osteitis in the newborn differs in many respects from osteitis in older children and is so closely related to neonatal sepsis that it is considered separately.

In the past, neonatal osteitis has been described in two forms—*benign* and *severe.* " Benign " is not a satisfactory description of a condition which may be characterised by recurrences and which not uncommonly results in permanent deformity. In the so-called benign form the disease usually affects only one bone, there is little systematic upset and even before the introduction of chemotherapy and antibiotics the prognosis was good. Unfortunately at the outset it is often impossible to say which form the disease will take.

Neonatal osteitis may in fact present as an acute or as a subacute infection. In the subacute form the disease most commonly occurs in the maxilla but any bone may be affected. Although the infecting organism is usually a coagulase-positive staphylococcus, severe toxæmia is unusual and the infant's life never appears to be in danger. Abscess formation and joint infection are common—probably due to the thin and porous infantile cortex and delicate epiphyseal cartilage. Sequestrum formation is rare and any sequestra are usually absorbed spontaneously. Bone deformities are quickly remedied by growth and full joint function may be restored early. Even before the introduction of antibiotics such cases responded well to minor surgical intervention.

In almost half the patients neonatal osteitis presents as an acute infection and one or more bones may be involved. The disease was formerly known as *generalised osteitis of the newborn*. There may be multiple swellings of the extremities and joint infection occurs early. The diagnosis is confirmed by blood culture and by radiographic changes (Fig. 15). In many patients there is gross deformity following joint infection, due to damage to the articular ends of the bones and not to adhesions in the joint (Fig. 16). The disease is rarely diagnosed before the nutrient artery is thrombosed so that extensive bone damage is common (see Hæmatogenous Osteitis, Chap. V). The mortality is almost 6 per cent., much higher than the mortality from hæmatogenous osteitis in older children and death occurs from septicæmia or pyæmia. Recurrences are common in the survivors and a patient may have metastatic foci in many bones.

Clinical Features.—Early diagnosis is usually difficult as the disease may present in several ways. As already stated, septicæmia in the newborn may present with pneumonia or gastroenteritis and only swelling of a limb draws attention to the fact that the infant is also suffering from osteitis. In other infants, excessive irritability, often increased by handling or relative immobility of a limb, may be the first signs of bone infection. Soft tissue abscesses are relatively rare in the newborn and swelling, particularly of a limb, is more likely to be from infection in bone. One must of course exclude the effects of birth trauma,

Treatment.—All staphylococcal infections in the newborn should be carefully treated. If apparently trivial lesions such as paronychia and umbilical sepsis are treated inadequately, pyæmic lesions may appear in bone. The infecting organism is cultured without delay and its

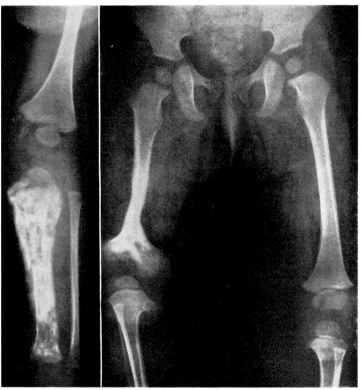

FIG. 15   FIG. 16

Fig. 15.—Neonatal osteitis of tibia.
Fig. 16.—Gross damage to lower femoral epiphysis and metaphysis
due to neonatal osteitis.

sensitivity to the different antibiotics assessed. Treatment is started with a wide-spectrum antibiotic of the tetracycline group or with a mixture of penicillin and streptomycin. Septicæmia is usually controlled within a few days but because of damage to the blood supply the antibiotic may not reach the metaphyseal focus and the risk of metastatic spread is great. Subperiosteal abscesses are evacuated and the wound sutured as in the older child (Chap. V). Joint infections are aspirated and the appropriate antibiotic instilled. The hip joints are most commonly affected and only too frequently the upper femoral epiphysis is gravely damaged.

The bacteriologist's report will give guidance as to the most suitable antibiotic but none should be administered continuously for long periods because of the risk of staphylococcal enterocolitis. For this reason, and to give the infant a chance to develop immunity to the infection, systemic administration of the antibiotic is stopped for a few days once toxæmia is controlled. Repeated short courses are given at intervals and it may be necessary to continue treatment for many weeks.

LYMPHADENITIS

Pyogenic Lymphadenitis.

As in the adult, the most common sites of adenitis are the cervical, inguinal and axillary glands. In the adult the primary focus is usually quite obvious when the patient presents with adenitis; in childhood the primary focus is often healed and forgotten by both patient and parents before the adenitis manifests itself. Adenitis in adult life frequently subsides without pus formation; in childhood pus formation is the rule and most infected glands break down and require incision.

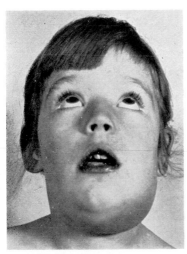

FIG. 17
Pyogenic submandibular adenitis.

The cervical glands are most commonly affected and the swelling may be in the anterior or posterior triangle or in the submandibular, submental, preauricular or post-auricular regions (Fig. 17). The organism is usually a coagulase positive staphylococcus, resistant to penicillin in more than half the patients. The infected glands are deep to the deep cervical fascia and the pus should be evacuated by Hilton's method before there is superficial fluctuation. The superficial inguinal lymph glands are frequently affected ; less commonly axillary adenitis occurs. Fluctuation occurs earlier in these regions. Popliteal adenitis may simulate infection of the knee joint or even osteitis of the lower end of the femur. Pre-auricular adenitis may be mistaken for parotitis, and post-auricular adenitis for acute mastoiditis.

Tuberculous Lymphadenitis.

In the first quarter of the present century tuberculosis of the cervical glands was one of the common surgical affections of childhood. In Scotland it is now becoming a surgical rarity, thanks to the widespread use of milk from tuberculin-tested cattle and of pasteurised milk. The incidence of human infection has been reduced by measures including the use of streptomycin and ancillary drugs and, more recently, by immunisation of infants and children with B.C.G. For the same reasons tuberculosis of the mesenteric lymph glands has ceased to be a surgical problem in childhood.

Primary Cutaneous Tuberculosis.

Primary tuberculous infection in a skin wound in a child differs from the *verruca necrogenica* (anatomical tubercle ; butcher's wart ; pathologist's wart) which occurs in a previously infected adult. There is usually a history of a cut or abrasion that has healed some time before the associated regional lymph glands became enlarged. The glandular enlargement is usually painless, but there may be sudden painful enlargement due to an associated pyogenic infection. In our patients the infection has followed cuts or abrasions, most commonly of the foot, but also of the shin, knee, hand and forehead (Fig. 18). The original wound may be healed on the surface, scabbed, or obviously infected when the glandular enlargement is first seen. If untreated, the regional lymph glands invariably soften and form an abscess. Abscess formation may occur any time from two weeks to six months from the time of infection of the wound.

Treatment.—When tuberculous infection is suspected, the wound of entry should be excised and the tissues examined histologically. There is usually subcutaneous tuberculosis with

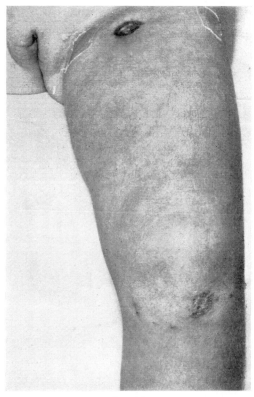

FIG. 18

Primary cutaneous tuberculosis of knee with secondary inguinal gland involvement.

some involvement of the skin. If the regional glands are still firm they should be excised. The Mantoux test is usually positive. The lung fields are X-rayed to detect evidence of hæmatogenous spread. Once the glands have softened to form an abscess, the pus is evacuated, the remains of the glands removed and the wound sutured.

Lymphadenitis following B.C.G. Vaccination.

Intradermal vaccination of the newborn with B.C.G. (the bacillus of Calmette-Guérin is a strain of bovine tuberculosis made innocuous by prolonged cultivation outside the body) is practised in most maternity units in the West of Scotland. In a significant number of infants, lymphadenitis of the regional

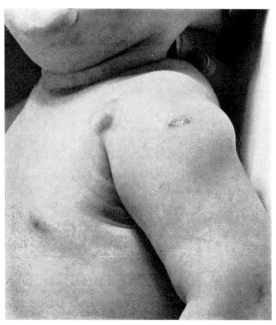

Fig. 19
B.C.G. vaccination with involvement of gland
in delto-pectoral groove.

glands develops at periods varying from one to nine months after vaccination. Depending on the site of vaccination in the arm, the glands may be affected in the axilla, the lower cervical group, the supraclavicular group or the gland in the delto-pectoral groove. The enlarged glands may be tender and may become fluctuant and the skin may be involved (Fig. 19). If the skin perforates, the gland is excised, but in most cases the parents can be assured that the glandular swelling will slowly resolve.

ABSCESS IN ABDOMINAL WALL

In infants and children it is not uncommon to find a tender swelling in the anterior abdominal wall and exploration usually reveals blood-stained pus. The abscess probably arises in a hæmatoma of the rectus muscle and this hæmatoma may spread deeply through the posterior rectus sheath. Whether infected or not, the extraperitoneal collection may be mistaken for a tumour or for an intraperitoneal abscess. In either case the swelling is exposed and the blood clot or pus evacuated.

CHAPTER V

Bone

GENERAL AFFECTIONS OF THE SKELETON

MOST of the conditions considered in this section are well recognised clinical entities but none is common. They are considered briefly as they may enter into the differential diagnosis of more common conditions encountered in infancy and childhood.

Osteogenesis Imperfecta (Fragilitas ossium).

This is a developmental condition characterised by fragility of skeletal bone; both sexes are affected. The sclerotics are usually deep blue in colour and otosclerosis may occur in those who live beyond the third decade. Prenatal cases are usually more severe and many patients die at birth or survive only a few weeks. Three types of osteogenesis imperfecta are described: (1) *Thick bone type*—severe prenatal cases born with stunted limbs (Fig. 20) and numerous fractures (Fig. 21). (2) *Slender fragile bone type*—all post-natal cases are of this type (Fig. 22). (3) *Osteogenesis imperfecta cystica*—there is pronounced honeycombing of bones (Fig. 23) and deformity is progressive with advancing years (Fig. 24). In types (1) and (3) the condition may be mistaken clinically for achondroplasia.

There is no treatment for the condition apart from protection of the child from injuries. Fractures are treated on general lines and union always occurs.

Osteopetrosis (Marble bones; Albers-Schönberg disease).

There is excessive radiographic density of the bones (Fig. 25) with or without fragility. As a result of the reduction of blood-forming bone marrow there is a tendency to anæmia which may be severe and fatal. There is a distinct familial incidence. There is no specific treatment.

51

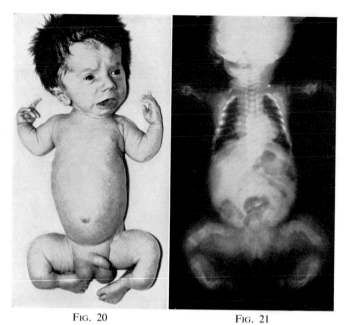

FIG. 20   FIG. 21

Fig. 20.—Baby with osteogenesis imperfecta.
Fig. 21.—Osteogenesis imperfecta (thick bone type), showing multiple
intra-uterine fractures.

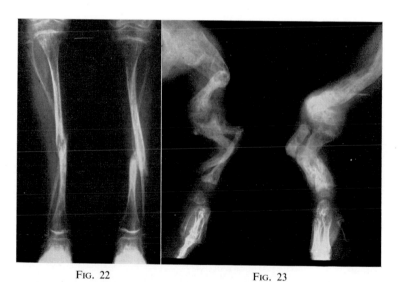

FIG. 22   FIG. 23

Fig. 22.—Osteogenesis imperfecta (slender bone type).
Fig. 23.—Osteogenesis imperfecta cystica ; gross deformity of arm bones.

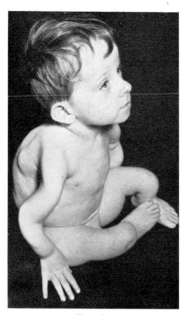

FIG. 24
Boy of 8 suffering from osteogenesis
imperfecta cystica.

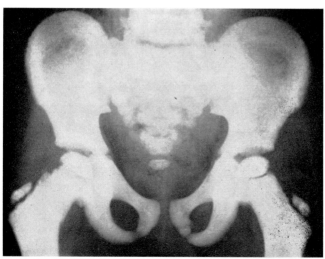

FIG. 25
Osteopetrosis showing loss of bone trabeculation.

Metaphyseal Aclasis (Multiple exostoses).

This hereditary condition is characterised by cancellous exostoses capped by cartilage, and by failure of the periosteum to mould the metaphysis (Fig. 26). The long bones are chiefly

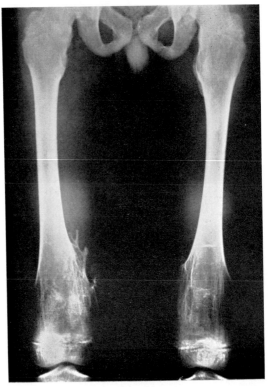

Fig. 26
Metaphyseal aclasis.

affected and a single exostosis may grow to a size sufficient to give rise to symptoms, from pressure on nerves or by causing deviation deformities. Exostoses which cause pain or deformity should be removed.

Dyschondroplasia (Ollier's disease ; multiple enchondromata).

In this developmental error there are rounded masses of unossified cartilage in the metaphyses and diaphyses of the long bones of the limbs and in the metacarpals and phalanges (Fig. 27). The lesions are essentially endosteal and not projections on the surface as in metaphyseal aclasis. There

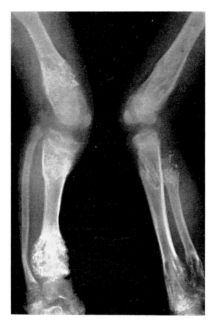

FIG. 27
Dyschondroplasia.

is no hereditary or familial influence in this condition. The enchondromata in the hands may lead to gross deformity (Fig. 28). Treatment is symptomatic.

Chondro-osteodystrophy (Morquio-Brailsford disease).

The outstanding features are dwarfism, kyphosis, knock knee, flat foot and progressive changes in the femoral head and acetabulum (Fig. 29). Clinically the condition may resemble achondroplasia or gargoylism. In Morquio's disease the skull and face are normal and there is no mental deficiency. There is no treatment.

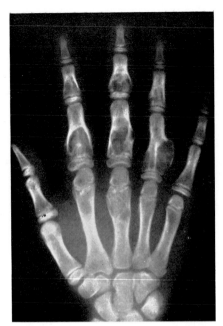

FIG. 28
Enchondromata in a child suffering from Ollier's disease.

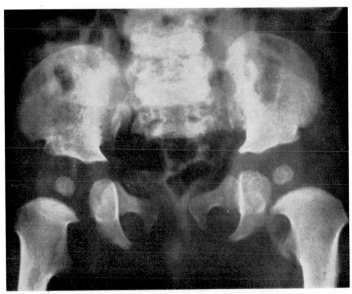

FIG. 29
Chondro-osteodystrophy with deformity of femoral heads and acetabula.

Achondroplasia (Chondrodystrophia fœtalis).

There is interference with endochondral ossification (Fig. 30) and the condition is characterised by short limb dwarfism, a

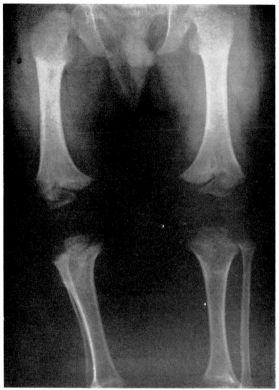

FIG. 30
Achondroplasia.

large head and "trident hands" (Fig. 31). No known treatment has any influence on the disease.

Myositis Ossificans Progressiva.

Swellings arise in association with connective tissue, fascia and tendons and progress to ossification. The muscles are only affected secondarily. There is characteristic shortening of the thumbs and great toes (Fig. 32). Interference with joint

4

movement may be temporarily alleviated by extirpation of a lesion. The condition becomes widespread and although only

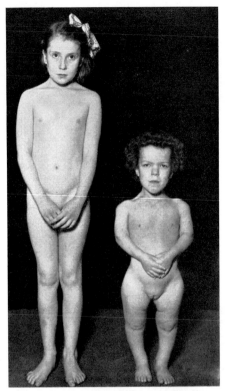

FIG. 31
Achondroplastic dwarf with normal child of the same age.

slowly progressive, is ultimately fatal. Joints are stiffened, the chest becomes immobile and the patient becomes bed-ridden and susceptible to intercurrent disease. Cortisone may alleviate pain and stiffness during periods of acute exacerbation.

Cranio-cleido-dysostosis.

In this condition there is deficient formation of the clavicles with imperfect ossification of the skull (Fig. 33). The patient can usually approximate the tips of the shoulders to each

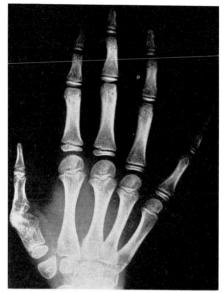

FIG. 32
Typical short thumb in myositis
ossificans progressiva.

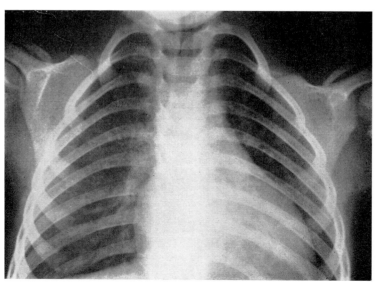

FIG. 33
Cranio-cleido-dysostosis showing deficient clavicles.

other below the chin (Fig. 34). There is no disability or discomfort and no treatment is called for.

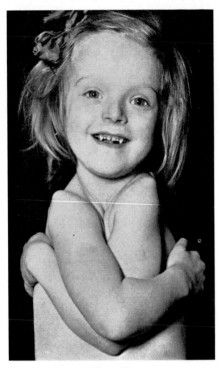

FIG. 34

Cranio-cleido-dysostosis. The tips of the shoulders can be approximated to one another below the chin.

Neurofibromatosis (von Recklinghausen's disease).

There are pigmented (*café-au-lait*) spots in the skin, cutaneous fibromata, multiple neurofibromata and in some cases skeletal changes (Fig. 35). The skeletal affections take the form of a resistant type of scoliosis and diminution in growth of a bone. The lesions may or may not be progressive. The scoliosis may eventually cause complete crippling in spite of intensive and heroic orthopædic treatment. Sarcomatous change may occur in more than one fibroma in later life.

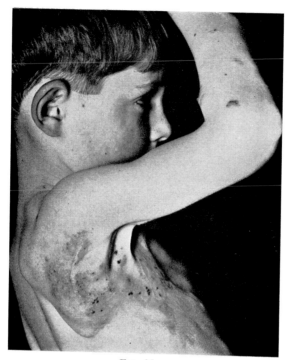

FIG. 35

Neurofibromatosis. Fibrous nodules, pigmentation, hypoplasia of the scapula and early scoliosis.

Arachnodactyly (Spider fingers; Marfan's syndrome) (Fig. 36).

The essential features are the extreme length of the digits, slender build with poorly developed muscles and hypermobility of the wrists, ankles and digits. Other deformities such as funnel sternum, foot deformities and calcaneal spurs may be present. There is a congenital dislocation of the lens in half the patients and congenital heart disease is found in one third. The patients die of intercurrent disease in adolescence or early adult life.

Fibrocystic Disease of Bone.

Osteitis fibrosa cystica due to hyperparathyroidism is not encountered in childhood but fibrocystic disease may appear

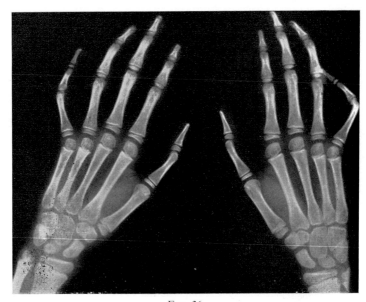

Fig. 36
Arachnodactyly.

in two forms: (1) *Bone cysts* and (2) *polyostotic fibrous dysplasia.*

SOLITARY BONE CYST.—This may appear in any long bone (Fig. 37) and may present with pain and swelling of the part. Pathological fracture may occur. The cyst is cured by simple curettage, a thin-walled cavity being filled with bone chips. The histology is similar to that in hyperparathyroidism but there are few osteoclasts and the original bone trabeculation disappears.

POLYOSTOTIC FIBROUS DYSPLASIA.—In this condition there are multiple lesions in the skeleton without general decalcification or disturbance of calcium metabolism (Fig. 38). In a third of the cases there are areas of pigmentation in the skin, with precocious puberty in females (Albright's syndrome). The major long bones are principally affected and the skull may be involved as in leontiasis ossea. Fractures are common but unite readily. The bone changes are arrested when growth ceases.

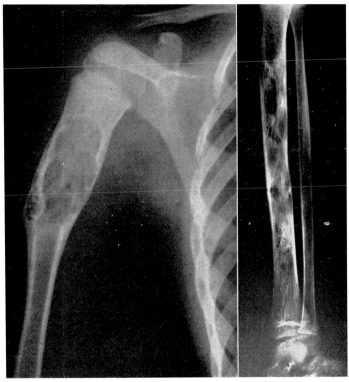

FIG. 37   FIG. 38

Fig. 37.—Multilocular cyst of the humerus.
Fig. 38.—Polyostotic fibrous dysplasia.

Infantile Scurvy.

The disease is characterised by hæmorrhages and disturbances in ossification and is due to lack of vitamin C. There is often visible and palpable swelling of a limb with pain and tenderness and accompanied by fever, and the condition may be mistaken for infantile osteitis. Most cases occur between 6 and 12 months and fortunately hæmatogenous osteitis is not common in this age group. In most patients with scurvy the bone lesions are bilateral and the child lies in the frog position with the thighs abducted and the knees flexed (Fig. 39). Hæmorrhage may occur at any site, but in infants swelling and hæmorrhage in the gums is most typical. The radiographic

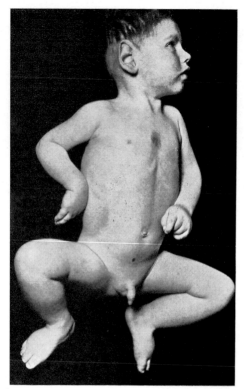

Fig. 39
Typical attitude of child with scurvy.

appearances are diagnostic and are due to subperiosteal hæmorrhages (Fig. 40).

The response to administration of vitamin C in the form of ascorbic acid is dramatic. There is marked improvement within twenty-four to forty-eight hours and all pain has gone within a week.

Rickets.

Deformities such as genu varum and genu valgum may occur in neglected cases of *infantile rickets, resistant rickets* or *cœliac rickets*. Most bones show a remarkable return to normality with medical treatment. Where severe deformities

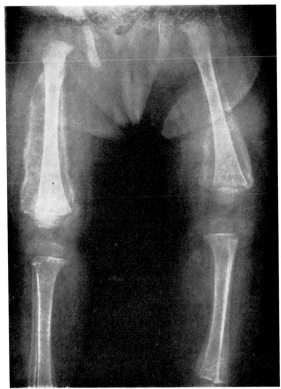

FIG. 40
Calcification in subperiosteal hæmorrhages in scurvy.

have occurred (Fig. 41) splintage may be necessary when the active phase of the disease is over. Rarely osteotomy may be required.

In *renal rickets* and one of the *Fanconi syndromes* (renal glycosuria with hypophosphatæmic rickets), orthopædic problems are completely overshadowed by the kidney lesions and their dire effects.

Reticulo-endotheliosis.

A number of conditions are grouped together on account of the fundamental pathology common to them all. They are *eosinophilic granuloma of bone, Hand-Schüller-Christian disease, Letterer-Siwe disease* and *Gaucher's disease,* and osseous lesions occur in all four. All four conditions are rare, but the first three may present with a diagnosis of abscess

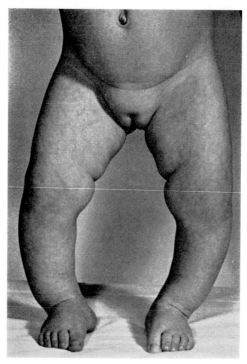

Fig. 41
Genu varum in infant recovering from resistant rickets.

or bone infection (Figs. 42, 43 and 44). Eosinophil granuloma and Hand-Schüller-Christian disease may be improved or even cured by X-ray therapy. There is at present no treatment which will benefit patients with Letterer-Siwe or Gaucher's disease.

Infantile Cortical Hyperostosis.

There is symmetrical periostitis affecting the clavicles, mandible, scapulæ, ribs and long bones (Fig. 45 and Fig. 183). The mandibular swelling gives the infant a characteristic

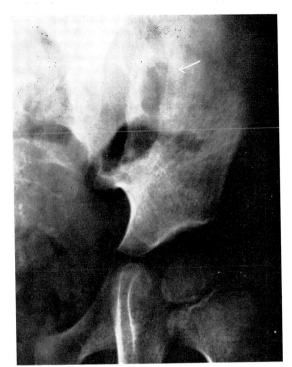

FIG. 42
Eosinophil granuloma of left ilium (arrowed).

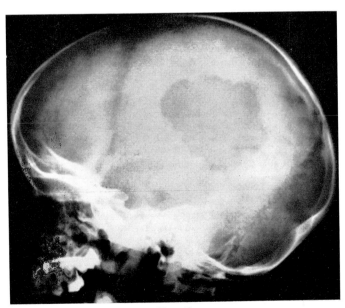

FIG. 43
Skull defect in Hand-Schüller-Christian disease. Patient presented
with an " abscess " of scalp.

67

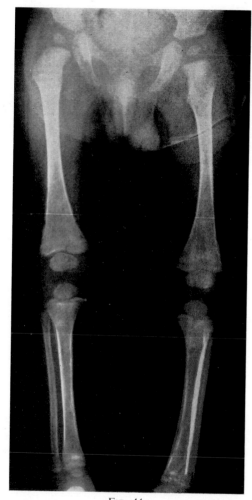

FIG. 44

Bone lesions in Letterer-Siwe disease. Condition
was first thought to be hæmatogenous osteitis.

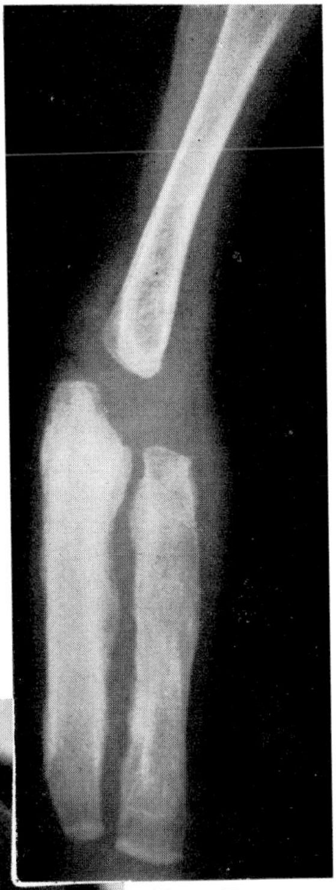

Fig. 45.—Subperiosteal new bone in infantile cortical hyperostosis. The patient was admitted with a diagnosis of hæmatogenous osteitis.

Fig. 46.—Facies in infantile cortical hyperostosis.

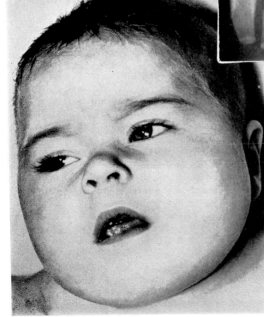

FIG. 45

FIG. 46

appearance (Fig. 46). The disease appears in the early months of life and in its early phase may closely resemble neonatal osteitis. The ætiology is unknown.

Complete recovery takes place spontaneously usually within a year but cure may be expedited by administration of cortisone.

Leukæmia.

Bone lesions are common in leukæmia in children and may take the form of decalcification, osteosclerosis or subperiosteal

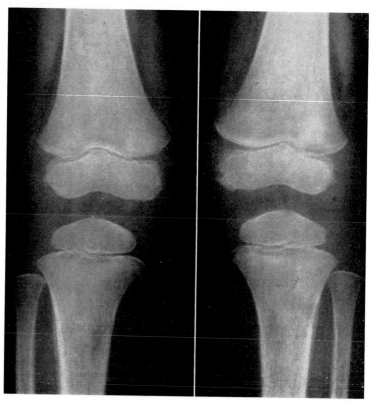

Fig. 47
Bone lesions in leukæmia.

shadows (Fig. 47). The bone changes may precede the typical blood and bone marrow picture. The patient may complain of pain in the limbs and the bone changes may be mistaken for low-grade osteitis.

OSTEOCHONDRITIS

This is a non-inflammatory derangement of the normal process of growth which occurs at various centres of ossification during the period of their greatest activity. Before puberty the common sites are the *femoral head* (Perthes' disease) and the *tarsal scaphoid* (Köhler's disease). Less commonly osteochondritis is seen in the medial tibial condyle (Blount's disease). These conditions will be considered more fully in Chapter XXIII. Osteochondritis of the tibial apophysis (Osgood-Schlatter's disease), of the calcaneal apophysis (Sever's disease), of the second metatarsal (Freiberg's infraction) and of the vertebral epiphyses (Scheuermann's disease) are rarely seen in a children's hospital.

FRACTURES

GENERAL CONSIDERATIONS

In Chapter I we have discussed how the response of the child's tissues to injury differs in many respect from that of the adult. Not only is the healing of fractured bones rapid but the soft tissues also recover speedily and completely from the effects of trauma and there is a welcome freedom from œdema, stiff joints and muscle dysfunction. A birth fracture is firmly united in about three weeks but as the child grows this speed of repair diminishes steadily until, by the time growth ceases in adolescence, the normal adult rate of healing is established. Similarly, should the fracture unite with angulation of the fragments, the resulting deformity will be corrected in due course—in an infant within a few months, in the older child within a year or so. Not only is angulation corrected, but should shortening of the limb result, the rate of growth of the fractured limb increases beyond its fellow until the limbs once more are equal in length. Indeed in some cases the correction is excessive and the fractured bone may for a time exceed its fellow in length but eventually equality is reached.

The free blood supply of the growing bone results in more extensive hæmorrhage at the site of the fracture and if the periosteum remains intact, a closed hæmatoma results. The biochemical changes in this hæmatoma are particularly active; decalcification and absorption of the bone ends proceed concurrently with very active deposition of new bone and the subsequent callus is much greater than in the adult. It is wise to warn the parents that the hard, visible and palpable swelling in their child's limb is not permanent and will soon disappear completely. Should the periosteum be torn, the blood extravasates extensively through the tissues and ecchymosis may appear at some distance from the fracture site.

Except in the bones of the skull and in the clavicles, which develop in membrane, primary and secondary centres of ossification appear in regular sequence. The radiologist or surgeon called upon to interpret the X-ray film of a suspected fracture must be familiar with the times of their appearance and of their fusion. Twin centres of ossification are not uncommon and their appearance on X-ray may be mistaken for fracture of a single centre. The occasional presence of small accessory bones should also be remembered as they too may simulate a fracture. The blood supply of the epiphysis is derived from the periosteal and articular vessels and never from the nutrient artery. Separation of an epiphysis is thus rarely followed by avascular necrosis with the exception of the femoral capital epiphysis.

The *incomplete* or *greenstick* fracture is particularly common and may be found in three forms:

1. The hairline crack in the cortex resulting from torsional strain and presenting with slight local pain and tenderness. The crack may easily be overlooked in the immediate X-ray films and only after a week or ten days the slight raising of the periosteum due to subperiosteal hæmorrhage and new bone formation suggests the diagnosis (Fig. 48, A and B). Not infrequently in a young child there is a slight rise of temperature and this may suggest an inflammatory cause for the local pain and tenderness, but there is no evidence of toxæmia and the signs and symptoms subside quickly with rest in bed.

2. The compression fracture in which the X-ray film shows a horizontal line of compressed cortex (Fig. 49, A and B).

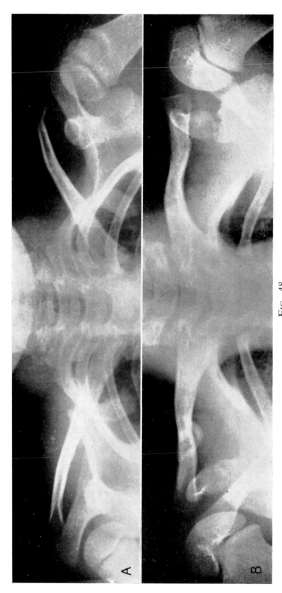

Fig. 48

Injury to right shoulder. A, Radiograph on day of accident shows no obvious fracture. B, Ten days later, callus and fracture line visible in right clavicle.

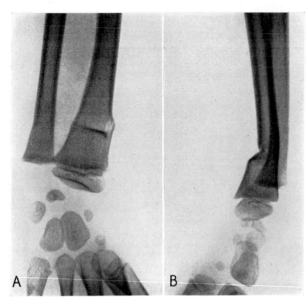

Fig. 49
Compression of cortex in fracture of radius.

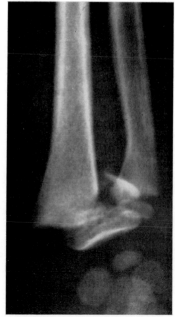

Fig. 50
Fracture-separation of lower radial epiphysis.

Deformity and abnormal mobility are absent and again the local pain and tenderness subside quickly with rest in bed and the application of a plaster splint.

3. The common and typical greenstick fracture in which the cortex is broken through on one side but only bent or incompletely broken at the opposite side (Fig. 227). Deformity, local tenderness and pain are present but there is no abnormal mobility or crepitus, the periosteum frequently remaining intact. It is impossible to correct the deformity without rendering the fracture complete.

Where the force of the injury has been applied at the end of a long bone, there may result not a fracture but a *separation of the epiphysis.* In the minor degrees of this injury the displacement is negligible and the exact diagnosis is evident only in the X-ray film. In the more severe forms, the epiphysis when displaced carries with it a small triangular fragment of the metaphysis and the injury is more accurately described as a fracture through the metaphysis (Fig. 50). The deformity is usually obvious but there is no undue mobility—and the crepitus if any is soft and muffled.

COMPLICATIONS

1. **Non-union.**—Non-union of the fragments is rare in children. Once the pain of the fracture has passed off, children find it difficult to " keep still " and minor degrees of movement of the fragments cannot always be avoided despite apparently adequate immobilisation. The effect is merely to increase the amount of callus and sometimes to delay union, but rarely to cause non-union. Refracture of a bone at the site of a recently united fracture is, however, not uncommon. Whereas the normal response of the adult to a recently healed fracture is to refrain from full freedom of use for a considerable time, the child, on the other hand, soon forgets the injury and indulges freely in the usual strains and stresses. A comparatively minor injury may thus cause a refracture at the same site. The repair process is always less active after a refracture and immobilisation must be effectively maintained for a longer period than after the original fracture. Failure to do so may be followed by non-union or fibrous union.

2. **Localised Traumatic Ossification.**—Where a muscle has been torn from its attachment, a mass of bone may form within the muscle, restricting its movement and limiting the range of movement of the neighbouring joint (Fig. 51). The

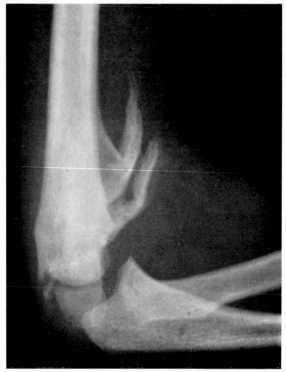

FIG. 51
Heterotopic ossification after supracondylar
fracture of humerus.

growing bone of the child is peculiarly liable to this complication, particularly around the elbow joint. It may follow dislocation without actual fracture. The possibility of its occurrence is increased by repeated attempts at reduction of deformity and also by misguided massage and *passive* movements before absorption of the callus. The only permissible physiotherapy after fractures or dislocations at the elbow joint should be active *voluntary* movements by the child, encouraged possibly by suitable incentives. This condition should not be mistaken for the subperiosteal ossification that results from a failure in the process of absorption of callus.

3. **Interference with the Circulation.**—This is not a common complication of fractures in childhood but it may follow injuries in the region of the elbow and forearm. The results of unrelieved arterial or venous obstruction are so disastrous for the child that comment in some detail is called for.

The mechanism of obstruction and the resulting pathological changes in the tissues are so varied that the clinical picture is often confusing. Irreversible changes may occur early as a direct and immediate result of the vascular damage and no treatment is effective in preventing this. On the other hand, warning of interference with the circulation is frequently presented in time to permit of treatment and prevent permanent damage. In teaching students the necessity for frequent inspection of the limb in all such fractures, the authors have felt justified in calling upon " apt alliteration's artful aid " and stressing the importance of *pain, pallor, paralysis, purple* colour and *absence of pulse* as indications for immediate action. In a darkened ward at night the lowered temperature of the fingers will indicate the need for a more thorough examination. There are two possibilities to consider :—

(*a*) *Arterial occlusion.*—The brachial artery may be occluded by pressure of bone fragments as a direct result of the accident and the pallor and absence of pulse form part of the immediate clinical picture. The same clinical picture may result from spasm of the vessel due to bruising or partial occlusion by a bone fragment. There is no effective method of differentiating between these two conditions. It has been suggested that gentle manipulation to relieve pressure followed by immersion of the sound arm in warm water will relieve spasm. The effect of this manœuvre may be slight or equivocal and time lost may render irreversible the damage to muscles and nerves. The only permissible treatment where the pulse is absent is immediate exploration of the fracture site. If the arterial occlusion or spasm is allowed to persist unrelieved, the collateral vessels may also be affected by the spasm and the ischæmia may affect not only the forearm muscles but also the median and ulnar nerves. Motor and sensory paralysis of variable degree follows with, later, flexion contractures of the fingers and wrists. A similar condition may affect the arteries of the leg.

(b) *Venous Obstruction.*—The clinical picture of venous obstruction develops more slowly. The pulse remains palpable and the presenting signs are cyanosis of the hand and increasing pain in the forearm. Voluntary extension of the fingers cannot be performed and passive extension causes extreme pain. This development may be spontaneous but more often shows itself after manipulation and the application of splints or plaster. It has been suggested that tissue œdema, coupled with slow and continuous hæmorrhage under the deep fascia, results in increasing pressure to the extent of causing ischæmia of the forearm muscles. The flexor group are usually most affected and permanent fibrosis and contracture result unless the pressure is relieved. Prophylactic elevation of the limb and the use of split or padded plasters may prevent the onset of the condition. If ischæmia is suspected, constricting splints and bandages are slackened. Multiple and early incisions through the deep fascia offer the best chance of limiting the muscle damage. Not infrequently the clinical picture suggests a combination of arterial and venous obstruction, with neurological signs and symptoms which baffle interpretation.

The onset of this complication of fracture is usually spontaneous but it may follow unskilled treatment. In a supracondylar fracture of the humerus forced flexion of the elbow, in the presence of uncorrected displacement of the fragments or even of marked swelling, may easily obliterate the pulse, either immediately or soon after manipulation. The mode of application of splints or plaster after manipulation of a forearm fracture may easily produce venous obstruction following reactionary swelling.

4. **Nerve Injury.**—Primary nerve injury as a complication of fracture in childhood is uncommon. Bruising of the radial or ulnar nerves may occur in supracondylar fracture of the humerus, and of the peroneal nerve in fracture of the upper end of the fibula. Recovery is usually rapid and complete.

5. **Damage to the Growth Area of a Long Bone.**—Separation of any epiphysis in a child is rarely accompanied by damage to the neighbouring growth area. Such damage, however, is not unknown and is due to crushing caused by the shearing

force applied at the junction of the metaphysis and the epiphysis. Despite complete reduction of the displacement, subsequent interference with the growth of the bone occurs and causes a most severe and intractable deformity and disability.

PATHOLOGICAL FRACTURES

Spontaneous and pathological fractures are not uncommon in childhood and they are met with in three groups of conditions.

1. **General Affections of the Skeleton.**—In *osteogenesis imperfecta, osteopetrosis* and *fibrocystic disease of bone* fractures occur with trivial violence. In untreated *rickets*, the bones fracture readily but such cases are now rare. Union occurs readily despite active rickets.

2. **Neoplastic Disease.**—Neoplastic disease sufficient to allow fracture is always malignant (primary or metastatic) and union rarely occurs before death.

3. **Generalised Decalcification of Bone.**—Following prolonged recumbency with immobilisation in a splint or plaster-of-Paris case there is decalcification of the bones of that limb. Greenstick fracture may readily result from careless handling of the child when the splint or plaster is first removed. Similarly in children suffering from severe palsy, as in poliomyelitis or spina bifida, decalcification of bone will occur. Fracture is not uncommon in such cases and occurs, not when the patient is wearing a splint or caliper but when he is in bed without support for the limb.

Hyperæmic decalcification may result from a local focus of chronic bone infection and it also occurs quite early in acute hæmatogenous osteitis (p. 89). Since the introduction of antibiotics in the treatment of pyogenic infection of bone, massive involucrum formation is no longer seen and hyperæmic decalcification may so weaken the bone that fracture may result from trivial violence (Fig. 52).

TREATMENT

First-aid Treatment.—As in the adult, the joint above and below the fracture should be immobilised before the child is moved from the scene of the accident. In the upper limb, the arm is held to the side of the body by a sling; the forearm is bandaged to a padded piece of wood or a folded newspaper. The leg is best immobilised in a Thomas splint but if no suitable splint is available the legs should be bandaged together.

The details of treatment will be described in the sections

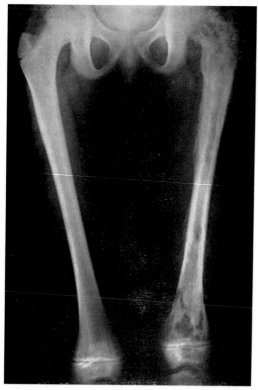

FIG. 52

Bipolar osteitis with pathological fractures of femoral neck and supracondylar region.

dealing with individual fractures but certain general observations demand emphasis here.

The speed of repair of the child's bone calls for the earliest possible correction of deformity. Callus develops so rapidly that within a few days accurate alignment of the fragments becomes impossible. Nevertheless should extensive swelling be present when the fracture is first seen it may be wiser to wait for twenty-four hours before attempting reduction, as it is desirable that correction should be attained at the first attempt. Repeated manipulations cannot be too strongly condemned. With each attempt fresh hæmorrhage occurs followed by increased swelling and not only is reduction increasingly difficult but there is a very real danger of producing heterotopic ossification. The capacity for the restoration of normal structure is so great that it is often wiser to be content with less than complete correction in the knowledge that nature will in due course make good the shortcomings of the surgeon.

Where traction is employed it should be remembered that the ratio of muscle power to body weight is high in the child. A relatively greater weight is thus required in the child to overcome muscle spasm and reduce shortening. Despite this, *skeletal traction should never be employed* as the child's bone will be cut through readily with consequent risk of damage to the epiphysis. Skin traction correctly applied will carry all the weight required.

Where immobilisation is called for, plaster of Paris offers the simplest and most effective method of splinting. It can be easily applied and accurately moulded to the varying contours of the limb, but it has a very real disadvantage in being inflexible when it dries. For that reason the plaster should take the form of slabs applied to the opposite sides of the limb and bandaged in place. Alternatively, a plaster cast may be applied to encircle the limb but the cast must then be split throughout its entire length. Either method is a safeguard against the possibility of vascular obstruction.

In children the field for the operative treatment of fractures is very limited. The condylar fractures at the elbow that will not yield to manipulation, call for open replacement to avoid gross disturbance of the carrying angle. Fractures of the olecranon and patella with wide separation of the fragments may require replacement and suture. There also some justification for operation in fractures of both bones of the forearm with rotation of the fragments.

Splints.—In any children's hospital, the provision of facilities for the making of splints is essential and our hospital is fortunate in having a large orthopædic appliance department. The immobilisation of fractures is most easily and efficiently carried out by means of plaster of Paris but cases may occur where the use of this material is unsatisfactory by reason of its weight. In fractures of the neck of the humerus, for example, a light-weight plastic or fibre splint is efficient and more comfortable. In certain cases where union is slow, a light splint of " Glassona " or some such material is desirable. In children suffering from congenital deformities or paralysis, the continuous alteration in size and girth demands the frequent adjustment and renewal of the splints.

DISLOCATIONS OF TRAUMATIC ORIGIN

The joint of a growing child is normally more flexible and is possessed of a greater range of movement than that of the adult. Actual dislocation is therefore relatively less common in childhood though minor sprains with or without effusion of fluid into the joint occur more frequently than is generally recognised. Reduction of the dislocation under general anæsthesia is usually obtained without difficulty and restoration of normal function is almost invariable. Physio-therapy is rarely necessary though appropriate exercises with suitable incentives may be useful for the timid child.

ACUTE HÆMATOGENOUS OSTEITIS

(Acute Hæmatogenous Osteomyelitis)

Definition.—*Acute osteitis is a sudden illness associated with severe toxæmia and definite evidence of inflammation of bone, the duration of the illness being days rather than weeks.* The term **osteitis** is preferred to **osteomyelitis** as the bone marrow plays only a small part in bone suppuration. The older terms periostitis, osteitis and osteomyelitis as denoting separate diseases should be abandoned and the inflammations of bone tissue alluded to as *osteitis*—a term which covers all the essential structures of a bone.

Ætiology

Organism.—The most common infecting organism is the *Staphylococcus pyogenes aureus.* Most pathogenic staphylococci coagulate rabbit plasma and are termed " coagulase positive." In a series of 212 consecutive cases of acute osteitis in the Royal Hospital for Sick Children, Glasgow, a coagulase-positive staphylococcus was the responsible organism in all but ten patients. Streptococcal osteitis is more common in infancy and usually gives rise to a subacute infection but a streptococcus was responsible for seven of the acute cases. Acute pneumococcal osteitis is rare but when it occurs it is clinically indistinguishable from staphylococcal osteitis.

Route of Infection.—The infection is commonly blood-borne from such septic foci as boils, septic abrasions, infected teeth and tonsils. In the neonatal period (p. 39) infection probably enters through the respiratory or alimentary tract, but it may enter through the umbilical cord. Direct implantation is only found in association with compound fractures and accidental wounds, and as an occasional complication of marrow transfusion.

Localising Factors.—The accepted ætiology is that a child suffering from a symptomless bacteriæmia arising from a septic focus is subject to some minor trauma to the delicate vascular metaphysis. There is a definite history of injury in almost half of our patients and evidence of a septic focus is found in more than a third. As osteitis never follows a simple fracture, one must postulate that solution in the continuity of a bone allows release of tension in the region of the fracture hæmatoma. In childhood, infection can lie latent for long periods and the initial lesion is often healed and forgotten for two or three weeks before the onset of the disease. The daily bumps and twists to which the normal child subjects himself may be similarly forgotten.

Social Incidence.—There is a definite class distinction manifest in the child who is affected by osteitis and the disease is rarely encountered in private consulting practice. Acute osteitis is uncommon in the great public schools although minor injuries and infected abrasions are common. The incidence of osteitis is low where the standard of cleanliness is high.

Age and Sex.—Acute osteitis is essentially a disease of childhood. Apart from neonatal osteitis (Chap. IV), the disease is relatively uncommon in the first two years of life. It is more common in boys and occurs most frequently during a period of active growth. Trauma is common during this period and boys probably injure themselves more frequently than girls.

BONES AFFECTED

The bones of the lower extremity are most liable to infection and the tibia and femur are by far the most common sites for osteitis. The upper metaphysis of the tibia and lower metaphysis of the femur are frequently subjected to injury and this may be an influential factor. Any bone in the body may be the seat of acute osteitis.

PATHOLOGY

In most patients, the disease appears to start as a septicæmia. The septicæmic phase may be of short duration or it may be prolonged for several days. The circulating organisms then settle in the vascular metaphysis of a long bone and there lead to an acute suppurative inflammation. Around this bone focus there is an outpouring of leucocytes and a tiny abscess forms, surrounded by a zone of intense hyperæmia. The infection extends to the cortex and periosteum close to the epiphyseal line and the periosteum is raised from the bone, first by œdema then by pus. The small periosteal arteries are obliterated and the blood supply to the cortex is impaired (Fig. 53). Superficial portions of the bone undergo necrosis and may later form sequestra. Since the periosteum is closely attached to the circumference at the epiphyseal cartilage, the infection does not spread into the joint at an early stage except in certain regions such as the hip and shoulder, where the metaphysis is intra-articular. The pus spreads inwards through the Haversian canals at different levels and invades the medulla (Fig. 54) giving the " spotty " character to the shaft infection which is clearly seen radiographically. Direct spread into the medulla occurs late. The nutrient artery may be occluded by œdema or by actual thrombosis, with death of large areas of the bone.

In the *untreated case*, the medulla is converted into oily pus owing to the destruction of the fatty tissue. The surface of the bone is bathed in pus and the bone loses its healthy shining appearance and becomes a dull opaque white. Necrosis of bone is usually greatest in the region of the metaphysis where thrombosis and tension destroy the living framework of the bone. Extensive necrosis is now seen only in museum specimens.

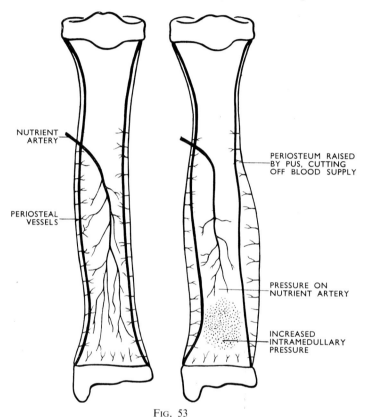

NUTRIENT ARTERY

PERIOSTEAL VESSELS

PERIOSTEUM RAISED BY PUS, CUTTING OFF BLOOD SUPPLY

PRESSURE ON NUTRIENT ARTERY

INCREASED INTRAMEDULLARY PRESSURE

FIG. 53

Diagrammatic illustration of interference with blood supply in hæmatogenous osteitis of a long bone.

The dead portion of bone is at first continuous with the living but demarcation is not long delayed and small portions of dead bone may be absorbed. Around the dead mass, vascular granulation tissue develops and before the dead bone is set free as a sequestrum, it shows an eroded worm-eaten appearance. New bone forms both on the surface and in the depths of the old bone. When the periosteum has been widely separated an extensive new case of subperiosteal bone—an *involucrum*—may develop. This involucrum is at first light and porous but as the blood supply diminishes it eventually becomes sclerosed.

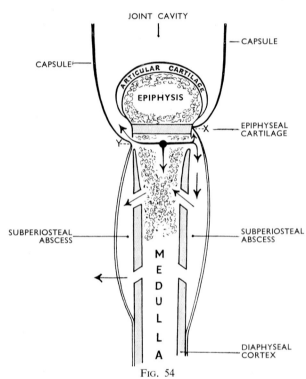

FIG. 54

Mode of spread of infection from a metaphyseal focus in hæmatogenous osteitis. X represents attachment of capsule and periosteum when metaphysis is extra-capsular : Y is point of fixation when metaphysis is intracapsular.

Its surface is rough and irregular and it is usually perforated by *cloacae* marking the position of sinuses through which purulent discharge escapes to the surface (Fig. 55).

At any stage, septic thrombi may give rise to emboli and pyæmia. The blood culture is positive and the septicæmia may be so overwhelming that death may occur before any extensive changes take place in the metaphysis. The adjacent joint may become filled with a sterile serous effusion or the process may rupture into the joint to cause a purulent arthritis.

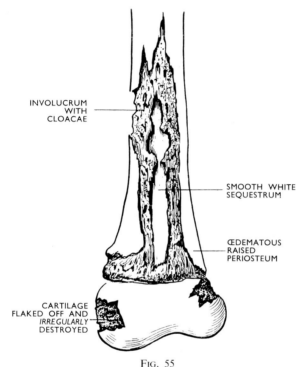

INVOLUCRUM
WITH
CLOACAE

SMOOTH WHITE
SEQUESTRUM

ŒDEMATOUS
RAISED
PERIOSTEUM

CARTILAGE
FLAKED OFF AND
IRREGULARLY
DESTROYED

FIG. 55

Chronic osteitis. Drawn from a specimen in the pathology museum, Royal Hospital for Sick Children, Glasgow.

CLINICAL FEATURES

In a typical case, the disease begins suddenly with acute pain in the affected limb but occasionally the acute symptoms are preceded by a variable period in which the child is in indifferent health. There is commonly a history of recent injury and a primary focus of infection may be found. The child is ill, flushed and restless, although the affected limb is kept absolutely still. The patient resents any attempt to examine the limb and is obviously apprehensive when anyone comes near the bed. The pulse is rapid, the temperature high, the tongue dry, the urine scanty and concentrated and the eyes are bright. In the more intense infections, toxæmia may be so severe that the child soon becomes delirious and the general symptoms may obscure the local condition.

Patience and gentleness should be exercised in the examination of the child. The affected limb lies with the related joint flexed to relax the adjacent muscles. In the early stages there is no swelling of the limb but by gentle palpation an area of maximum tenderness is found over the affected metaphysis. Associated with subperiosteal effusion, swelling of the limb occurs but redness does not appear until the periosteum ruptures. The neighbouring joint becomes swollen, at first due to a sympathetic effusion ; later the swelling may be due to pus in the joint. The associated lymphatic glands are neither enlarged nor tender until pus bursts into the soft tissues. A general examination of the patient is carried out, paying particular attention to the heart, lungs and pleura. A white blood count usually reveals a high polymorphonuclear leucocytosis and the erythrocyte sedimentation rate is markedly raised. Apart from soft tissue œdema there are no radiographic changes in the first ten days of the illness and radiography has little to offer in the early diagnosis of acute osteitis.

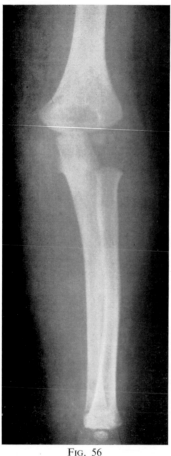

FIG. 56

Osteitis of ulna. Radiographic appearances on day of admission— soft tissue œdema only.

RADIOGRAPHIC CHANGES

During the first few days, soft tissue œdema is seen (Fig. 56). About the tenth day there is usually evidence of raising of the periosteum and about the fourteenth day a translucent area of decalcification can be seen in the affected metaphysis. These

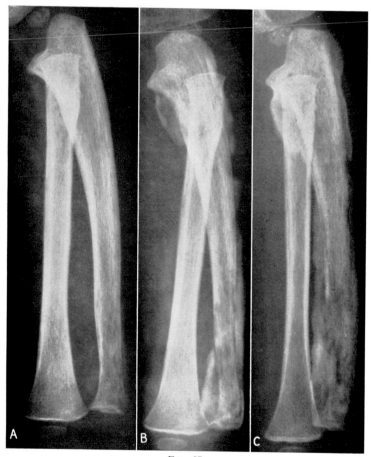

FIG. 57

Same patient as Fig. 56. A, Raised periosteum and patchy decalcification of lower ulna. B, Subperiosteal new bone formation. C, Gross involucrum and sequestrum in lower ulna.

appearances, however, may be delayed for three or four weeks, particularly in the upper femur and metatarsal bones. From this time onwards new subperiosteal bone is seen and this bone spreads for varying distances along the shaft. About twenty-one days, patchy decalcification is evident in the metaphysis (Fig. 57)

6

and usually this decalcification is progressive over a period of weeks or even months. The appearance of decalcification may be exaggerated by the generalised decalcification which is seen in an immobilised limb. After four weeks sequestrum formation is shown by the appearance of areas of increased density.

DIFFERENTIAL DIAGNOSIS

Certain conditions are liable to be confused with acute osteitis. They are as follows: *Cellulitis, acute rheumatism, simple fracture* (generally greenstick), *acute poliomyelitis,* other forms of *septicæmia, pyogenic arthritis.* Early administration of sulphonamides or antibiotics may make accurate diagnosis more difficult.

1. **Cellulitis.**—Cellulitis may closely simulate acute osteitis. The area of redness is usually more widespread; the pain and toxæmia are less than in osteitis and the tenderness is more diffuse. Cellulitis only appears in osteitis when there is pus under the periosteum or in the soft tissues and occurs relatively late in the disease.

2. **Acute Rheumatism.**—Acute rheumatic fever is essentially a polyarticular disease, but in the early stages painful swelling of a large joint may simulate osteitis. On careful examination the pain will be found to be localised to the joint and not to the adjoining metaphysis. Although fever is high toxæmia is less than in osteitis.

3. **Simple Fracture.**—The swelling and pain of a greenstick fracture in younger children may be confused with acute osteitis but fever is rarely marked and toxæmia is absent. Radiography may be necessary to confirm the diagnosis.

4. **Acute Poliomyelitis.**—In the early stages of acute poliomyelitis with loss of function, tenderness in a limb and pyrexia, the condition may be mistaken for acute osteitis. During an epidemic of poliomyelitis it is not uncommon for patients with acute osteitis to be treated as cases of poliomyelitis. In poliomyelitis the tenderness is in the muscles, rather than in the bone.

5. **Septicæmia.**—When the toxæmia of osteitis conceals the local signs, the condition resembles any other form of septicæmia—pneumococcal or meningococcal.

6. **Pyogenic Arthritis.**—In this condition joint symptoms predominate, muscle spasm is intense and slight movements cause extreme pain. Primary pyogenic arthritis is a rare disease of childhood and in all cases of joint infection a focus in the adjacent metaphysis should be suspected, although radiography may not reveal the bone focus for two to three weeks. Traumatic synovitis of the hip (Chap. XXIII) is common in childhood and may closely simulate a pyogenic bone or joint lesion.

TREATMENT

The aim of treatment is to control septicæmia and to reduce tension in the local focus. The relief of tension eases pain, lessens absorption and preserves the blood supply of the bone. If the infecting organism is penicillin-sensitive and penicillin therapy is instituted early, these objects should be achieved without surgical intervention. Unfortunately, pus is usually present under the periosteum or in the soft tissues by the time the patient reaches hospital and surgical intervention is usually necessary.

Although treatment should begin promptly and should not be delayed until laboratory data are available, the introduction of antibiotics has increased rather than lessened the surgeon's responsibility for precise diagnosis. Having made a provisional clinical diagnosis of the site of the disease, a complete general examination is carried out paying particular attention to the pericardium, to the respiratory tract and to the remainder of the skeleton. Venous blood is taken for culture and penicillin administration is started without waiting for the bacteriological report.

Treatment is considered under three headings; general treatment of the patient, penicillin administration and operative procedure.

General Treatment.—The affected limb is immobilised and if the child is toxic and dehydrated an intravenous drip is set up. Even if pus is obviously present in the soft tissues, the extremely ill child is not taken to the operating theatre at once. Penicillin is administered (after removing blood for culture) and in very ill patients an intravenous drip may be set up and penicillin may be given by this route. In the absence of redness and gross œdema of the part it is hoped that local pain and the signs of toxæmia will abate or at least not become more severe. If the pain and toxæmia do not abate in twenty-four to forty-eight hours, either there is pus under tension in the bone or under the periosteum, or the organism is not sensitive to penicillin. Exploration soon settles the first point; until the bacteriologist's report on sensitivity is received one cannot be certain about the second and under such circumstances a combination of penicillin and streptomycin is injected or administration of penicillin is stopped and one of the broad-spectrum antibiotics of the tetracycline group is substituted. On theoretical grounds and from clinical experience we consider that it is undesirable to combine bactericidal and bacteriostatic antibiotics.

Immobilisation.—The immobilised limb must be available for inspection and is never enclosed in a plaster case during the first fourteen days of treatment. An unsuspected soft tissue abscess may form under the plaster and evacuation of pus may thus be unduly delayed. A sling or abduction splint is used in osteitis of the humerus, the forearm bones are immobilised in a plaster-of-Paris gutter, skin traction is used for pelvic and upper femoral lesions and a posterior plaster-of-Paris gutter or padded Cramer wire splint for all other lesions of the lower limb. Immobilisation is continued after the acute phase to avoid pathological fracture as the bone becomes progressively decalcified. During this period, a sling is used for the upper limb, a walking caliper for femoral lesions and plaster of Paris for other lesions of the lower limb. Immobilisation is continued until radiographic examination shows satisfactory recalcification and this may take several months.

Penicillin Administration.—Our aim is to maintain a constant therapeutic level of penicillin in the blood and in the bone. Penicillin is given by intermittent intramuscular injections and, using a scheme based originally on a dose of 5,000 units per lb. body weight each twenty-four hours, a therapeutic level can be maintained in the blood (Table III). Injections are given at four-hourly intervals.

Administration of penicillin is continued for twenty-one days or until marrow culture is reported sterile (whichever is the longer). The penicillin level in the marrow bears no constant relationship to the level in the blood stream and marrow puncture is essential to confirm a therapeutic level in the marrow. The frequent intramuscular injections of penicillin cause pain and unhappiness to many of the children. The long-acting preparations of penicillin give therapeutic blood levels for twenty-four hours or longer and, given at night, allow an exhausted child a complete night's rest once toxæmia is controlled.

TABLE III

Scheme of daily Penicillin and Tetracycline Dosage used as a Guide to the Resident Staff (Royal Hospital for Sick Children, Glasgow)

Age Group	Penicillin	Tetracycline (in divided doses by mouth)
Birth to 1 month . .	...	25 mg.
1 month to 6 months . .	...	50 mg.
6 months to 2 years . .	25,000 units or	100 mg.
2 years to 5 years . .	50,000 units or	150 mg.
5 years to 10 years . .	75,000 units or	200 mg.
10 years to 12 years . .	100,000 units or	250 mg.

Except in the neonatal age group (p. 43) the problems of osteitis due to a penicillin-resistant staphylococcus has not yet become serious. In a series of 100 consecutive cases of acute osteitis outwith the neonatal period, the organism was resistant to penicillin in only one instance. A penicillin-streptomycin preparation was given to this patient. In this preparation 0·1 gm. of streptomycin sulphate is combined with every 100,000 units of penicillin.

Operative Procedures.—Once an abscess has formed it cannot be sterilised by the general administration of antibiotics owing to the deficient blood supply, and so long as cases of acute osteitis continue to arrive at hospital with pus under the periosteum or in the soft tissues, surgery cannot with impunity be discarded.

Aspiration.—In spite of reports to the contrary we have found that aspiration is rarely successful in evacuating pus in acute osteitis. The pus may be too thick to pass through the needle or through the nozzle of the syringe. Even if pus is located by needle and successfully aspirated, there is often a considerable quantity of residual pus.

Incision.—Even if pus is obviously present in the soft tissues on admission to hospital, general penicillin administration is started and the limb is immobilised for a few hours before the patient is taken to the operating theatre. Operation is usually undertaken within an hour after an intravenous or intramuscular injection of penicillin, so that a high level is present in the blood stream during the operation. The incision is made over the most superficial part of the bone and should be of adequate length. Pus is evacuated as completely as possible, the soft tissues are insufflated with penicillin-sulphathiazole powder or Polybactrin powder spray [1] and the wound is sutured with deep silk or silkworm gut sutures round a wide-bore needle inserted into the subperiosteal cavity. When the suturing is complete penicillin is instilled down the indwelling needle, the needle is withdrawn and a dry dressing applied. One must be prepared occasionally to reopen a wound, as the cavity may refill from the metaphyseal focus. After operation the limb is immobilised in the appropriate manner. It must never be enclosed in plaster of Paris during the acute phase, but must always be available for inspection. Bone drilling should rarely be necessary, but less harm will be done by bone drilling followed by primary suture of the skin than by incomplete relief of tension. If pus is present in the soft tissues or under the periosteum, the tension in the bone has probably been relieved. At a later stage if one suspects that the blood supply to the bone is inadequate, drill holes without elevating the periosteum will eventually give an alternative blood supply to the metaphysis and also allow local instillation of penicillin.

Guttering and saucerisation have no place in the modern treatment of acute osteitis. Diaphysectomy should never be necessary although in extensive infection of a rib, removal of the rib in whole or in part may be the simplest form of treatment.

Treatment of Arthritis.—Pyogenic arthritis in an associated joint is treated by aspiration and local instillation of penicillin.

---

[1] Neomycin, Polymixin and Bacitracin (Calmic Ltd.).

If the organism is reported resistant to penicillin, streptomycin or tetracycline is instilled. With the exception of the hip joint, it should rarely be necessary to open a joint, but even after open evacuation followed by instillation of the appropriate antibiotic, primary suture should be followed by a mobile joint. Except in the neonatal group, there is a recovery to full function in almost every patient.

Sympathetic effusion may occur in an associated joint. The diagnosis is confirmed by aspiration of straw-coloured fluid. It is wiser to instill penicillin prophylactically while awaiting the bacteriologist's report.

Marrow Puncture.—The duration of penicillin administration is controlled by the results of marrow puncture. By examining the aspirated fluid one can find if penicillin is in fact reaching the focus of infection and penicillin therapy is continued until the marrow fluid is reported sterile. Marrow puncture is performed with full aseptic precautions in the operating theatre, under a light general anæsthetic, on the fourteenth and twenty-first day of treatment. If the aspirated fluid is not sterile, therapy is continued and marrow puncture repeated until the marrow fluid is reported sterile.

RESULTS

Since the introduction of penicillin and other antibiotics, the response to treatment, although not immediate, is dramatic. The blood culture, if initially positive, becomes sterile within three days and although the patient may remain seriously ill for some days, improvement is slowly progressive from the time treatment starts. Even with associated joint involvement, a full recovery of function may be expected in the affected limb if the organism is penicillin-sensitive, if subperiosteal pus is evacuated early and if there is no gross interference with the blood supply to the affected metaphysis. An increasing incidence of penicillin-resistant staphylococci has been reported from many centres, but in Glasgow, apart from neonatal infection, resistant organisms are still rare in osteitis of childhood. Other antibiotics have been used successfully in the treatment of osteitis caused by a penicillin-resistant staphylococcus. Although streptomycin and the tetracyclines have proved satisfactory in controlling septicæmia they do not appear to be as effective as penicillin in controlling the local manifestations of the disease in either bone or joint.

Delay in evacuation of pus, inadequate penicillin dosage or insufficient duration of treatment may all lead to cavitation or sequestrum formation and if these conditions are not treated early, to limb lengthening. The common complications are: *pyogenic arthritis, sequestrum formation, limb lengthening* and *pathological fracture.*

Complications.

Although metastatic lesions have become rare, the occasional case of pericarditis serves as a reminder that penicillin has not lessened our responsibility for thorough examination and precise diagnosis.

PYOGENIC ARTHRITIS.—Arthritis is still a common complication of acute osteitis and almost all joint infections are from direct extension from an adjacent bone focus. Metastatic joint infections have become rare since the introduction of antibiotics.

SEQUESTRUM FORMATION.—So long as patients continue to arrive at hospital in the late stages of the disease, there will be interference with blood supply with death of portions of the bone. Without a blood supply, parenteral penicillin will fail to reach such dead fragments and the infected sequestrum will remain and give rise to future trouble including overgrowth of the affected limb. The treatment of sequestra will be considered in the section on chronic osteitis.

LIMB LENGTHENING.—Before the introduction of penicillin in the treatment of osteitis, gross limb lengthening was common and was due to the continuing hyperæmia caused by the presence of an infected sequestrum. Although sequestrum formation is much less common in penicillin-treated cases, it does occur and measurable increase in length is still seen (Fig. 58). When one of two paired bones is diseased, the increase in length affects both bones equally (Fig. 59), always providing that there has been no damage to the epiphyseal cartilage. The hyperæmia presumably affects the soft tissues and increases the blood supply throughout the segment. Irregular growth occurs when there is damage to one part of the epiphysis. The increase in length may be as much as 3 cm. and the lengthening usually

becomes obvious six to twelve months after the onset of the
disease.

Although limb lengthening is most commonly a sequel to hæmatogenous

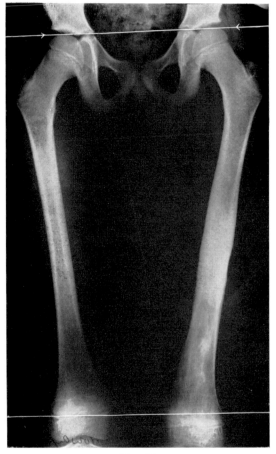

FIG. 58

Healed osteitis of left femur showing increase in length
and girth two years after onset of the disease.

osteitis it may occur in the following conditions in childhood ; simple
and compound fracture of the femur, arteriovenous fistulæ, severe
lacerations and burns of the leg and synovial tuberculosis of the hip.
In all these conditions there is the common factor of increased blood
supply.

In osteitis the growth stimulus, over-activated by the increased blood supply, gradually passes off and in the actively

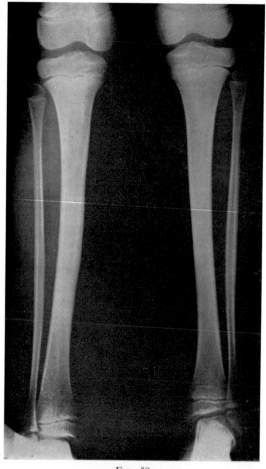

FIG. 59

Osteitis of right tibia.   Radiography eighteen months after onset shows sclerosis of tibia and increase in length of both tibia *and* fibula.

growing child a moderate increase in length (up to 2 cm.) is rectified within five years.   In all patients the overgrowth is rectified by the time adult life is reached.   Presumably growth ceases earlier in the overgrown limb.   The growing child can compensate for a long lower limb by such secondary defects as scoliosis and genu valgum (Fig. 60). Such deformities develop insidiously over a period of years if suitable raising is not applied to the footwear of the normal leg.

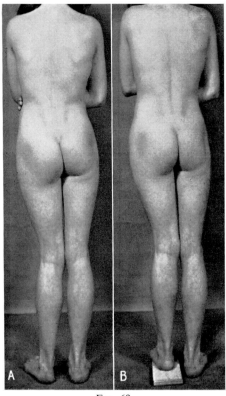

FIG. 60

Osteitis of right femur four years after onset. A, Lengthening of right leg with secondary scoliosis and genu valgum. B, Deformity partially corrected by 2 cm. block under foot on sound side.

PATHOLOGICAL FRACTURE.—The most striking radiographic change in penicillin-treated osteitis is the progressive decalcification and relative absence of involucrum (Fig. 52). To prevent pathological fracture in the decalcified and unsupported bone, immobilisation must be continued long after the period of acute infection is passed.

OTHER COMPLICATIONS.—Metastatic foci seldom arise after penicillin administration has begun but those already present on admission will not subside without surgical intervention. Metastatic foci which commonly occurred before the introduction of penicillin were distant subperiosteal abscesses, infection of distant joints and soft tissue abscesses. Foci were also common in pericardium, lungs, serous cavities and kidneys. Multiple small pyæmic abscesses may form within forty-eight hours of the onset of the bone infection.

RECURRENCES.—Recurrent infection is invariably due to residual cavitation with or without sequestration. Sclerosis of bone may render such cavities or sequestra almost invisible in X-ray films. Recurrences may present with local pain and swelling, with sinus formation or with a metastatic focus.

These problems will be considered in the section on chronic osteitis.

CHRONIC OSTEITIS

In most patients chronic osteitis is a legacy of previous acute hæmatogenous osteitis. Rarely chronic osteitis arises insidiously, due to a staphylococcus of attenuated virulence.

1. Chronic Osteitis following Acute Osteitis.

The principal pathological features of the chronic phase are the presence of unabsorbed sequestra and unobliterated cavities containing infected granulation tissue, pus or necrotic bone. The rigidity of the wall of the bone cavity prevents collapse and natural healing and the cavity slowly becomes surrounded by dense sclerotic bone. A sinus may lead to the surface and this may discharge pus continuously or intermittently. Small sequestra are usually retained and serve to keep up infection.

The condition may be painless but there is sometimes dull boring pain, usually worse at night. The condition is subject to an occasional acute excacerbation which may occur many years after the condition is apparently cured. The recurrence may also manifest itself by a metastatic focus at some distant site, either in bone or in soft tissues.

2. Chronic Osteitis arising insidiously.

This type of infection is uncommon in childhood. Scanty or avirulent organisms carried by the blood stream are deposited, usually at a metaphysis, and give rise to a low-grade inflammatory reaction. This area becomes surrounded by a proliferative defensive reaction, and a *Brodie's abscess*, surrounded by an

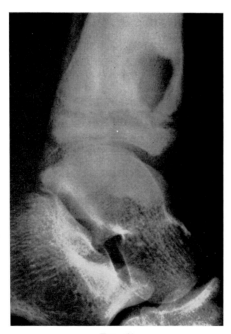

FIG. 61
Brodie's abscess in lower end of tibia.

area of dense sclerosis, results (Fig. 61). The abscess at first lies close to the metaphysis but may move away from it as the bone grows.

The condition may remain unrecognised for a long time, but eventually there is pain of a dull aching or boring character, especially at night. The neighbouring joint may be the seat of recurring effusion. The diagnosis is established by radiography.

TREATMENT

Parenteral penicillin has little value in eradicating chronic infection from a bone even if the responsible organism is penicillin-sensitive. Retained sequestra and unobliterated bone cavities must be treated surgically, but each operation must be preceded by at least two days of parenteral penicillin (or streptomycin and penicillin if the organism is penicillin-resistant). The indications for surgical intervention are pain in the bone, pain or swelling in an associated joint and sinus or abscess formation. The cavity or sequestrum is localised as accurately as possible by radiography and an appropriate incision is made excising widely any sinus which may be present. The cortex overlying a cavity is opened with a gouge and any sequestra are removed. Infected granulations are removed by curette and swabbing, and cortical bone is removed until the walls of the cavity slope gently (saucerisation). The cavity and soft tissues are then frosted with penicillin-sulphathiazole powder or Polybactrin and a wide-bore needle is inserted into the cavity. The wound is closed around the needle and the appropriate antibiotic is instilled and the needle withdrawn. The limb is immobilised as in acute infection and immobilisation is continued long enough to avoid risk of fracture when saucerisation has been extensive.

Radiography may reveal only sclerosis with no definite evidence of sequestrum formation or cavitation. In such cases symptoms may be relieved by making multiple drill holes and instilling a suitable antibiotic.

TRAUMATIC OSTEITIS

Any open wound communicating with a bone, or a compound fracture, may lead to osteitis. Traumatic osteitis has been uncommon during the past twenty-five years and since the introduction of chemotherapy and antibiotics it has become a surgical rarity (Fig. 62). In recent years there have been reports of osteitis following transfusion into the bone marrow. This method of transfusion has no advantages over intravenous transfusion other than technical simplicity and is very rarely justified.

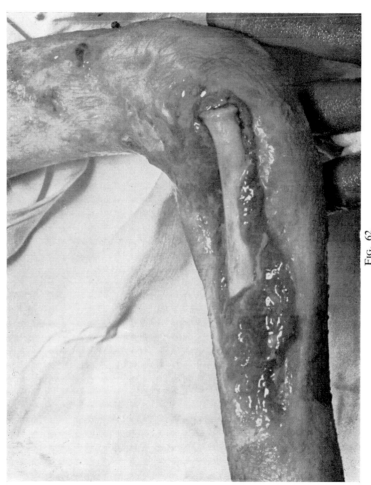

Fig. 62

Traumatic osteitis in a boy of 10 years—the result of mauling by a leopard.

The principles of treatment of traumatic osteitis are the same as in hæmatogenous osteitis.

TUMOURS OF BONE

Exostoses and enchondromata have been considered as congenital malformations (p. 54).

Osteoid Osteoma.—This is a small tumour of endochondral bone which occurs usually in the long bones of the extremities. There is characteristic boring pain and there may be swelling, tenderness or even local redness. The radiographic appearances are typical (Fig. 63). The differential diagnosis is from Brodie's abscess, tuberculosis or fibrocystic disease. Histologically the tumour consists of irregular spicules of osteoid tissue.

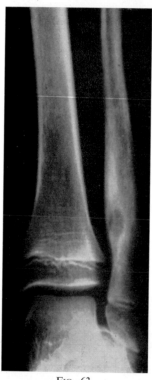

FIG. 63

Osteoid osteoma of lower fibula.

Treatment.—The tumour will recur if not completely removed and the cavity *must not* be merely curetted. The tumour must be excised completely, if necessary by partial diaphysectomy. The relief from pain is dramatic.

Sarcoma.—This may be round cell, reticulum cell or chondrosarcoma (Figs. 64, 65, 66 and 67). If the tumour can be removed completely the prognosis is better than in young adults. No example of Ewing's tumour has been seen at the Royal Hospital for Sick Children, Glasgow. Radiographic appearances indistinguishable from Ewing's tumour have been seen in metastases from a sympathicoblastoma.

Secondary Metastases in Bone. — Sympathicoblastoma, Hodgkin's disease, leukæmia and lymphosarcoma may all involve the skeleton.

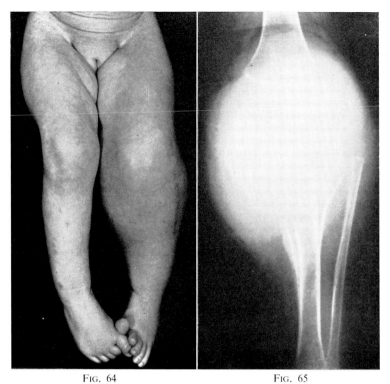

FIG. 64   FIG. 65

Fig. 64.—Reticulum-cell sarcoma in a girl aged 1 year.   Patient alive and well
eight years after amputation.
Fig. 65.—Radiographic appearance in patient shown in Fig. 64.

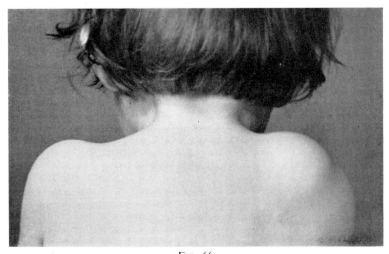

FIG. 66
Sarcoma of scapula.

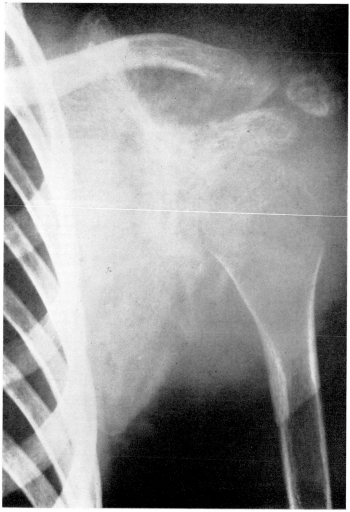

FIG. 67
Sarcoma of scapula showing sun-ray spicules.

CHAPTER VI

Hæmangioma and Lymphangioma

HÆMANGIOMA

THERE are many different classifications of the hæmangiomata, usually according to their histological features: *capillary, cavernous* or *compact.* This classification is unsatisfactory because of the great diversity of vascular tissue in each case. Probably they are all *hamartomatous* in origin, that is, they are malformations of vaso-formative tissue, misplaced or unused during fœtal development, rather than true tumours.

These lesions may be obvious at birth or soon after, or they may not appear until later life. They occur most commonly in the skin and subcutaneous tissue but may be situated in almost any tissue (liver, breast, tongue, kidney and brain).

The classification used here is essentially practical, based on the appearance of the lesion and treatment advised.

1. FLAT.

(*a*) **Spider Nævus.**—These lesions may appear after birth or later, in association with cirrhosis of the liver. They have a bright red central core with intradermal vessels radiating for a few millimetres.

Treatment.—Many disappear spontaneously but if they do not, they can be treated by diathermy needle under general anæsthesia.

(*b*) **Salmon Patch.**—This is a superficial capillary hæmangioma, light pink in colour, most commonly seen on the nape of the neck and forehead and bridge of the nose. The colour varies with temperature changes and deepens when the child cries or strains.

Treatment.—Most lesions have almost disappeared by school age. If they are still unsightly they can be treated with carbon dioxide snow or thorium X paint.

(*c*) **Port-wine Stain.**—There is a thin layer of capillary tissue in the dermis causing a purplish discoloration which does not blanch readily on pressure. On the face the lesions

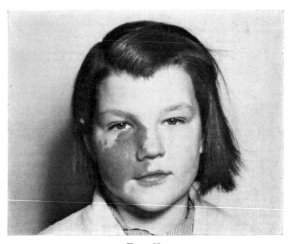

Fig. 68
Port-wine stain.

are very unsightly (Fig. 68) and may be associated with intracranial lesions (Sturge-Weber syndrome).

Treatment.—This type seldom regresses but the disfigurement can be partially concealed by cover cream or pancake make-up. Only in the last resort is surgical excision with grafting undertaken.

2. RAISED.

(*a*) **Superficial.**—Capillary tissue with subcutaneous extensions forms a bright red, slightly raised and lobulated mass—**strawberry birth mark**. These lesions may grow rapidly in infancy and ulceration may occur with sepsis and unsightly scarring. There is also a risk of hæmorrhage—for example, from a comb catching in a scalp lesion. They are most common about the face and scalp but may occur anywhere (Fig. 69).

Treatment.—Strawberry birth marks may increase in size during the first six months of life, they then become stationary and many disappear spontaneously before the age of 7, leaving little or no mark. Unfortunately it is difficult to persuade the parents to wait for spontaneous regression and treatment is usually undertaken. With the exception of lesions of the perineum and vulva and breast in the female, these lesions are best treated by radium under the supervision of an experienced radiotherapist. If the anxious parents will not wait even the six to twelve months which radium treatment may require,

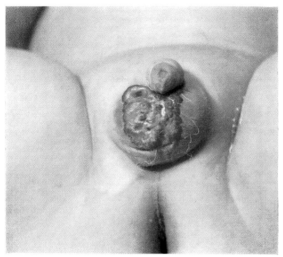

FIG. 69
Strawberry birth mark of scrotum.

the lesion can be excised. Visible scars should be avoided, particularly in girls.

(*b*) **Deep.**—The **cavernous hæmangioma** is usually subcutaneous, lifting the skin and showing a light blue discoloration. These lesions may communicate with the underlying systemic veins into which the blood can be squeezed, to return on release of pressure and fill up the hæmangioma like a sponge.

Treatment.—Many of these lesions react well to radium ; others are treated by excision, diathermy or injection of a saturated solution of saline.

(*c*) **Diffuse Hæmangiomatous Giantism.**—The vessels in these lesions are of adult type and do not react to radiotherapy. They may present as a deeply placed solitary mass or a whole limb may be riddled with hamartomatous tissue with thousands of small arteriovenous shunts (Fig. 70). In time the shunts cause pressure on the right heart and may kill the patient in later life. Hæmorrhage (which may terrify the parents) can occur following slight trauma to a cutaneous lesion.

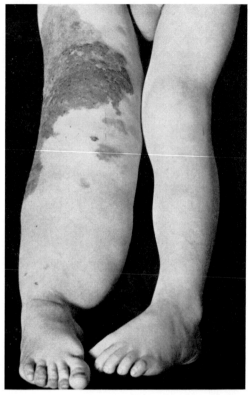

FIG. 70
Diffuse hæmangiomatous giantism of leg.

Treatment.—All forms of treatment are unsatisfactory. There are too many arteriovenous shunts to ligate individually and ligation of the main artery or even amputation may not save the patient's life in the later stages.

Birth marks are usually unsightly and have unfortunate psychological effects upon both the patient and the parents.

It is convenient at this point to consider another form of birth mark—the mole.

PIGMENTED AND HAIRY MOLE (Nævus)

These common lesions vary from small brown moles (benign melanomata) to large hairy pigmented areas which may cover large areas of the face, limb or trunk (Fig. 71).

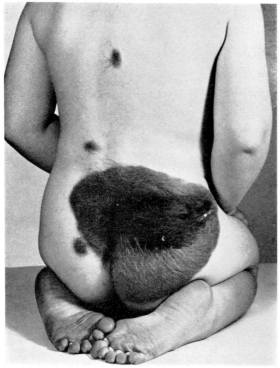

FIG. 71
Pigmented hairy moles.

Treatment.—There is rarely any indication for removal of a pigmented nævus which has been present since birth. If the area is subject to constant trauma, wide surgical removal may be undertaken. Large pigmented areas can be treated by serial excision or by complete excision and skin grafting. There is no risk of malignant change if serial excision is undertaken in childhood.

LYMPHANGIOMA

A lymphangioma is similar to a hæmangioma except that the spaces and channels contain lymph. *Capillary lymphangiomata* occur in the lips (*macrocheilia*) and tongue (one form of

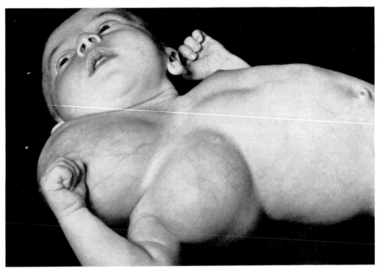

FIG. 72
Lymphangioma involving neck and axilla.

macroglossia). *Cavernous lymphangiomata* are seen in the skin and mucous membranes and some pathologists consider that the cavernous lymphangioma is the same lesion as the *cystic lymphangioma* (*hygroma*). In the neck, axilla and groin the cystic spaces may be several centimetres in diameter and such a lesion is called a *cystic hygroma*. Occasionally an angioma partakes of the nature of both hæmangioma and lymphangioma —*hæmolymphangioma*.

Clinical Features.—Most cystic hygromata appear in the posterior triangle of the neck and occupy the supraclavicular fossa. The condition also occurs in the axilla and the lesion may extend from one region into the other (Fig. 72). The

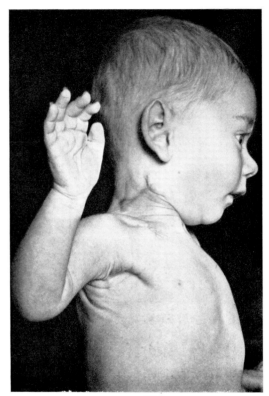

FIG. 73
Same patient as Fig. 72, two weeks after
excision of lymphangioma.

swelling may be present at birth and most lymphangiomata become apparent during the first year of life. The overlying skin is normal in texture and there is a bluish tint from the underlying fluid. The mass can be transilluminated but hæmor-rhage or infection may alter the size and consistency of the swelling. The chief complaint is of disfigure-ment, and important structures are rarely affected by pressure. In macrocheilia there is chronic enlargement of the lip ; in macro-glossia the enlarged tongue may protrude from the mouth (Fig. 74). Superimposed infection may give rise to considerable swelling with consequent interference with swallowing and breathing.

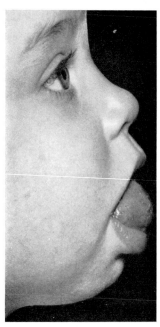

FIG. 74

Macroglossia due to lymphangio-matous infiltration of tongue.

Treatment.—A hygroma may undergo spontaneous regression but this is exceptional. Regression may follow infection. Macrocheilia and macroglossia may respond to radiotherapy but plastic surgical procedures may be necessary. Sclerosing agents (5 per cent. sodium morrhuate) injected into the mass, at first cause increase in size but within three days the swelling may shrink markedly. Large cervical and axillary masses are sometimes cured by radium but if this form of therapy is unsuccessful, the resultant fibrosis makes subsequent surgery more difficult. Although many large hygromata in the neck and axilla can be completely excised (Fig. 73) fibrous lymph-angiomatous extensions among the nerves and great vessels may render complete removal impossible.

CHAPTER VII

The Œsophagus

CONGENITAL ATRESIA OF THE ŒSOPHAGUS

EMBRYOLOGY.—At an early period the primitive stomach is separated from the primitive pharynx by a mere constriction which becomes elongated to form the œsophagus. A median ventral groove is converted into a diverticulum which becomes separated from the œsophagus to form the trachea. With the growth of the embryo the œsophagus lengthens and like the rest of the alimentary tract its lumen is temporarily obliterated. The lumen is later re-established and errors in re-canalisation result in the various forms of œsophageal atresia (Fig. 75).

Surgical Anatomy.—In most cases the anomaly is Type 1 as shown in Fig. 75, A. The upper œsophageal pouch ends blindly and there is a tracheo-œsophageal fistula from the lower œsophagus which enters near the bifurcation of the trachea (Fig. 76). The œsophageal ends are separated by a variable distance ; in some infants, the ends may be quite close to each other and in others they may be several centimetres apart. In the Type 2 deformity, where the lower œsophagus has no connection with the trachea, the lower pouch is very short, scarcely protruding above the diaphragm.

Almost one-third of these patients have congenital anomalies elsewhere in the body which may in themselves be a serious threat to life. The two most common associated anomalies are congenital heart disease and malformations of the anus and rectum. About one-quarter of the patients are born prematurely, probably due to the common co-existence of œsophageal atresia and hydramnios.

Clinical Features.—In most patients the symptoms are constant and diagnostic and the condition should be suspected and identified in the early hours of life in the full-term child, preferably before the first feed. In the premature baby where feeding is delayed, the diagnosis may not be made for a day or two. What appears to be excess saliva dribbles as a froth from the infant's mouth. There are attacks of choking and cyanosis and these attacks are precipitated by attempts at feeding. When the airway is cleared the general condition is

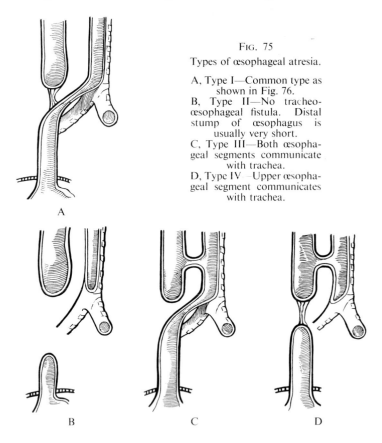

FIG. 75

Types of œsophageal atresia.

A, Type I—Common type as shown in Fig. 76.
B, Type II—No tracheo-œsophageal fistula. Distal stump of œsophagus is usually very short.
C, Type III—Both œsophageal segments communicate with trachea.
D, Type IV—Upper œsophageal segment communicates with trachea.

good, but subsequent attempts at feeding are always followed by respiratory distress. The feeds are rejected and often partially aspirated.

Whenever the anomaly is suspected the patency of the œsophagus should be investigated. This is done by gently attempting to pass a No. 8E urethral catheter through the mouth into the stomach. (If a smaller catheter is used it may curl up in the œsophageal pouch and thus appear to pass into the stomach. Every maternity unit should carry a stock

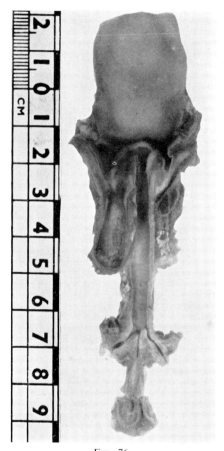

FIG. 76

Autopsy specimen showing Type I œsophageal atresia. There is a blind upper
pouch and a fistula arising from the
bifurcation of the trachea.

of radio-opaque catheters and an attempt should be made to pass a catheter into the stomach of every infant born from a hydramniotic sac). In œsophageal atresia the catheter will be arrested 10 to 12 cm. from the alveolar margin. Final confirmation of the diagnosis is obtained radiologically by

passing a small urethral catheter through the nose or mouth
and instilling 1 to 2 ml. of lipiodol (iodised oil); this will
outline the blind œsophageal pouch. A lateral film is also
taken to demonstrate, if possible, the presence of a fistula which

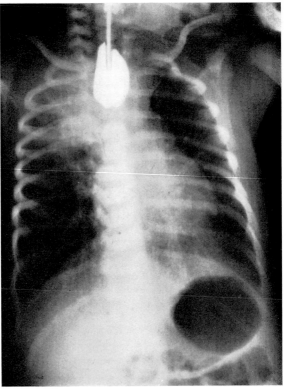

FIG. 77

Œsophageal atresia, Type I. The upper œsophageal pouch
is outlined by instilled lipiodol : gas in the stomach indicates
the presence of a tracheo-œsophageal fistula.

occasionally extends forward from the pouch into the trachea.
The film must include the upper abdomen as gas in the stomach
indicates the presence of a tracheo-œsophageal fistula (Fig. 77).
The lipiodol is withdrawn by aspiration at the end of the
radiographic examination. Barium mixtures should *never* be
used for this investigation as the barium may overflow and

cause severe reaction in the lungs. Radiography will also demonstrate the state of the lungs. Most of these infants have some pneumonitis by the time they are admitted to hospital.

Treatment.—If œsophageal atresia is not recognised and treated, the baby will die of pneumonia and starvation. Although surgical treatment must be carried out as soon as possible, many hours may be profitably spent in improving the condition of the infant. The lung condition is treated by antibiotics and by nursing the baby in a semi-sitting position in an incubator, to reduce reflux from the stomach. Frequent suction is applied to a catheter passed into the œsophageal pouch. Glucose in quarter-strength saline may be given intravenously. Vitamin K (Synkavit, 1 mg.) is injected intramuscularly.

Operation.—Under endotracheal general anæsthesia, the œsophagus is exposed by a transpleural approach through the fourth or fifth interspace on the right side. The intravenous drip is then changed from glucose-saline to blood. The tracheo-œsophageal fistula is ligated and divided, the pouch is mobilised and opened and end-to-end anastomosis of the two ends of the œsophagus is performed using fine silk. Post-operatively, the infant is nursed in an incubator and is fed through an indwelling polythene tube or through a gastro-stomy performed at the conclusion of the thoracic procedure. Both these feeding methods prevent soiling of the suture line during healing. In the immediate post-operative period hypothermia is common (Chap. II), and by regulating the temperature of the incubator the patient's temperature is brought up to normal levels within a few hours. Some degree of stenosis may develop at the site of anastomosis and œsophageal dilatation may be required at intervals for a few months.

In the rare cases where no tracheo-œsophageal fistula exists, primary end-to-end anastomosis is impossible without bringing the stomach into the thorax. It is alternatively possible to exteriorise the upper pouch in the neck above the left clavicle and to perform a gastrostomy. An intrathoracic œsophagus is constructed at a later date using a free loop of the right colon or transverse colon.

ŒSOPHAGEAL STENOSIS OR STRICTURE

Œsophageal strictures may occur in any part of the œsophagus and are of four types: (1) *Congenital*; (2) *post-operative*; (3) *following peptic œsophagitis*; (4) *following chemical burns.*

Congenital Œsophageal Stenosis.

Most of these malformations are discovered in the first year or two of life. The dominant symptoms are regurgitation of part of each feed and failure to gain weight, usually starting at the time of weaning. The œsophagus above the obstruction becomes dilated. The diagnosis is confirmed by radiography following a barium swallow. Many cases diagnosed as congenital stenosis or stricture are actually examples of stricture following peptic œsophagitis in the first month or two of life (*vide infra*).

Treatment.—Under general anæsthesia, the lesion should be examined by œsophagoscopy to assess the character of the stricture and the state of the mucous membrane at and above the narrow segment. Most patients can be treated satisfactorily and safely by dilatation using gum elastic bougies. Quite young children can be taught to pass the bougies themselves. It is usually necessary to continue dilatation for many months.

Post-operative Œsophageal Stricture.

Following anastomosis in the surgery of œsophageal atresia, almost one-third of the survivors require dilatation for a stricture at the operation site (p. 119). Dysphagia may occur within a few weeks of œsophageal anastomosis or may be delayed for several months. The stricture is gently dilated with graded gum elastic œsophageal bougies.

Stricture following Œsophagitis.

Peptic ulceration occurs when there is relaxation of the cardia and reflux of gastric juices (cardio-œsophageal chalasia) and where there is a hiatus hernia. Peptic erosion sets up an inflammatory reaction in the lower œsophagus, causing spasm and later fibrosis and cicatricial contraction.

The symptoms are those of œsophageal obstruction—dysphagia, regurgitation, vomiting (which may be blood-stained) and loss of weight. A gastrostomy may be necessary as a life-saving measure. The treatment of the œsophagitis is considered under the causal condition (*cardio-œsophageal chalasia*, p. 123, *hiatus hernia*, Chap. XVII).

Stricture following Chemical Burns.

Caustic soda is the most frequent of the various injurious chemicals which a child may swallow. Sodium hydroxide in various proprietary forms is used for cleaning toilets, drains and floors, and the colourless or pale white fluid is drunk by the thirsty child in mistake for water or milk. The lye solutions cause burns of the lips, mouth and œsophagus. The hydrochloric acid of the gastric juice quickly neutralises any caustic fluid which reaches the stomach. Stricture may occur in any part of the œsophagus.

Treatment : First-aid.—If readily available, vinegar, lemon or orange juice may have some neutralising effect. Sipping of small quantities of olive oil helps to sooth the painful lips and mouth. Sedatives should be administered in generous doses.

In Hospital.—It is impossible to predict what course of therapy will be necessary for any given patient. At first all food and drink will be refused but after a day or two, water will usually be taken. If water can be swallowed then milk is given for nourishment and for its soothing effect on the mucous membrane.

A dilute barium swallow may help to assess the degree and extent of the burn. When the acute stage has passed it may be possible to dilate any resulting stricture with bougies. If the stricture is very narrow a temporary gastrostomy is performed to maintain nutrition.

DUPLICATIONS OF ŒSOPHAGUS

Duplications of the alimentary tract are discussed in Chapter XI. Cysts of the foregut arising in the posterior mediastinum are usually lined with gastric mucosa and have been called " gastric thoracic cysts." They should be differentiated from bronchiogenic cysts which are lined with ciliated epithelium and are situated in the lung or in association with a main bronchus. Œsophageal duplications lie along one side of the œsophagus and balloon into the pleural cavity.

Clinical Features.—Duplications of the œsophagus usually present with repeated hæmoptysis or hæmatemesis. On X-ray, the outline of the cyst may be seen and a barium swallow shows indentation or displacement of the œsophagus. As duplications may be multiple, a thoracic cyst may be associated with an intestinal duplication. Vertebral anomalies such as anterior spina bifida and hemivertebræ are frequently associated with thoracic duplication.

Treatment.—The cysts are excised through a transpleural approach. Although densely adherent to the œsophagus, duplications rarely communicate with it. If the œsophagus is opened at operation, the opening is closed with inverting silk sutures and a mediastinal drain inserted.

CARDIOSPASM (ACHALASIA OF THE CARDIA)

Cardiospasm is a condition in which there is dilatation, hypertrophy and lengthening of the œsophagus without any apparent mechanical obstruction. The condition is not common in childhood and consequently diagnosis may be long delayed.

Clinical Features.—The symptoms are dysphagia, regurgitation and retrosternal discomfort. The child is usually underweight, has a worried look and may be labelled "neurotic." Radiography following a barium swallow shows the dilated and elongated sac with narrowing of the lower end of the œsophagus into a smooth rounded symmetrical cone (Fig. 78).

Treatment.—Medical treatment with antispasmodic drugs produces only temporary relief and repeated dilatation appears to increase the associated psychological upset in the affected children.

Heller's operation is simple and gives dramatic results. The operation is based on the principle of Ramstedt's [1] operation for congenital pyloric stenosis (p. 131). Through a paramedian incision, the lower œsophagus is exposed and liberated and the

[1] Conrad Ram(m)stedt spelt his name with two "m's" until after the First World War, when he changed it to one "m." Both spellings are therefore correct. We have decided to adopt the one with the single "m".

longitudinal and circular muscles (which are *not*, however, hypertrophied) are divided by a longitudinal incision until

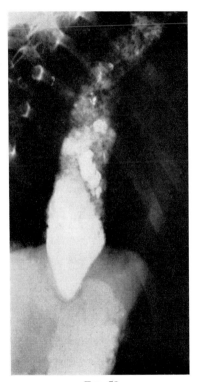

FIG. 78
Cardiospasm. Dilated œsophagus
outlined with dilute barium.

the semi-transparent mucosa bulges outwards freely. Although the symptoms are relieved in a dramatic fashion it is many months before the dilated œsophagus returns to normal proportions.

CARDIO-ŒSOPHAGEAL CHALASIA

Normal infants may vomit liquor amnii or blood swallowed during delivery (Chap. IX). If vomiting persists for the first two days in spite of gastric lavage and there is no evidence of intracranial injury or infection, one should suspect the existence of obstruction. Among the babies who vomit, there is, however, a small group with a neuromuscular disturbance

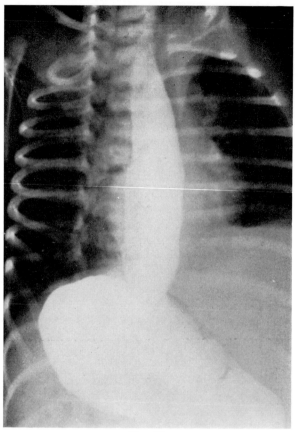

FIG. 79
Cardio-œsophageal chalasia showing regurgitation of
barium from stomach into lax œsophagus.

in the œsophagus and cardia. Their symptoms may suggest pyloric stenosis or closely simulate sliding hiatus hernia. Investigation shows that there is a failure of the cardio-œsophageal sphincteric action and the lesion has been termed " chalasia." The pædiatric surgeon must know of the condition although no operative treatment is required.

Clinical Features.—The baby appears normal at birth but within a week he starts to vomit. Vomiting becomes more frequent and occurs during or immediately after each feed ; it is effortless and not usually projectile and the vomitus is very rarely bile-stained. Untreated, the baby fails to gain or loses weight. There may be blood in the vomitus from œsophagitis. Apart from varying degrees of dehydration and malnutrition there is nothing abnormal detected on clinical examination.

Following a barium swallow, radiography shows the barium flowing freely back up the œsophagus when the stomach is compressed or the head tilted down (Fig. 79).

Treatment.—Relief from vomiting is obtained by maintaining the baby in a sitting position. The infant is kept in this position by bolstering him up with pillows or by the use of a small padded chair. It may be necessary to retain the baby in this posture for several months. Thickening feeds by adding cereal may help to prevent regurgitation. The œsophageal function always returns to normal in time. Very rarely a temporary gastrostomy may be required because of severe œsophagitis.

CHAPTER VIII

The Stomach

CONGENITAL HYPERTROPHIC PYLORIC STENOSIS

THIS is the most common condition requiring surgical intervention in infancy. Early in the century the mortality was 75 per cent. ; it is now less than 1 per cent. There is no satisfactory explanation for the condition and the various theories are only of academic interest. Some workers do not believe that the lesion is congenital.

Pathology.—There is hypertrophy of the smooth circular muscle fibres of the pylorus, giving rise to a bulbous or fusiform mass about the size of a small hazel-nut (20×15 mm.). The pyloric tumour is pale in colour and of firm rubbery consistence. The mucosa is pushed inwards, decreasing the pyloric lumen. On section, the muscle is grey-white in colour and feels almost like cartilage. There is an abrupt termination of the pyloric sphincter at the distal end and the duodenum assumes its full size at once (Figs. 80 and 81). It is important to remember this anatomical point during operation as it is only too easy to open the duodenum accidentally where it balloons out just beyond the pylorus. During the first week of life the pyloric mucosa is essentially normal. Later, forcing of the curds through the narrow pyloric lumen leads to œdema of the mucosa and further reduction of the lumen. This explains why projectile vomiting is rarely seen until the infant is a week or two old, although the pyloric stenosis has been present since birth. There is also some hypertrophy of the muscular coats of the stomach and increase in the mucosal rugae (Fig. 80).

Clinical Features.—The symptoms are those of high obstruction with loss of fluid and electrolytes, especially hydrochloric acid. Eighty per cent. of patients are male and 50 per cent. are first-born children. The cardinal signs are

126

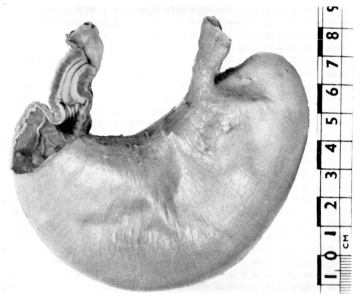

FIG. 80

Pyloric stenosis showing dilated and hypertrophied stomach.
Pylorus and antrum cut in longitudinal section.

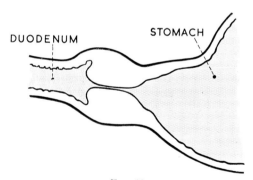

FIG. 81

Longitudinal section of stomach in pyloric
stenosis to show how muscular hypertrophy of
pylorus tapers off gradually on gastric side but
ends abruptly at duodenum.

projectile vomiting and *palpable pyloric tumour*. The stools are infrequent and scanty, and as the condition progresses the patient shows evidence of dehydration and starvation with wrinkling of the skin. *Visible gastric peristalsis* is no longer regarded as a diagnostic feature.

Vomiting.—Vomiting seldom occurs before the eighth day.

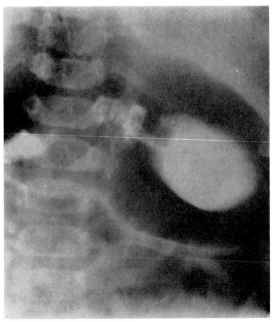

FIG. 82

Pyloric stenosis. Radiography shows " string sign " in pyloric canal and indentation of duodenum by pyloric tumour.

It starts as a simple regurgitation after feeds but gradually becomes more forceful and projectile. The vomitus rarely, if ever, contains bile. The infant is constantly hungry and is eager for a feed immediately after vomiting. If vomiting is long continued or severe, *alkalosis* will develop. Urinary chlorides are diminished or absent.

Visible Peristalsis.—During or after feeding, waves of gastric peristalsis may be seen passing from left to right across the epigastrium.

Pyloric Tumour.—Seated comfortably on the left of the patient, the clinician rests the fingers of the left hand gently on the abdomen. The finger tips feel slowly around the right upper quadrant. Palpation should be carried out while the infant is having a feed, and with patience the rounded tumour, about the size of a hazel-nut, should be felt in almost every case. If the tumour cannot be palpated, and particularly in older infants when the diagnosis is in doubt, it is occasionally necessary to confirm the diagnosis radiologically. With a small quantity of barium it is possible to visualise the pylorus accurately and to demonstrate the characteristic narrowing of the lumen (Fig. 82).

Differential Diagnosis.

1. *Poor Feeding Regime.*—Vomiting may be caused by unnecessary or careless handling after feeds; or may be due to excessive air swallowing caused by underfeeding, nasal obstruction or from the use of a teat with too small or too large a hole.

2. *Intracranial Injury.*—Injury or hæmorrhage from birth trauma may cause vomiting which is small in amount and unrelated to feeding. There may be convulsions, spasticity and a bulging fontanelle, and fluid from spinal or subdural tap may provide the diagnosis.

3. *Other Forms of Obstruction.*—In œsophageal atresia regurgitation starts on the first day of life. In atresia of the duodenum or intestine vomiting starts within a day or two of birth and the vomitus usually contains bile. Vomiting due to malrotation of the bowel may start at any time, the vomitus contains bile and the diagnosis is confirmed by radiography.

4. *Chalasia of the Œsophagus.* — Apart from vomiting, there are no signs of pyloric stenosis. Radiography shows regurgitation of barium from the stomach up into the œsophagus.

5. *Infection.*—Vomiting may accompany any of the common infections, *e.g.*, gastro-enteritis, upper respiratory infection, pyuria and septicæmia.

Treatment.—Treatment may be either medicinal or by operation. Medical treatment includes gastric lavage and oral administration of an alcoholic solution of atropine methyl nitrate (eumydrin) twenty minutes before a feed. It is now the practice in the Royal Hospital for Sick Children, Glasgow, to advise operation in every established case of pyloric stenosis. Excessive dehydration is corrected by hypodermoclysis or intravenous infusion and the stomach is washed out with saline four hours before operation. Body heat is conserved during operation by wrapping the limbs in gamgee and by keeping the theatre temperature up to 70° or 75° F.

The anæsthetic may be local or general. If a local anæsthetic is used, the infant is bandaged to a padded cross. It is difficult to ensure deep pre-operative sedation with safety and the infant is soothed on the operating table with a teat containing glycerine or dilute brandy and sugar. Infiltration of the abdominal wall slightly prolongs the surgeon's work and the infant may struggle when the abdomen is open. When a trained pædiatric anæsthetist is available, the patient is given $\frac{1}{250}$ gr. atropine half an hour before operation. A urethral catheter is passed through the nose or mouth into the stomach and left in place throughout the operation. When the infant is anæsthetised the abdomen is opened through an upper abdominal incision and the pylorus delivered and inspected. A Ramstedt pyloro-myotomy is performed by making a longitudinal incision through the serous and muscular layers (Fig. 83, A). Any remaining fibres are separated with blunt forceps until the intact mucosa bulges up to the level of the serosa (Fig. 83, B). Great care is taken to avoid puncturing the mucosa of the duodenum at the distal end of the wound. Should this happen the perforation is closed with a catgut suture. Bleeding points are secured and the pylorus returned to the abdomen. The incision in the abdominal wall is closed in layers with very fine silk.

After operation any hypothermia is corrected by warming the child. It is desirable to have a standard feeding regime; the type of fluid or feed makes little difference, but feeding should start three or four hours after operation. Small quantities of 5 per cent. glucose saline are given at half-hourly intervals for two hours. Milk feeds are then started and slowly increased. The patient is nursed in isolation to avoid cross infection. For the same reason the infant is discharged from hospital as soon as circumstances permit—usually about six days after operation.

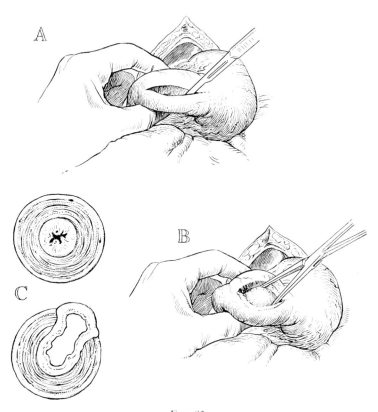

FIG. 83

Ramstedt's pyloromyotomy. A, Incision on anterosuperior aspect of pylorus through serosa and outer part of thickened muscle. B, Spreading edges of severed muscle, allowing submucosa to bulge up between muscle edges. C, Cross-section of hypertrophied pylorus before and after pyloromyotomy. Mucosa pouts through gap in muscle, thus providing an adequate lumen.

PEPTIC ULCER

Although rare in infancy and childhood, gastric and duodenal ulcers may cause serious or even fatal illness. In one fatal case in our small series, death followed perforation of a chronic duodenal ulcer in an infant of 5 weeks. Secondary (Curling) ulcers associated with severe infections or extensive burns have become very rare since the introduction of antibiotics.

Clinical Features.—Peptic ulcer may be relatively asymptomatic and the lesion may only be discovered at autopsy. Some of the vague abdominal pains which are so common in childhood may be due to undiagnosed peptic ulcer. While the disease may run a " silent " course in infancy, in the older child the clinical picture is similar to that in adult life. There is epigastric pain or discomfort, relieved by eating ; pain at night is common. Vomiting an hour or two after food may follow pylorospasm or actual scarring. There may be evidence of malnutrition. The disease may first present with recurrent or severe hæmorrhage or with perforation into the peritoneal cavity. Severe bleeding and perforation are more common in young infants ; in children, the disease resembles the more chronic recurring form seen in adults, and barium-meal examination may be diagnostic. A fractional test meal is of no value.

Treatment.—The condition may be arrested, if not cured, by rest and a modified ulcer regime. Mechanical obstruction is relieved by posterior gastrojejunostomy, but in two of our patients ulceration has recurred within five years. Perforation carries a high mortality as the diagnosis of an uncommon event is often delayed ; operative treatment should be confined to simple suture of the opening. Hæmorrhage is poorly tolerated and blood loss should be replaced early.

TRICHOBEZOAR

The formation of a hair ball may be followed by poor health and vague abdominal pain as the gastric lumen becomes partially occluded by a dense mass. A history of hair eating is rarely given spontaneously by the parents. A mass may be palpated in the epigastrium. The diagnosis is confirmed by X-ray after a barium swallow.

The hair ball (Fig. 84) may be passed spontaneously piece-meal, but gastrotomy may be required.

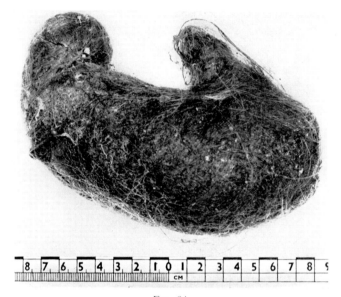

FIG. 84
Trichobezoar.

CHAPTER IX

Intestinal Obstruction in the Newborn

VOMITING IN THE NEWBORN

VOMITING in the newborn may have no serious significance, but it may be a sign of the utmost gravity. Persistent vomiting in the first day or two of life should always suggest the possibility of obstruction. It is rare for the vomitus to contain bile unless there is a mechanical obstruction. In pyloric stenosis vomiting seldom starts before the end of the first week of life and the vomitus very rarely contains bile. For the convenience of the student the more common causes of neonatal vomiting are divided into two groups. The patients in the second group usually present as surgical emergencies.

Group I.

Irritation of the Stomach.—Vomiting may follow gastric irritation caused by meconium, liquor amnii or blood swallowed at the time of birth. It is particularly common in babies who have suffered from asphyxia. Blood from a crack in the mother's nipple may also cause irritation of the stomach. In this group vomiting usually ceases spontaneously, but it may be necessary to wash out the stomach with saline or a weak solution of sodium bicarbonate to get rid of the foreign material. Mucus from the posterior nares may also lead to continuous gastric irritation and to vomiting.

Intracranial Injury.—Persistent vomiting may be due to intracranial injury or hæmorrhage from birth trauma or hæmorrhagic disease. Vomiting is small in amount and unrelated to feeding. There may be convulsions, spasticity, a bulging fontanelle, and spinal or subdural tap may provide the diagnosis.

Infection.—Vomiting with or without diarrhœa may be an early sign of infection. Upper respiratory and urinary infection, meningitis, peritonitis and septicæmia may all manifest themselves by vomiting in the neonatal period.

Cardio-œsophageal Chalasia (p. 123).—Persistent vomiting occurs in this condition and the diagnosis is confirmed by radiography. The cardia is continually relaxed and barium regurgitates from the stomach up into the œsophagus. Vomiting is quickly relieved by thickening the feeds and propping the infant upright during and after feeding.

Group II.

The following conditions present as surgical emergencies in the neonatal period and they are considered more fully in later sections.

Atresia of the duodenum and intestine causes vomiting in the first day or two of life. (In atresia of the œsophagus there is excess salivation and regurgitation of feeds rather than actual vomiting.) Similar symptoms are caused by *annular pancreas* and by *meconium ileus* associated with fibrocystic pancreas. *Malrotation of the intestine* and *neonatal Hirschsprung's disease* may manifest themselves in the neonatal period. Other forms of intestinal obstruction in the early days of life are incarcerated *external* and *internal herniæ*, obstruction from *vitello-intestinal remnants* and the various forms of *imperforate anus*.

It may be very difficult indeed to decide if the condition calls for surgical intervention, and the co-operation of the pædiatric radiologist is invaluable in the investigation of difficult cases. The presence or absence of gas in the alimentary tract and dilated coils of bowel or fluid levels may be revealed on straight X-ray. Localisation of obstruction should be possible without the administration of barium by mouth. (Vomited barium may be aspirated with serious lung complications.) A barium enema may help to differentiate congenital megacolon (Hirschsprung's disease) from volvulus neonatorum. Mechanical obstruction of the duodenum or intestine may be rapidly demonstrated by radiography following the insufflation of intragastric oxygen or administration of an aerated drink.

All the conditions listed in this group call for surgical intervention—usually within the first two or three days of life. It is fortunate that during the early days of life the infant is endowed with marked resistance to trauma and stress and this is reflected in his metabolic response to surgery (Chap. II).

INTESTINAL OBSTRUCTION IN THE NEWBORN

Two important causes of neonatal obstruction, *congenital megacolon* and *malformations of the anus and rectum*, are more conveniently considered in Chapter XI, but many of the general remarks on the difficulties in diagnosis of intestinal obstruction which follow are equally applicable to these two conditions.   In this chapter we shall concern ourselves in particular with *atresia* and *stenosis* of the intestine and colon, *annular pancreas*, *meconium ileus* and *malrotation of the intestine* and *colon*.

Diagnosis.—Although most of the developmental anomalies which lead to neonatal obstruction are amenable to surgical treatment, delay in diagnosis is responsible for a mortality which is still too high. *Vomiting* is the most reliable sign of obstruction in the newborn.   It usually starts on the first day of life and becomes progressively more frequent.   Obstruction above the ampulla of Vater is rare, so that the vomitus almost invariably contains bile. *Bile-stained vomiting in the absence of an organic cause is exceedingly rare and all newborn children who vomit bile should be admitted to hospital.*   The character of the *stools* is of great importance and can be misleading.   Even in atresia the infant may pass stools, but instead of the usual tarry appearance of meconium the stools are scanty, dry and grey-green in colour.   Meconium is composed of (1) dead cells from the intestinal lining; (2) secretions from the stomach, intestine, liver and pancreas; (3) amniotic fluid with vernix caseosa.   Meconium from a normal child will therefore contain squamous epithelial cells swallowed with the amniotic fluid. In atresia of the intestine or colon these cornified cells will not be present. *Abdominal distension* may be present, but in the early stages it may be difficult to differentiate from the naturally protuberant abdomen of the newborn.   Further delay in diagnosis is often caused by the apparent well-being of the baby. Until vomiting has continued for some time or until there are secondary vascular changes in the affected bowel, the general condition of the baby remains remarkably good.   Most cases of neonatal obstruction can be diagnosed by plain radiography of the abdomen. Absence of gas, distended coils or fluid levels may indicate the need for laparotomy. A barium meal is rarely necessary and may be dangerous. Further details of the radiographic appearances will be considered later.

Most of the embryological events which are related to the developmental anomalies of the alimentary tract take place between the fifth and tenth weeks of intra-uterine life. Rather than consider the entire sequence at this point it is more convenient to consider the embryology of each anomaly separately.

ATRESIA OF THE INTESTINE AND COLON

Shortly after the fifth week of intra-uterine life the lumen of the intestine becomes obliterated by proliferation of the epithelium. Vacuoles appear and as they coalesce the lumen is reformed by the twelfth week. If development is arrested during the second and third months of fœtal life there may arise anomalies varying from *stenosis* (narrowing) to *atresia* (discontinuity). It has been suggested that atresia is caused by some vascular catastrophe *in utero*.

Intestinal atresia may take the form of a diaphragm occluding the lumen (Fig. 85, A), or there may be a blind-ending cul-de-sac, usually joined to the collapsed distal loop by a thin fibrous band (Fig. 85, B). Rarely there may be multiple atresias, the isolated blind segments joined to one another by fibrous threads like a string of tiny sausages. Proximal to the obstruction the intestine is dilated and may be 3 or 4 cm. in diameter. The intestinal wall is greatly thinned and the deficient blood supply leads to ischæmia. There may be gross distension of the blind sac even before birth, and perforation may occur before or shortly after birth. Only rarely will the sac survive without perforation beyond the third day after birth. Distal to the obstruction the bowel is unexpanded and is rarely more than 4 or 5 mm. in diameter. The unexpanded colon is not much larger.

Duodenal Atresia (Fig. 85, A and B).

In our experience the atresia is commonly distal to the ampulla of Vater and the vomitus contains bile. In atresia above the ampulla of Vater the vomitus consists only of gastric contents and there is likely to be delay in diagnosis. Vomiting usually starts on the first day of life and becomes progressively

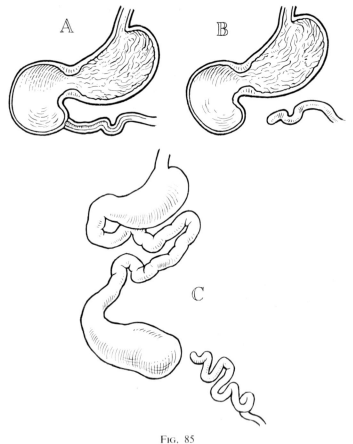

FIG. 85

Atresia of bowel. A, Diaphragm occluding duodenum. B, Common type of duodenal atresia. C, Jejuno-ileal atresia.

more intense as subsequent feeds are taken. There is a little abdominal distension, limited to the epigastrium, and gastric peristalsis may be seen passing from left to right. The stools may be misleading and may resemble normal meconium, but they contain neither stratified epithelial cells nor, later, milk curds. As in other forms of obstruction there may be fever due to dehydration, but if the temperature is above 102° F., rupture of the cul-de-sac with peritonitis should be suspected.

More than a third of the patients are mongols. There is no explanation for this association of anomalies.

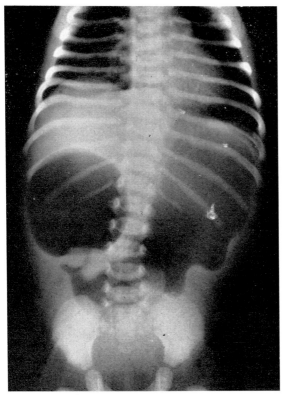

FIG. 86

Radiographic appearances in duodenal atresia.

Radiography.—Plain films of the abdomen may show distension of the stomach and duodenum with a complete absence of gas in the rest of the abdomen. If the diagnosis remains in doubt, improved pictures can be obtained by careful instillation of intragastric oxygen or by giving the infant a small drink of aerated water or lemonade (Fig. 86). As has already been stated, the administration of barium is unnecessary and dangerous.

It is usually impossible to differentiate duodenal atresia from annular pancreas before operation. Malrotation with duodenal ileus will present a similar clinical picture, but a skilled pædiatric radiologist can differentiate the two conditions.

Treatment.—Dehydration is corrected, if necessary, by intravenous glucose saline, but the danger of over-hydration must be borne in mind. Vitamin K (Synkavit, 1 mg.) is administered and an appropriate antibiotic given parenterally. A urethral catheter is passed into the stomach, and under general anæsthesia the abdomen is opened by a transverse supra-umbilical incision or by an incision through the right rectus muscle. The obstruction is relieved by a *duodeno-jejunostomy*, except in the rare case of atresia of the first part of the duodenum, when a gastrojejunostomy is performed. A fine polyvinyl tube is passed down from the nose through the anastomosis so that nutrition can be maintained during the first few post-operative days when œdema may occlude the stoma. The abdomen is closed in layers with fine silk and the infant is returned to an incubator. Sterile water can be given by mouth for the first twelve hours, and thereafter feeding is continued through the indwelling polyvinyl tube. Small feeds are given by mouth after the third or fourth day, and if they are tolerated, the tube can be removed.

Duodenal Stenosis.

It is usually impossible to distinguish the symptoms from those of duodenal atresia. In rare cases the lumen may be large enough to sustain life for weeks or even months. In such cases vomiting and failure to gain weight may be the presenting symptoms. The principles of treatment are as for duodenal atresia.

Jejuno-ileal Atresia (Fig. 85, c).

Vomiting usually starts on the first day and the vomitus contains bile. Quite early the vomitus may become malodorous (the so-called fæcal vomit). The stools are absent or scanty and misleading, as already described. Abdominal distension is usually marked and generalised, but if the child has swallowed no amniotic fluid or if it is premature and has not been fed, distension may not be evident until the infant is twenty-four or forty-eight hours old. There may be visible peristalsis. Dehydration fever may raise the temperature to 102° F.; a higher temperature indicates peritonitis or lung infection.

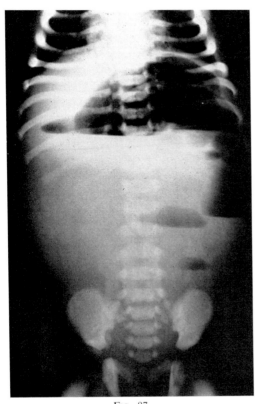

FIG. 87

Radiographic appearances in jejuno-ileal atresia— dilated coils of small bowel and fluid levels.

Radiography of the abdomen shows dilated intestinal coils containing fluid levels and absence of gas in the large bowel (Fig. 87).

The differential diagnosis is from meconium ileus, malrotation and neonatal Hirschsprung's disease.

Treatment.—Fluid loss is replaced and antibiotics and vitamin K are administered. With an indwelling gastric tube in position, the abdomen is opened under general anæsthesia. There is usually free fluid in the peritoneal cavity, and if this is cloudy or foul smelling a perforation should be looked for. The distended proximal loop must be handled with great care and delivered gently from the wound. Even if this blind loop appears to be quite viable it should be resected (Fig. 88, A),

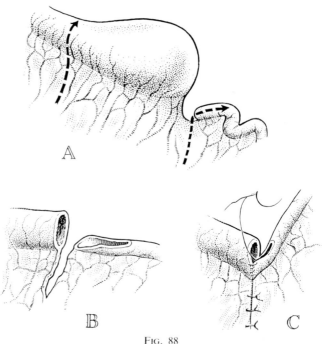

FIG. 88

Technique of repair in jejuno-ileal atresia. A, Resection of distended and devitalised proximal blind loop and very oblique section of unexpanded distal bowel. B and C, Oblique end-to-side anastomosis.

and after distending the unexpanded distal bowel by instilling saline through a hypodermic needle, an oblique end-to-side anastomosis is performed (Fig. 88, B and C).

After operation the baby is nursed in an incubator and antibiotics are continued. Sterile water is given for twenty-four hours and then small milk feeds are given and very slowly increased in quantity. It is rarely necessary to give fluids intravenously after operation.

Jejuno-ileal Stenosis.—This condition is rare and the principles of treatment are those of atresia.

Atresia in Other Sites.—We have only encountered atresia of the colon on one occasion (in the ascending colon). The condition was treated successfully by side-to-side anastomosis. Multiple atresias are uncommon, but a rapid search for their presence should always be made. If such lesions are found, an anastomosis should be made beyond the most distal block.

Most cases which have been diagnosed as stenosis of the colon or microcolon are examples of meconium ileus or neonatal Hirschsprung's disease.

MECONIUM ILEUS

Neonatal obstruction arising from impacted meconium presents one of the most serious problems of early life. Apart from the problem of relieving the intestinal obstruction in the early days of life, there is the medical problem of supervising the nutritional state for many years and of preventing or controlling recurrent respiratory infections.

The intestinal obstruction is only part of a widespread disturbance affecting the pancreas and the mucus-secreting glands of the alimentary and respiratory tracts. There is *fibrocystic disease of the pancreas*, in which the ducts are greatly dilated, the lining cells are flattened and there is a great increase in interacinar and interlobular connective tissue. There is no diminution of islet-cell activity or insulin formation, but the discharge of pancreatic juice into the duodenum is reduced in amount and enzyme content. The mucus-secreting glands of the alimentary and respiratory systems are also altered and their secretion is diminished in amount and is thick and sticky. As a result of the altered pancreatic physiology and widespread mucoviscidosis, the secondary effects are threefold. Firstly, the meconium in the lower ileum is dark, putty-like and exceedingly sticky and leads to intestinal obstruction (meconium ileus). Secondly, there is greatly altered absorption from the bowel leading to abdominal distension, wasting of the body and a chronically disturbed nutritional state. Thirdly, the alteration in the respiratory tract makes the child prone to recurring respiratory infection.

In meconium ileus the middle or lower ileum above the seat of obstruction is often distended and may undergo volvulus formation and may perforate. If perforation occurs before birth there is a widespread sterile peritonitis with numerous adhesions (*meconium peritonitis*). In meconium ileus the cæcum and colon are unexpanded and contain hard, pellet-like concretions.

Clinical Features.—Within a day or two of birth the baby starts to vomit, the abdomen becomes distended and there may be visible peristalsis. The putty-like masses in the ileum may be palpated in the lower abdomen, but otherwise the clinical picture closely resembles that of ileal atresia.

Radiography reveals distended loops of small bowel with fluid levels. The inspissated meconium may give a mottled or granular appearance.

Treatment.—Occasional mild cases of meconium ileus respond to treatment with enemata, gastric lavage and instillation of pancreatic enzymes. Most patients present with acute intestinal obstruction and may be treated by a Mikulicz resection and double ileostomy. The distended loop of ileum is exteriorised, the abdomen closed and the loop removed. The proximal ileostomy is used for decompression of the bowel above; the distal ileostomy allows instillation of pancreatic enzymes and flushing out of the terminal ileum and colon. Should the infant survive, a crushing clamp is applied to the adjoining limbs and the ileostomy closed within two or three weeks.

Once the immediate surgical problem has been solved the patient requires long-continued medical supervision. The diet is supplemented by pancreatic enzymes, water-soluble vitamins and daily oral antibiotics. In children who survive the first six months, respiratory infections are less frequent, but a very guarded prognosis must always be given.

DUODENAL OBSTRUCTION FROM ANNULAR PANCREAS

In this uncommon condition there is a ring of pancreatic tissue surrounding and constricting the second part of the duodenum. There may be atresia of the duodenum at the level of the pancreatic ring. In the neonatal period the condition presents like duodenal atresia or stenosis and the diagnosis is usually only made at operation. The duodenal obstruction is relieved by *duodeno-jejunostomy*.

MALROTATION OF THE INTESTINE AND COLON

Embryology.—The alimentary canal is at first a simple tube suspended in the midline of the abdominal cavity. It consists of three portions: (1) the *foregut*, extending to the first part of the duodenum and having a digestive function; (2) the *mid-gut*, from the ampulla of Vater to the middle of the transverse colon with an absorptive function; (3) the *hind-gut*, from the transverse colon to the rectum, excretory in function. Between the sixth and tenth weeks of intra-uterine life the alimentary tube grows so rapidly that it cannot be accommodated in the cœlomic cavity. Most of the mid-gut is extruded into the base of the umbilical cord forming a temporary physiological hernia. At the apex of this loop is the remains of the obliterated vitello-intestinal duct (Fig. 89, A). The peritoneal cavity grows, and about the tenth week the mid-gut is withdrawn into the abdomen, where it rotates in a counter-clockwise direction (facing the fœtus) so that the cæcum passes from the left side of the abdomen to the epigastrium. Rotation progresses and the cæcum passes from the right upper quadrant until it finally ends in the right lower quadrant. The ascending and descending mesocolons fuse to the posterior wall of the abdomen, anchoring the mesentery from the ligament of Treitz to the ileocæcal angle (Fig. 89, B, C and D).

Malrotation.

Arrests of development lead to lack of attachment of the mesentery to the posterior abdominal wall, to reversed or incomplete rotation of the cæcum or to a completely rotated but mobile and unattached cæcum. There are two important consequences: (1) *obstruction of the duodenum*; (2) *mid-gut volvulus*.

Obstruction of Duodenum.—When the cæcum is incompletely rotated it lies below the distal half of the stomach, and peritoneal bands run from it to the postero-lateral abdominal wall (Fig. 91).

9

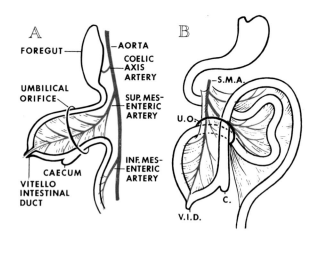

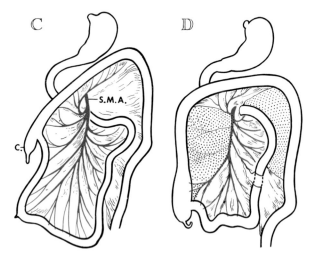

FIG. 89

Normal development, rotation and fixation of mid-gut
(*after* Dott). A is a lateral view; B, C and D are anterior
views. In D, shaded areas indicate fixation of the mesenteries
of the ascending and descending colons to the posterior wall.

These folds or bands lie across the second part of the duodenum and obstruct it by external pressure.

Volvulus of Mid-gut.—In malrotation the mesentery of the small intestine is poorly fixed to the posterior abdominal wall, and the bowel from the duodeno-jejunal flexure to the mid-transverse colon can readily twist on its narrow pedicle. This mid-gut volvulus almost invariably occurs in a *clockwise* direction and the twist may be anything from half a turn to two complete turns. When a volvulus occurs two serious conditions are established. (1) There is *obstruction* at the duodeno-jejunal junction and in the transverse colon. (2) The torsion occludes the superior mesenteric vessels and *infarction* of the entire mid-gut may occur.

It is important to realise that duodenal obstruction and mid-gut volvulus can coexist. After reduction of the volvulus one must also look for the duodenal obstruction. Occasionally there are further obstructing bands, most commonly at the third part of the duodenum.

Clinical Features.

Anomalies of intestinal rotation usually present in the neonatal period and are the most common cause of intestinal obstruction in the newborn. A few patients have no trouble until later childhood or even adult life.

In Infancy.—Duodenal obstruction leads to bile-stained vomiting in the neonatal period. As the obstruction may be incomplete or intermittent, normal meconium or curd-containing stools may be passed and the motions are occasionally blood-stained. Abdominal distension may not be marked. If there is an associated mid-gut volvulus there will be generalised distension and scanty stools. Dehydration occurs and there may be moderate fever. High fever may indicate infarction of the mid-gut loop. Radiography shows a distended stomach and duodenum, but unlike the picture in duodenal atresia there may be a few bubbles of gas in the lower intestine. Sometimes there is gross distension of the jejunum or ileum. The cæcum may be shown to lie high in the epigastrium. The differential diagnosis is from atresia and neonatal Hirschsprung's disease.

In Childhood.—The symptoms may be intermittent and the

child may have periodic attacks of abdominal pain, nausea and vomiting. The diagnosis of malrotation may be made on

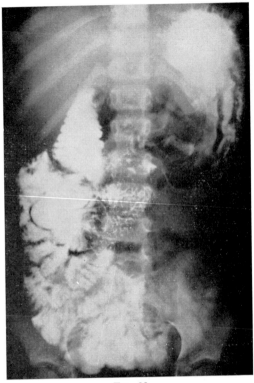

FIG. 90

Malrotation. Barium meal shows duodenal ileus
and small bowel lying on right side of abdomen.

radiographic examination (Fig. 90). A few cases are referred to the surgeon with a diagnosis of gastromegaly.

Treatment.

Dehydration is corrected and the stomach emptied with a rubber urethral catheter. Under general anæsthesia the abdomen is opened through a long right rectus incision. If the cæcum and ascending colon lie in the upper right quadrant and there is no volvulus, the duodenal obstruction is relieved by dividing the avascular peritoneal fold which runs laterally from the cæcum (Fig. 91, C and D). The cæcum is then displaced to the left. Further bands at the duodeno-jejunal flexure may require to be divided. If a volvulus is present the entire mid-gut

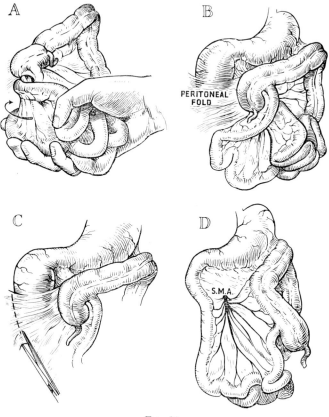

FIG. 91

A, Reduction of volvulus. B, Cæcum now lies high on right side and a peritoneal fold occludes duodenum. C, Division of avascular peritoneal fold which, as shown in D, frees duodenum, and cæcum and ascending colon come to lie in the midline or on the left side of the abdomen.

is delivered from the abdomen and the twist unwound, usually in a counter-clockwise direction. The cæcum and ascending colon must then be freed and transferred to the left (Fig. 91).

In the older child the appendix should be removed, but in the ill neonate appendicectomy is not advisable.

MECONIUM PERITONITIS

This form of chemical peritonitis has already been mentioned in Chapter IV as it may be followed by bacterial peritonitis if the perforation of the bowel is still present after birth.

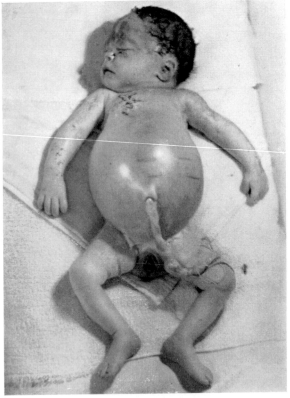

Fig. 92

Newborn child with meconium peritonitis due to
volvulus and antenatal perforation of bowel.

Meconium peritonitis usually follows antenatal intestinal obstruction, and perforation of the bowel proximal to the obstruction may occur before birth in bowel atresia, volvulus, meconium ileus and neonatal Hirschsprung's disease. In a few patients there is no evidence of intestinal obstruction and in these cases there is probably some abnormality in the bowel wall. The perforation may be sealed off, but the chemical peritonitis gives rise to tiny scattered foreign-body reactions which may become calcified.

The clinical features are those of neonatal intestinal obstruction—bile-stained vomit, abdominal distension and constipation (Fig. 92). The calcification following extrusion of the meconium may be demonstrated radiographically.

Treatment is by laparotomy and relief of the intestinal obstruction as described in the preceding paragraphs and in Chapter XI (Hirschsprung's disease).

CHAPTER X

Abdominal Pain in Infancy and Childhood

ACUTE ABDOMINAL PAIN

ABDOMINAL pain in infancy and childhood must always be a source of anxiety to the family doctor, and he meets with many difficulties in diagnosis not encountered in hospital practice. Although an error in diagnosis may lead to catastrophe, the doctor must not alarm parents unnecessarily. Abdominal pain is common in childhood and to the lay public there is little difference in the pain caused by a green apple and the pain from a " green appendix." The usual household remedy for abdominal pain is a dose of a popular laxative and only too frequently this has been given before the patient has been seen by the family doctor. The use of purgatives is the most certain method of converting uncomplicated appendicitis into diffuse peritonitis. As in hospital, the doctor may be faced with an irritable child who resents all attempts to examine him. In addition, anxious parents hovering around the bed do not simplify the situation. The very young patient can give no history at all and that given by a young child is rarely reliable. In the excitement of the occasion even intelligent parents give an incoherent history which cannot be relied on.

While attempting to gain the patient's confidence and co-operation much may be learned from inspection alone. The general appearance, the lustre or sunkenness of the eyes, the type of respiration and the position of the child may all help to guide the doctor to an accurate diagnosis. Grunting respirations may indicate a respiratory infection, but similar respirations are common in a young child with pus in the abdomen. Details of the actual examination of the child will be considered later. The differential diagnosis of appendicitis will also be considered fully, but it is convenient at this point to list a few guides to diagnosis.

If the patient has diarrhœa he or she is probably suffering from some irritant poisoning, either chemical or bacterial. One must always remember, however, that abdominal pain and diarrhœa may be presenting signs in inflammation of a pelvic appendix and in the now rare primary peritonitis. The " diarrhœa " may be due to the administration of a purgative, given to cure the pain caused by an inflamed or obstructed appendix. Many of the popular laxatives may themselves induce colic in the child.

If there is no diarrhœa the problem can be considered tentatively in two age groups. (1) In infants in the first year of life appendicitis can occur but is uncommon. Intussusception is the most common surgical catastrophe in the alimentary tract, but the average family doctor is unlikely to see more than three or four cases in a professional lifetime. Inflammation of a Meckel's diverticulum is uncommon and is seldom diagnosed before laparotomy. In ileocolitis diarrhœa may be delayed for twenty-four hours after the onset of pain. (2) After the first year the most serious common cause of abdominal pain is appendicitis. It has been said that all children with abdominal pain followed by vomiting and with a low-grade pyrexia *have* appendicitis until it is proved that they are suffering from something else—and then they have appendicitis as well! The commonest cause of abdominal pain is acute non-specific mesenteric adenitis associated with an upper respiratory infection, but unless the family doctor has time to return to re-examine the child this may be a very courageous diagnosis to make outside hospital. Other conditions which may give rise to difficulty in differential diagnosis are urinary infections, infective hepatitis, muscular strains of the abdominal wall and renal colic. Abdominal pain may be the presenting feature in tuberculosis of the thoracic spine and may precede the coma in diabetes mellitus. In recent years a subacute form of intussusception has become more frequent in children over the age of 2 years (p. 182), and recurrent colic may continue for three or four days before the child becomes really ill.

RECURRENT ABDOMINAL PAIN

Recurring and unexplained abdominal pain presents a difficult problem to the family doctor and to both the pædiatric physician and surgeon. The pain may amount to little more than discomfort or it may be accompanied by nausea or vomiting. Relatively little is found on abdominal examination. It may be difficult to assess the severity of the pain, and the clinician should endeavour to find out how far the symptoms interfere with the child's daily life. What is the duration of each attack? Is the child ever sent home from school because of the pain? Does it interfere with games or does it become worse when there are household chores to be done or messages to be collected? Does the pain ever waken the child from sleep? The possibility of *constipation* should be eliminated, and if there is any question of incomplete evacuation a gentle laxative such as a mixture of liquid paraffin and milk of magnesia should be administered daily for a period of two or three weeks. The history and examination may suggest *threadworm infestation* (p. 166). The spine is examined and X-rayed to exclude tuberculosis. Radiography may reveal calcification in tuberculous mesenteric lymph glands or calculus formation in the renal tract. The stools are examined for occult blood in an attempt to exclude peptic ulcer, Meckel's diverticulum or the presence of a polyp. Intravenous pyelography may demonstrate hydronephrosis or other renal anomaly. Barium meal and barium enema may reveal such lesions as polypi, peptic ulcer or malrotation. Radiography rarely reveals any pathology in the appendix.

If the investigations are all negative and the symptoms are sufficiently severe, laparotomy may be justified.

The term " *abdominal migraine* " covers a group of patients who suffer from recurrent attacks of abdominal pain, vomiting and headache. (*A child suffering from appendicitis very rarely complains of headache.*) In young children abdominal symptoms predominate, but as age advances abdominal pain and vomiting are less marked and headache is more prominent. Some cases are allergic in origin; in others there is definite evidence of nervous tension. In many instances there is a history of migraine in the parents or near relatives. The stools may be pale during the attack and the condition may be regarded as a bilious attack or cyclical vomiting. Treatment is directed to relieving nervous tension (in the parents as well as in the child), and some patients are benefited by small doses of pheno-barbitone. A food idiosyncrasy may be discovered and dealt with and some children have no further abdominal symptoms when given a low-fat diet.

In the female, recurrent abdominal pain may precede the onset of the first menstrual period by many months.

APPENDICITIS

Acute appendicitis is the most common lesion requiring intra-abdominal surgery in childhood. While it is the same disease in the child and in the adult, the reactions of the child are often quite different. The disease runs a more rapid and more deadly course, the criteria for establishing a diagnosis are different, and a somewhat different therapeutic approach is required. Since there is no mortality following the operative treatment of simple acute appendicitis, the success of therapy depends almost entirely on early diagnosis.

Pathology.—Simple catarrhal appendicitis is rarely seen at operation and it may be that many children recover from mild attacks of appendicitis. There is marked variation in the anatomy of the appendix and it varies in length, in position and in its course. The appendix is attached to the postero-medial quadrant of the cæcum and from this point it may pass in any direction. In childhood the appendix lies in a retrocæcal position in over 70 per cent. of patients. The course of the appendix is more important than its position, and although some pathological appendices run straight, the majority show angular bends, hair-pin bends and corkscrew twists. These bends are usually the site of obstruction and generally occur at the junction of fixed and mobile portions of the appendix. Obstructive appendicitis is common in childhood, the obstruction being caused by a kink, a concretion or the scar of a previous attack of inflammation. When inflammation occurs there is an accumulation of purulent exudate within the lumen and a miniature closed-loop obstruction is established. The blood supply to the organ is diminished by distension or by thrombosis of the vessels, and gangrene occurs early in the disease. Fluid is poured into the peritoneal cavity and within a few hours this fluid is invaded by bacteria, from perforation of the appendix or from organisms traversing the inflamed but still intact appendix. The peritoneal infection may remain localised by adhesions between loops of intestine, cæcal wall and parietal peritoneum. Even in very young children there may be very efficient enclosure of the inflamed organ in a protective omental sheath. If the walling-off reactions have not appeared in time, there may be diffuse infection of the peritoneal cavity. Administration of a purgative increases intestinal and appendicular peristalsis and perforation and dissemination of infection are more likely to occur.

Appendicitis may present as (1) *simple acute appendicitis*; (2) *appendicitis with local peritonitis*; (3) *appendix abscess*; (4) *appendicitis with diffuse peritonitis*. There is no mortality from the first three conditions adequately treated and the only deaths are in patients with diffuse peritonitis.

Clinical Features.—Appendicitis is rare in the first year of life but becomes more common from the second year onwards. The disease is more common in males than females. Over the age of 5 or 6 years the picture is similar to that in the adult —abdominal pain, followed by nausea and vomiting. The pain usually begins centrally and later shifts to the right iliac fossa. If the appendix is retrocæcal, abdominal pain and tenderness may be slight and the tenderness localised to the right loin. If the appendix lies in the pelvis, tenderness may again be slight or absent or elicited only on rectal examination. Under the age of 3 years the clinical picture may be rather different and the clinical features and the technique of examination will be discussed in some detail.

APPENDICITIS IN THE YOUNG CHILD

In many instances the onset is vague and the initial symptoms may be of a general nature. Only a third of the younger patients are seen within twenty-four hours of onset of abdominal symptoms, and the appendix has ruptured in a high percentage of all young patients before admission to hospital. The diagnosis is made late in too many cases, and *the chief reason for delay in diagnosis is failure to suspect appendicitis in a child of under 3 years of age.* The early symptoms are seldom suggestive of an intra-abdominal catastrophe. In spite of his limited powers of expression, the young child usually conveys to his parents that he has *pain* or *discomfort* in the abdomen.

Unfortunately he can rarely give accurate information about the type of pain or its situation. Although often not severe the pain appears to come in spasms, the child being relatively bright between attacks. The pain appears to be central abdominal until a late stage of the disease, and even a co-operative child invariably points to the umbilicus as the seat of his pain. As in older children an appendix abscess may form silently, and psoas spasm causing flexion of the hip and a limp may distract attention from the abdomen and direct it to the hip joint. *Vomiting* is an almost constant symptom. It may occur only once or twice early in the disease or it may be repeated and persistent. It may follow or precede the pain. The child is usually *fevered* and the temperature is commonly between 99° F. and 102° F. Temperatures above 102° F. suggest upper respiratory infection or diffuse peritonitis. A history of *constipation* is uncommon, and in a quarter of the patients there is a history of *diarrhœa*. This may be due to a pelvic peritonitis, but only too frequently a purgative has been given by the parents before the family doctor is called.

Technique of Examination.—One is usually dealing with a crying, alarmed and unco-operative child and much patience is required in the examination of young children. Much may be learned from inspection alone and, while attempting to gain the child's confidence, the general appearance, the lustre or sunkenness of the eyes, the type of respiration and the position of the legs are noted. The seat of the pathology and the degree of toxicity and dehydration may often be assessed by these observations. Grunting respirations may indicate a respiratory infection, but similar respirations are common in an infant or child with pus in his abdomen. The activity of the alæ nasi is more marked in respiratory infection. The tongue is usually dry and furred and there is often a typical " coliform " smell from the breath. One should not attempt to examine the throat at this stage.

Having gained the child's confidence as far as possible the bedclothes should be gently drawn down and the abdomen exposed. When asked to point to the sore place the child, if co-operative, will invariably point to the umbilicus. More commonly he vigorously denies feeling any pain, but strenuously resists all attempts to examine his abdomen. Movement or restriction of movement of all or part of the abdomen is noted. The child is encouraged to flex the thighs, a warm hand is laid gently on the abdomen and the bedclothes are drawn up again to cover the examining hand. It is sometimes wiser to carry out palpation *before* inspection. Both children and adults feel particularly vulnerable when the bedclothes are drawn down. A gentle, almost caressing touch often reveals more in the way of local rigidity than later, more detailed, palpation. Starting well away from the right iliac fossa, the hand is allowed to rise and fall as the child breathes. The patient's face is carefully observed as the gentle fingers palpate the suprapubic region, the right iliac fossa and the right loin. Attempts to push away the examining hand are noted. As in the older child the seat of maximum tenderness varies according to the position of the appendix. When the appendix is retrocæcal or lying deep in the pelvis there may be no evidence of abdominal tenderness. Only when satisfied that nothing further can be learned from gentle palpation of the abdomen and loins should one attempt to elicit rebound tenderness. Finally, a gentle digital rectal examination is made ; tenderness may be elicited or a mass felt.

The chest is examined and, lastly, the ears and throat are inspected. While examining the chest one should also examine the spine to eliminate, if possible, tuberculous disease of the vertebræ.

LABORATORY DATA

Leucocytosis is usually present. Unfortunately leucocytosis is often found in many conditions from which one must differentiate appendicitis. Children with diffuse peritonitis may show no leucocytosis.

A specimen of urine should be obtained and any sediment examined to rule out infection of the urinary tract. The urine is also examined for bile because infective hepatitis, too, may simulate appendicitis.

DIFFERENTIAL DIAGNOSIS

Upper Respiratory Infection.—The temperature is usually higher than in appendicitis, the face is flushed and there is more marked circumoral pallor. The common cold, sinusitis, acute tonsillitis and pharyngitis may all be associated with acute non-specific mesenteric adenitis. There may be a cough and an increased respiratory rate, but percussion and auscultation of the chest may reveal no abnormal signs. Radiography may be of help when the diagnosis is in doubt.

Acute Non-specific Mesenteric Lymphadenitis.—This is the most common condition to be differentiated from acute appendicitis. Enlargement and tenderness of the mesenteric lymph nodes almost invariably accompany respiratory infection. The condition is common in the prodromal phase of the exanthemata, but appendicitis *can* occur during the course of any of the common fevers. The abdominal pain may be generalised or localised to any region where the enlarged glands are located. The largest glands are in the root of the mesentery, but large tender glands in the mesentery of the terminal ileum may cause pain and tenderness in the right iliac fossa. Nausea is common, but vomiting is not an outstanding feature. Fever may be absent but may be high in the presence of upper respiratory infection. Tenderness is not so acute as in appendicitis and is often equal in both iliac fossæ.

Appendicitis is usually a progressive disease, and in mesenteric adenitis observation for several hours will show that the condition is stationary or even subsiding. If any reasonable doubt persists about the possibility of appendicitis, laparotomy should be performed.

Constipation.—Constipation can cause abdominal pain, nausea or vomiting, and with tenderness over the distended cæcum the condition may be mistaken for appendicitis. The temperature may be slightly elevated. Fæcal masses may be felt in the left colon or on digital rectal examination. In hospital a soap and water enema should be given and the child re-examined at short intervals. A satisfactory evacuation of the colon and rectum will bring rapid relief in patients whose symptoms are caused by constipation. In acute appendicitis evacuation of the bowel by enema will do little harm if the child is under constant observation in hospital.

Pyelonephritis (Pyelitis).—Infection of the kidney and renal pelvis can usually be differentiated by a higher temperature, white cells in the urine and by tenderness over one or other kidney. It may be difficult to differentiate pyelitis from inflammation in a retrocæcal appendix.

Gastro-enteritis.—In gastro-enteritis and dysentery there may be severe abdominal pain, and the pain and tenderness may be most marked over the distensible cæcum. When vomiting occurs the differential diagnosis from pelvic appendicitis or appendicitis with pelvic peritonitis may be difficult. There may be a history of similar symptoms in other members of the family or a history of diarrhœa in the district or in the school. Digital rectal examination may help to eliminate the presence of an inflamed pelvic appendix or pelvic peritonitis.

Infective Hepatitis.—Jaundice may occur in epidemic form, and a mistake in diagnosis should not be made at this time. The pre-icteric phase may last a week, and in sporadic cases it may be difficult to eliminate the presence of an inflamed highly placed appendix. The temperature is 100° to 101° F., the child complains of headache (rare in appendicitis), nausea and vomiting, and abdominal pain and tenderness. On examination the liver may be enlarged and tender. During the icteric phase the jaundice may not be obvious if the patient is first seen at night and examined by artificial light. The urine will not show the presence of bile until shortly before the appearance of clinical jaundice. Infective hepatitis is usually benign in childhood, but if an erroneous diagnosis is made and the child subjected to a general anæsthetic and laparotomy, the patient is more ill than usual and recovery is delayed.

Acute Distension of the Gall-bladder.—Acute cholecystitis is rare in childhood, but in association with mesenteric adenitis the cystic lymph node may be enlarged and may obstruct the cystic duct. An acute hydrops of the gall-bladder may simulate inflammation in a highly placed appendix. The condition responds to simple cholecystostomy.

Iliac Adenitis.—Streptococcal or staphylococcal infection of the leg, anus or perineum may give rise to inflammation of the lymph glands in the iliac fossa without involving the inguinal glands. The outstanding feature may be either *abdominal pain* or *restriction of hip movement*. There is fever, abdominal pain or discomfort referred to one or other iliac fossa. Nausea and vomiting are not marked features of the condition. There is flexion deformity of the thigh due to spasm of the ilio-psoas,

If the child is not ill he will walk with a limp and will probably present as an orthopædic problem (Chap. XXIII).

On examination there is lower abdominal tenderness and there may be a tender palpable mass above the inguinal ligament. On rectal examination there may be only tenderness, but later a tender swelling will be felt on one side of the pelvis. The primary focus may be found. On the right side the condition may be difficult to differentiate from appendix abscess, and a final diagnosis may not be made until an incision is made down to the peritoneum. The inflammation may subside with bed rest and local application of heat. If suppuration occurs the pus must be evacuated and the abscess cavity drained extraperitoneally by an incision above the inguinal canal.

Primary Peritonitis.—Since the introduction of chemotherapy and antibiotics primary peritonitis has become a rare disease except in the neonatal period or when it arises as a complication of *nephrosis*. The responsible organism is a hæmolytic streptococcus or a pneumococcus, and although the disease may occur in any age group, two-thirds of the cases occur in the first four years of life. It is difficult to determine the route of invasion, but the bacteria usually reach the peritoneal cavity by the blood stream and a positive blood culture is found in almost half the patients suffering from primary peritonitis. Many textbooks suggest that there is an ascending infection via the uterus and tubes, but this fails to explain the mode of infection in males, who are as commonly affected as females. Rarely there may be an infection from the gastro-intestinal tract. The transdiaphragmatic lymphatics have been suggested as a route of infection, but it is more likely that both pneumonia and peritonitis could occur in a pneumococcal septicæmia.

There is a diffuse infection of the visceral and parietal peritoneum with exudation of fluid between the intestinal loops. The mesenteric lymph glands are swollen and injected. In streptococcal infection the exudate is thin and cloudy and in pneumococcal peritonitis the fluid is thick and soapy to the touch. Like the rest of the viscera the appendix may be red and injected on its outer aspect.

The disease is equally common in males and females. There may be a preceding respiratory infection and the abdominal signs may be masked by the respiratory infection or by the diarrhœa associated with pelvic peritonitis. There is diffuse abdominal pain, vomiting, dehydration and high fever. Diarrhœa is present in half the patients during the first day of illness, but is usually followed by constipation. The abdomen may be board-like, but in young children it is often " doughy." There is usually some abdominal distension. On rectal examination there is diffuse tenderness. The white cell count ranges from 20,000 to 50,000.

If the patient is known to be suffering from nephrosis, treatment is by chemotherapy and antibiotics. In other patients the diagnosis can only be suspected and the abdomen is opened through a small incision. If the peritoneal exudate is odourless the peritoneal cavity is drained and chemotherapy instituted. If the pus has a " coliform " odour the inflamed appendix is delivered and removed.

Tuberculous Peritonitis.—Acute infection of the peritoneum may follow rupture of a caseous lymphatic gland or rupture of a tuberculous pyosalpinx. It is now exceedingly rare for tuberculous peritonitis to present as an acute abdominal emergency. Should the abdomen be opened in a suspected case of appendicitis and tuberculous peritonitis found, the wound is closed without drainage. With prolonged bed rest and streptomycin the prognosis is good.

Renal Colic.—Severe abdominal pain and vomiting may occur during the passage of a calculus, blood or pus down the ureter. Blockage of the ureteropelvic junction by stricture, stone or an aberrant vessel causes abdominal pain and nausea. The pain and tenderness are maximal in the flank. Red or white cells may be found in the urine. Intravenous pyelography may confirm the diagnosis. Renal colic may also be caused by simple crystalluria (Chap. XVI).

Acute Regional Ileitis.—Chronic regional ileitis (Crohn's disease) is rare in childhood, but at operation the terminal ileum may be found to be acutely inflamed and thickened and free fluid may be present. There is no evidence of tuberculosis and the peritoneal fluid is sterile. The condition presents with all the symptoms of acute appendicitis. After operation recovery is uneventful and X-ray later reveals no evidence of spasm or obstruction. The condition does not recur during childhood.

Pyogenic Mesenteric Adenitis.—This is an uncommon condition, usually caused by a hæmolytic streptococcus. One or more glands show abscess formation and peritonitis occurs early. The diagnosis is made only at operation.

Inflammation of *Meckel's diverticulum* and *intussusception in older children* may simulate acute appendicitis. These conditions are considered in Chapter XI. In four of our patients with *torsion of the omentum* a pre-operative diagnosis of acute appendicitis was made.

Tuberculosis of the thoracic spine may present with acute abdominal pain, but appendicitis and Pott's disease may co-exist. In infancy and childhood *diabetes mellitus* may progress very rapidly and the patient may first present in the stage of pre-coma with a history of constipation and anorexia and upper abdominal pain. If the odour of acetone in the breath is not detected, the routine examination of the urine will show the presence of sugar and ketone bodies. The onset of *menstruation* may simulate appendicitis, and many girls have recurring attacks of lower abdominal pain, sometimes for a year before menstruation actually begins. *Hæmatocolpos* (Chap. XVI) is a rare cause of difficulty in diagnosis.

TREATMENT OF APPENDICITIS

The treatment of acute appendicitis is early operation. In the toxic child with peritonitis a few hours may be profitably spent in combating toxæmia and dehydration. In such cases penicillin with streptomycin or, more recently, tetracycline is given pre-operatively.

The incision is planned to give the best access to the appendix with the minimal disturbance of the peritoneal cavity. It is usually of the grid-iron type or made through the lower right rectus. A Penrose or " cigarette " drain is inserted into the peritoneal cavity through the incision in all patients with peritonitis. An excellent drain can be made by inserting a central core of loose gauze into a section of Paul's tubing.

If an appendix abscess has formed prior to admission to hospital the patient's powers of resistance are good and the prognosis is excellent. In adults expectant treatment is usually adopted in such cases, but in children early appendicectomy and drainage is preferable. If appendicectomy cannot be performed without breaking down dense adhesions the abscess is drained and appendicectomy deferred for six or eight weeks.

Anæsthesia is given with minimal ether, using nitrous oxide or cyclopropane, often combined with some relaxant drug such as Flaxedil. A rubber tube is passed into the stomach before the operation starts.

Toxic patients and those with abdominal distension due to an ileus are nursed in an oxygen tent. We are convinced that a high oxygen atmosphere not only helps to combat abdominal distension but also has a sedative effect on many patients. Post-operative vomiting is treated by repeated gastric aspiration. The double lumen Miller-Abbott tube cannot be used in young children. The Fowler position has not been used by us during the past ten years ; there have been no subphrenic collections of pus following appendicitis in our patients during this period. Sulphonamides, penicillin, streptomycin and the tetracyclines have been administered to controlled cases of peritonitis during the past ten years. In our opinion tetracycline or penicillin-streptomycin are the most efficacious drugs available in the treatment of peritonitis. Tetracycline is administered intra-muscularly if gastric decompression is being employed The usual post-operative sedative is opoidine, $\frac{1}{12}$ gr. to $\frac{1}{6}$ gr. according to the age (p. 17).

Drainage of the Peritoneal Cavity.—The peritoneal fluid which accompanies an inflamed but unruptured appendix does not necessarily contain bacteria, and if the fluid is odourless it may be safe to close the abdomen without drainage. If there is any question of the fluid being infected with bacteria a " cigarette " or Penrose drain should be inserted through the wound down to the pelvis. In adult patients with diffuse peritonitis it is fashionable to close the peritoneal cavity without drainage ; in childhood one must never hesitate to insert a " cigarette " drain. Stiff rubber tubing may erode the intestine and should never be used.

Should appendicitis occur during the course of one of the infectious fevers (we have seen acute appendicitis complicating measles on several occasions), the child should be admitted to an isolation hospital with suitable operating facilities.

POST-OPERATIVE COMPLICATIONS

Pyelophlebitis and thrombophlebitis are now almost unknown in childhood, but the other complications of appendicitis are the same as in the adult—*residual abscess, intestinal obstruction, atelectasis and pneumonia, wound infection* and *fæcal fistula.*

Residual Abscess.—A localised abscess may form after the subsidence of a diffuse peritonitis and is most commonly pelvic. Fever may fail to resolve after appendicectomy, or after being low or normal for a day or two the temperature may start to rise. There is usually lower abdominal pain and tenderness and there may be frequency of micturition, diarrhœa or even retention of urine. There may also be abdominal distension due to an associated ileus affecting the terminal ileum. On digital rectal examination a tender swelling is felt. Many pelvic collections resolve; very occasionally the pus may be evacuated spontaneously through the rectum. It may be possible to insert a finger through the original incision and by very gentle finger dissection open the abscess, evacuate the pus and insert a Penrose drain; but it may be wiser to attempt evacuation through a separate incision according to the site of the residual abscess.

Subphrenic collections are rare and present the same problems as in the adult.

Intestinal Obstruction.—Post-operative intestinal obstruction is usually due to impaired function in matted coils of ileum lying bathed in pus in the pelvis and usually occurs within four or five days of operation. Treatment is by sedation, continuous gastric suction and intravenous fluids. The patient is nursed in an oxygen tent which will diminish gaseous abdominal distension. A true paralytic ileus may result from a diffuse peritonitis. The above treatment is combined with intravenous antibiotics.

From the seventh day onwards, the obstruction is usually due to mechanical occlusion. It may be caused by matted and adherent coils of bowel or organising fibrous bands. The treatment in such cases is prompt surgical relief of the obstruction.

Respiratory Complications.—Mild atelectasis is not uncommon and infection of the collapsed area should be prevented if possible by chemotherapy and breathing exercises. Since the routine use of the Fowler position has been abandoned, serious lung complications have been rare. The child is encouraged to move around in bed.

Wound Infection.—Soft tissue infection only occurs in patients in whom the wound has been closed without drainage. Evidence of infection may be obvious within a day or two of operation but may be delayed for several weeks. There is a rise in temperature, local tenderness and eventually redness and swelling. The pus may be liberated by the removal of one or two stitches, but it may be necessary to insert a pair of sinus forceps.

Fæcal Fistula.—This complication is fortunately rare and is usually due to necrosis of the cæcal wall. It may also follow evacuation of a residual abscess or attempts to relieve post-operative obstruction. The wall of the inflamed ileum is very easily damaged by the exploring finger. The fistula usually closes spontaneously with conservative treatment. If there is an obstruction distal to the fistula there may be rapid wasting from loss of fluids and nourishment. The skin around a small bowel fistula is rapidly excoriated by digestive juices. These cases may present very difficult nursing and biochemical problems.

Pelvic peritonitis in the young female may lead to sterility in adult life.

THREADWORMS AND THE APPENDIX

It is not uncommon for both adults and children to harbour threadworms without noticeable symptoms. Many signs and symptoms have been ascribed to the presence of threadworms, and these include weight loss, poor appetite, nausea, vomiting and abdominal pain. It is almost impossible, however, to prove the relationship of the helminth to the symptoms. Mechanical obstruction of the appendix by a bolus of parasites occasionally causes acute appendicitis, but threadworms are found in only about 2 per cent. of acutely inflamed appendices. Some 40 per cent. of children in Scotland suffer from threadworm infestation, so that it is hardly surprising that the parasites are found in 25 per cent. of appendices removed as an interval procedure for recurring abdominal pain. In these patients there is almost invariably enlargement of the mesenteric lymph nodes. The relationship of threadworms to appendicitis has been a frequent subject of discussion, and opinion is by no means uniform in the matter. If a child with a proved threadworm infestation has symptoms suggestive of the chronic appendicular syndrome the appendix should be removed. The administration of a vermifuge will seldom empty an appendix of worms.

CARCINOID TUMOUR OF THE APPENDIX

Argentaffinomas are very rare in childhood, but a carcinoid tumour may obstruct the lumen of the appendix and lead to obstructive appendicitis. There is no secretion of 5-hydroxy-tryptamine before puberty, and flushing of the skin is not seen. The tumours appear to be benign and solitary, but in the present state of our knowledge the post-operative follow-up should include repeated assay of the urine for 5-hydroxy-indole acetic acid.

CHAPTER XI

Intestine, Colon, Rectum and Anus

DUPLICATIONS OF THE INTESTINE AND COLON

(ENTEROGENOUS CYSTS)

DUPLICATIONS are spherical or elongated hollow structures, lined with some form of alimentary mucous membrane and intimately adherent to the alimentary tube. They may arise at any level from the base of the tongue to the anus and are most commonly seen in relation to the small bowel (Fig. 93). The lining mucous membrane is not necessarily the same as that of the adjoining part of the alimentary tube, *e.g.*, a duplication at the base of the tongue may be lined with colonic epithelium ; ileal and rectal cysts may be lined with gastric mucosa. There is no satisfactory embryological explanation for the occurrence of alimentary duplications, but they are probably the final result of an abnormal extension of the lumen of the gut produced on its posterior aspect by incomplete separation of the notochord. Interference with anterior fusion of the vertebræ leads to vertebral anomalies which are often associated with duplications. Duplications of the œsophagus are considered separately in Chapter VII, but it must be remembered that developmental anomalies are frequently multiple and thoracic and intestinal duplications may co-exist.

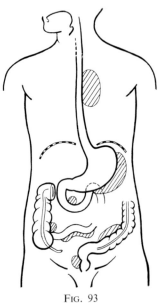

FIG. 93

Sites of duplication of the alimentary tract.

It is important to emphasise the firm adherence of the duplication to the adjoining bowel. There may be a furrow between the duplication and the bowel, but on attempting dissection the muscle layers will be found to be continuous

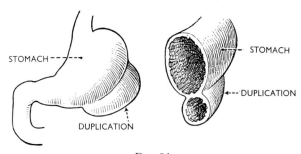

Fig. 94

Relationship of serous, muscular and mucous coats in a duplication and in the adjoining stomach.

(Fig. 94). The contained fluid is usually clear, colourless and mucoid in consistency. As in other developmental cysts there may be an increase in pressure with distension, necrosis and

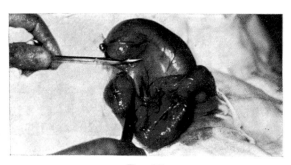

Fig. 95

Duplication of stomach and duodenum—treated by gastro-gastrostomy and excision of duodenal cyst.

sloughing of the lining and the fluid may become hæmorrhagic. Duplications vary in size from a small grape to an enormous dilatation. They also vary in shape: (1) saccular dilatations which rarely communicate with the adjoining bowel (Fig. 95); and (2) tubular structures which not infrequently communicate at one end with the bowel (Fig. 96).

10 B

Clinical Features.—Although duplications are commonly found in infancy and childhood they may be discovered at any period of life. Duplications below the diaphragm may present in four ways: (1) they may grow in size and cause *intestinal obstruction*; (2) increase in tension within the cyst may cause *abdominal pain* ; (3) the duplication may encroach on the vessels in the mesentery and cause *necrosis, sloughing* and *bleeding* in the adjacent bowel ; (4) a duplication lined with gastric mucosa may

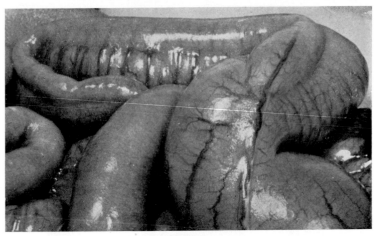

Fig. 96

Tubular duplication of ileum.

develop *peptic ulceration* and may *perforate* into the peritoneal cavity or into the adjoining bowel.

Radiography may demonstrate a space-filling shadow and a barium series may show indentation of the lumen of the stomach or bowel or evidence of obstruction.

If bleeding from the rectum is the presenting symptom the condition simulates peptic ulceration in a *Meckel's diverticulum.* If swelling is the outstanding feature the two most difficult conditons to eliminate are *omental* and *mesenteric cysts.*

Treatment.—As the bowel and duplication have a common wall and sometimes a common blood supply, it is usually impossible to separate one from the other without injuring the bowel or impairing its blood supply. In most cases the treatment of choice is resection of the duplication along with the adjacent gut, and re-establishment of continuity by primary anastomosis. In duplications of the stomach and duodenum it may be possible to excise the cyst or it may be necessary to resect a portion and marsupialise the remainder.   In one large duplication of stomach we opened the cyst and performed a gastro-gastrostomy.   After

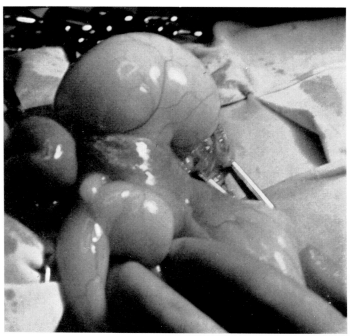

Fig. 97
Mesenteric cyst which caused volvulus.

excising a portion of the cyst wall to ensure that it was in fact lined with gastric mucosa, the opening in the cyst was sutured.

OMENTAL CYSTS.—These arise from congenitally misplaced lymphatic tissue.   They vary greatly in size, are thin-walled, rounded or lobulated and contain serous fluid.   The cysts may be small and lie in the substance of the omentum or they may largely replace this structure.

Clinical Features.—There is a slowly enlarging abdominal swelling with little associated discomfort.   The mass can be

moved from side to side.   Radiography after administration of
barium shows a mass in front of the intestine.

Treatment.—Excision presents no difficulties.

MESENTERIC CYSTS.—Mesenteric cysts arise from any part of
the mesentery or mesocolon.   Like omental cysts they also arise
from misplaced lymphatic tissues ; they occur most commonly
at the jejunum or ileum.   The cyst lies between the peritoneal
leaves of the mesentery and may obstruct the adjacent intestine
(Fig. 97).   They are thin-walled and the contents may be serous
or chylous.   There is always a line of cleavage between the cyst
and the adjacent bowel.   The condition may be associated with
malrotation of the gut.

Clinical Features.—There is slow enlargement of the abdomen
with mild abdominal pain or signs of intestinal obstruction.
Radiography following barium shows an opaque shadow
displacing bowel.

Treatment.—Mesenteric cysts can usually be dissected out
from the mesentery.   The vessels are gently displaced to avoid
interfering with the blood supply of the adjoining bowel.   It
may, however, be impossible to remove the cyst without
jeopardising the blood supply of the adjacent intestine, and in
such cases bowel resection is necessary.

MECKEL'S DIVERTICULUM

Meckel's diverticulum is found in about 2 per cent. of all
routine autopsy examinations in general hospitals.   Most of
these people have lived their allotted span without any symptoms
referable to the diverticulum.   Remnants of the vitello-
intestinal duct may, however, lead to dramatic surgical
catastrophes in the first few years of life.

EMBRYOLOGY

In the early weeks of intra-uterine life the apex of the mid-
gut loop has a wide communication with the yolk sac.   This
opening is narrowed to form the vitello-intestinal duct and the
duct and its accompanying artery and veins are normally
obliterated.   Vestiges of the duct or its vessels may persist.

PATHOLOGY

1. **Vitello-intestinal Fistula.**—The vitello-intestinal duct fails to close and small intestinal contents are discharged at the umbilicus (Fig. 98).

2. **Meckel's Diverticulum.**—The duct closes at the umbilical end but remains open at the intestinal end (Fig. 99). The diverticulum (half an inch to two inches long) arises from the antemesenteric border of the ileum, one to three feet proximal

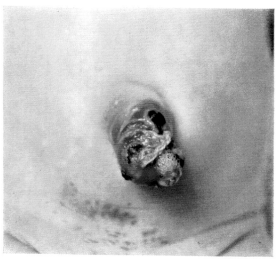

FIG. 98
Vitello-intestinal fistula. Note fæces
and gas bubbles.

to the ileocæcal valve, and generally has a small mesentery containing the patent remains of the vitelline vessels. It may terminate in a thin cord attached to the umbilicus. This cord represents the fibrous remnants of the vitelline duct or its vessels and it may occasionally acquire a new attachment elsewhere. The umbilical portion of the duct may remain to form an *enterotoma* and, more rarely, both ends may close leaving an *omphalo-mesenteric cyst* (entero-cystocele).

Although the vitelline duct is embryologically related to the ileum, its remnant is not necessarily lined throughout with ileal

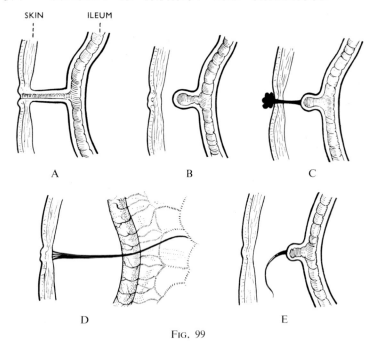

SKIN   ILEUM

A   B   C

D   E

FIG. 99

Common anomalies of the vitello-intestinal duct.

A, Patent vitello-intestinal fistula.
B, Meckel's diverticulum.
C, Umbilical polyp associated with Meckel's diverticulum.
D, Remnant of vitelline vessels.
E, Diverticulum with free cord which may ensnare any part of bowel.

mucosa.   In 25 per cent. of diverticula there is heterotopic tissue
—gastric, duodenal, colonic or pancreatic.

COMPLICATIONS

Complications from a Meckel's diverticulum can present in
many ways (Table IV).

Simulation of Appendicitis.—When the diverticulum presents
with acute abdominal pain due to diverticulitis the signs and
symptoms are usually indistinguishable from appendicitis.   The
diverticulum has commonly perforated and peritonitis is present
when the patient is first seen.   The diverticulum has a thinner
wall than the appendix and therefore perforates earlier.   When
the signs and symptoms are more severe than expected from the

short duration of the illness, a tentative pre-operative diagnosis of inflammation of a Meckel's diverticulum rather than appendicitis may be made.   The illness usually begins with central abdominal colic and vomiting, followed by pyrexia and lower abdominal pain.

When a diagnosis of acute appendicitis has been made and when at operation the appearance of the appendix is not in keeping with the clinical picture, the ileum should be delivered and a Meckel's diverticulum looked for.   It may be possible to excise the diverticulum alone, but occasionally it may be necessary to resect a portion of the adjoining ileum along with the diverticulum followed by direct anastomosis or, if the child is very ill, by a Mikulicz procedure.

TABLE IV

Findings in 100 successive Cases of Meckel's Diverticulum removed at Operation (Royal Hospital for Sick Children, Glasgow)

Abdominal pain simulating appendicitis .	30 cases
Intestinal obstruction	21 ,,
Intestinal hæmorrhage	14 ,,
Intussusception	9 ,,
Umbilical fistula	7 ,,
Umbilical cyst or polyp	3 ,,
Perforation from foreign body (fish-bone) .	1 case
Incidental finding at operation . .	15 cases

Recurrent attacks of abdominal pain simulating a chronic appendicular syndrome may originate from a Meckel's diverticulum.   The symptoms in such cases may be due to some disturbance of peristalsis caused by the presence of the diverticulum.

Intestinal Obstruction.—This is the most serious complication of Meckel's diverticulum and the infant or child is always gravely ill.   The obstruction may occur in the neonatal period or at any time throughout life, most commonly about the fourth or fifth year.   It is usually caused by a fibrous cord from the diverticulum which may hang free or which may be attached to the umbilicus, to the mesentery or to any part of the bowel or peritoneum.   A loop of bowel may become ensnared by the cord or may rotate around it as in a volvulus.

Adequate pre-operative preparation is essential as it may be necessary to resect the gangrenous portion of bowel and perform an anastomosis.

Intestinal Hæmorrhage.—Bleeding arises from peptic ulceration from heterotopic gastric mucosa. There may be the sudden passage of a blood-stained stool in a *young* child in whom there has been no previous symptoms. The bleeding may be copious, and while the first stool may be dark in colour subsequent ones are usually bright red. The red cell count may fall to alarmingly low levels in a short space of time. Bleeding from a Meckel's diverticulum may be unaccompanied by pain or there may be mild discomfort, in sharp contrast to the severe colic which accompanies the bleeding in intussusception. Although there are usually scant abdominal signs the ulcer may perforate soon after the onset of bleeding and there may be evidence of peritonitis. The perforation may occur in the heterotopic mucosa or in the adjoining normal mucosa.

In older children there may be a longer history of rectal bleeding of a less dramatic type. There are recurring attacks of varying duration and frequency, with the passage of black stools or small amounts of red blood, often accompanied by mild abdominal colic.

Simple excision of the diverticulum may be possible, but if there is thickening around the base there should also be a wedge-shaped excision of the diverticular base. It may even be necessary to resect a short piece of ileum to ensure complete removal of heterotopic gastric mucosa or aberrant pancreatic tissue.

Intussusception.—There are no distinguishing features in intussusception started by a Meckel's diverticulum. As in idiopathic intussusception the clinical picture is one of recurring abdominal colic with pallor and vomiting during the paroxysms of pain. The abdominal symptoms may be present for many hours before blood appears in the stools. The intussusception may be enteric or ileocolic in type (p. 188).

Umbilical Fistula.—Shortly after separation of the cord an infant may pass fæces and flatus through the umbilicus and the diagnosis can be made with certainty (Fig. 98). More commonly there may be a history of repeated discharge from the umbilicus. Instillation of lipiodol and X-ray may show a communication with the intestine, thus excluding a patent urachus. The track should be excised completely at an early age as the ileum may prolapse through the umbilicus and cause intestinal obstruction.

Umbilical Cyst or Polyp.—An umbilical polyp (Fig. 100) may be associated with purulent discharge and excoriation of the skin.   If cautery and ligation do not cure the discharge the

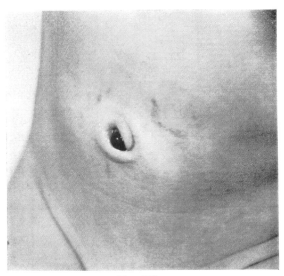

Fig. 100
Umbilical polyp.

abdomen should be opened and any underlying fibrous band, cyst or diverticulum removed.

Incidental Finding at Operation.—A diverticulum which has not given rise to symptoms, but which is discovered in the course of a laparotomy, should be excised if the condition of the patient is satisfactory.   A Meckel's diverticulum is always a potential source of future trouble, and if it can be removed without any appreciable risk to the patient this should be done.

INTUSSUSCEPTION

In intussusception one portion of the bowel is invaginated into an adjacent distal segment (Fig. 101).   In infancy and childhood retrograde intussusception is very rare.   The outer layer is called the *intussuscipiens*; the entering and returning layers together form the *intussusceptum*. In adults there is usually some mechanical cause for the intussusception (polyp, carcinoma, or submucous lipoma). In infants there is rarely any demonstrable cause, but in older children a Meckel's diverticulum or a polyp may form the apex.

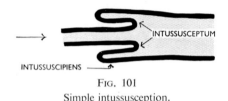

FIG. 101
Simple intussusception.

In many textbooks on general surgery will be found a section headed "*Intestinal Obstruction*," and prominent in the list of causes "*Intussusception*." This association of the idea of intestinal obstruction with intussusception is an important factor in causing delay in diagnosis. To wait for all the signs of intestinal obstruction is to court disaster.

ÆTIOLOGY

Age.—Most cases of intussusception (over 70 per cent.) occur during the first year of life. The condition is rarely seen under the age of five weeks but can occur in the neonatal period. The greatest incidence is between the fourth and eighth months. Change from milk to a more solid diet may alter peristalsis in such a way as to initiate intussusception. An associated enteritis may also disturb normal peristalsis. Enlarged mesenteric glands are almost always found at operation and although the glands may be secondary to the intussusception, they may also be associated with a preceding lymphoid hyperplasia (*vide infra— Season*). Only rarely is a definite mechanical factor found to be responsible for initiating the invagination.

Sex.—Males are more commonly affected than females. The mortality in females is almost twice that in males. The infant with intussusception is usually a vigorous, well-nourished baby boy. It has been suggested that in vigorous male infants with strong musculature the tonicity of the bowel muscle is greater than its ability to relax. It is in the fine fat baby boy, however, that lymphoid tissue is best developed (*vide infra—Season*).

Season.—The seasonal incidence has been stressed by many authors. In Great Britain the peak periods occur in spring and December; in America the peaks are in mid-summer and December. It has been suggested that Easter and Christmas are seasons of injudicious feeding with consequent gastro-intestinal disturbances. Whatever the season, intussusceptions certainly tend to occur in small " epidemics." There is no relationship between intussusception and seasonal diarrhœa, but an almost constant relationship with upper respiratory infections. As non-specific mesenteric adenitis usually follows upper respiratory infection and mesenteric adenitis is common in intussusception, it is reasonable to assume that the lymphoid hyperplasia involves *Peyer's* patches and the collar of lymphoid tissue which is so marked in the terminal ileum of infants.

Mechanism.—Any swelling of the ileocæcal valve or lymphoid tissue in that region readily comes in contact with the segment of cæcum immediately distal to the swelling and is treated as a foreign body or as intestinal contents. This appears to be the most reasonable explanation of the method of formation of ileocæcal and ileocolic intussusception. The age, sex and seasonal incidence accord with this conception. In enteric intussusception the origin is probably in a swollen Peyer's patch. In infancy the colic mucosa is thrown into folds which project into the lumen of the relatively narrow colon. The folds are studded with small lymphoid follicles and if these lymph nodes become swollen, the folds project farther into the lumen of the bowel and simulate a foreign body.

CLASSIFICATION

There is still confusion in the terminology of the intussusception which commences in the neighbourhood of the ileocæcal valve. Even an experienced pædiatric surgeon may have difficulty in naming with certainty the type of intussusception which he has just reduced. In the *ileocæcal* type the apex is formed by the ileocæcal valve and usually includes the base of the appendix (Fig. 102, A). If the mesentery of the cæcum and ascending colon has failed to become obliterated the cæcum is mobile and the apex of the intussusception may reach the sigmoid or even the rectum with relatively slight interference with the blood supply.

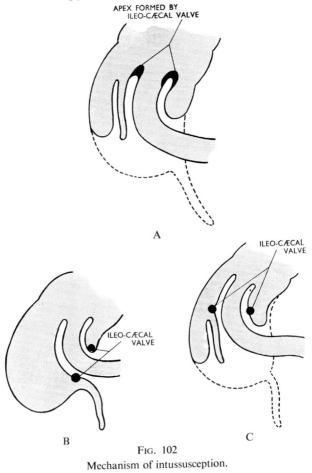

FIG. 102

Mechanism of intussusception.

A, Ileocæcal.
B, C, Ileocolic.

The exact origin of the *ileocolic* type is in some doubt. If the cæcum and ascending colon are relatively fixed the ileum may prolapse through the ileocæcal valve and can, in fact, advance at its own expense—that is, with a shifting apex. If the cæcum and ascending colon are more mobile the advance then continues at the expense of this portion of the bowel (Fig. 102, B and C). As the ileum advances through the ileocæcal valve its mesentery soon becomes constricted ; the blood supply is obstructed with consequent œdema and congestion. The peritoneal surfaces of the inner and middle layers become adherent and any further progress is at the expense of the cæcum and colon. The obstruction of blood supply may be followed by gangrene of the intussusceptum before there is time for the obstruction of the lumen of the bowel to manifest itself.

Ileocæcal and ileocolic intussusceptions occur with equal frequency and constitute about 90 per cent. of all intussusceptions. *Colic* intussusceptions (colon into colon) constitute 4 per cent. and the remaining 6 per cent. are *enteric*. Enteric intussusception usually occurs in older children.

CLINICAL FEATURES

In infancy most cases of intussusception show a remarkable uniformity of symptoms. The patient is usually a healthy and vigorous boy of 3 months or more who has previously given no cause for anxiety on account of his health. The onset is dramatic, as the child, without warning, screams loudly, drawing up his knees as though in extreme abdominal pain. Mothers with experience of peevish and crying children recognise the cry as quite unlike anything they have heard before. The attack ceases as suddenly as it began and in a few moments the child seems at peace and may fall asleep. The mother is reassured by the apparent quick recovery and frequently postpones sending for the doctor. After a lapse of time, varying from a few minutes to several hours, a further similar attack occurs and the doctor is hurriedly summoned. Again the attack ceases as suddenly as before and the doctor may find nothing abnormal on examination. If, however, the attack has been severe or prolonged the child may seem unduly quiet or even listless, paler than usual and he may be perspiring freely. Abdominal examination is not resented and reveals a small swelling about the size of a golf ball to the right of the umbilicus or in the right hypochondrium. There is no distension, no apparent tenderness nor guarding of the muscles, but the stimulus of palpation may precipitate a fresh attack and the swelling is felt to harden and become more prominent just before a fresh outcry from the child renders further palpation impossible. Rectal examination yields a trace of blood on the examining finger and the diagnosis is established beyond a doubt. It is a typical picture that presents itself in the majority of cases. Why, then, should there be any difficulty or delay? The chief reason seems to be the difficulty in detecting the tumour. No textbook description of intussusception seems complete without a reference to a " sausage-shaped tumour," and whoever first coined the phrase must bear a heavy responsibility. The simile is apt only in cases where a persistent mesentery has allowed the intussusception to travel along the colon and so acquire the slightly curved and elongated outline of a sausage. In the early stages the mass is small and may be hidden under the edge of the liver, which in infants extends well beyond the costal margin. Furthermore it is uncommon for the tumour to reach and project from the anal sphincter and justify the differential diagnosis from prolapse of the rectum so popular with students.

The next most important factor in causing delay in diagnosis is undoubtedly the association of the idea of intestinal obstruction with intussusception, and for this the textbooks are largely to blame. The classification of intussusception as one of the causes of acute intestinal obstruction suggests to the student that the two conditions are always associated. The triad of colic, vomiting and abdominal distension is expected, and the absence of the two latter engenders hesitation. Vomiting is not conspicuous. The child may vomit after each bout of colic, but it is only in the later phases that the frequent retching and vomiting of bile associated with obstruction presents itself. Distension likewise is later in developing, and to wait for such signs is to wait too long. The diagnosis must be made before the onset of abdominal signs and even when no tumour can be detected.

In 20 per cent. of patients with intussusception, particularly over the age of 2 years, the picture is not so typical. Colic may not be an outstanding feature and blood may not be passed per rectum for many hours after the onset. In enteric intussusception the passing of blood is often a late sign. The child is usually peevish and difficult to examine and great patience may be required in carrying out adequate examination of the abdomen. If no mass is felt and intussusception is still suspected, the child should be admitted to hospital, where there should be no hesitation in administering a short general anæsthetic. If the hand is lubricated with soap the mass is more easily felt, and with a finger in the rectum a thorough bimanual examination of the abdomen can be made. The mass may be almost entirely concealed under the liver and can only be felt after very careful palpation. If the intussusception is not very tightly impacted, the " tumour " may feel very soft and slide readily from under the examining finger as the intussusception is partially reduced. It should be remembered that relaxation of spasm of the gut under anæsthesia may render the mass less prominent. The diagnosis can sometimes be made on the appearances in a straight X-ray film.

For the first forty-eight hours there is usually a direct relationship between the duration of symptoms and the mortality. Older children may suffer from a subacute condition of longer duration, the intussusception coming and going with relatively little vascular obstruction. Blood may never be passed per rectum in these patients.

DIFFERENTIAL DIAGNOSIS

Volvulus may present a somewhat similar picture but there is no intermission of the pain ; the shock is more severe, to the stage of collapse. Palpation of the abdomen is usually easier and reveals a large ill-defined swelling. *Gastro-enteritis* is perhaps the commonest cause of difficulty, but the onset is less dramatic and the colic rarely quite so severe or such as to cause shock. The rectum contains loose fæces mixed with blood. The temperature is usually elevated and vomiting may be a prominent feature. Palpation of the abdomen reveals no tumour but a generalised tenderness. It must always be remembered, however, that the swollen mucous membrane in enteritis may so stimulate peristalsis as to produce a true intussusception. Such a sequence may easily escape notice until the general condition of the child has so deteriorated that laparotomy becomes hazardous. In older children, of the age of 3 years or more, *Henoch's purpura* may cause difficulty.

Here again the onset is slower, the colic never quite so severe but more continuous, the blood in the rectum is accompanied by loose motions and there is usually evidence elsewhere of hæmorrhagic effusions. There may indeed be a palpable tumour in the abdomen, caused by local hæmorrhage into the wall of the bowel and closely simulating an intussusception.

No doubt in some cases the diagnosis may be difficult, but let it be repeated—a healthy infant of 6 months who has severe recurrent colic, severe enough to produce signs of shock, pallor, listlessness, perspiration, subnormal temperature and a quick, soft pulse and from whose rectum the examining finger displays blood-stained mucus, has an intussusception whether a tumour is palpable or not. This is the stage at which the diagnosis should be made. To await further signs or symptoms is to court disaster. Should the child not be treated within the first few hours after the onset the clinical condition becomes increasingly grave. With every attack of colic surgical shock becomes more pronounced and, later, signs of toxæmia and intestinal obstruction develop. The pulse rate increases and the quality deteriorates, the eyes become sunken and the tongue dry. Vomiting now becomes marked and abdominal distension is present.

TREATMENT

The treatment of intussusception is early operation. Reduction can be effected by colonic injection of saline, air or barium, but the procedure is only justified where there are no suitable facilities for surgery.

The criticisms of *conservative treatment* are :—

1. Delay in operation following unsuccessful attempts at reduction by hydrostatic pressure.

2. Danger of perforation. This risk is slight if the pressure of the enema is never more than three feet of water.

3. Uncertainty of reduction. If a saline enema is used the girth of the abdomen increases when the fluid passes into the small bowel. If a barium enema is used the barium is seen to pass high into the small bowel under the fluorescent screen. In either method the fluid cannot always be persuaded to pass beyond the ileocæcal valve, and if any doubt exists the abdomen must be opened.

4. The causal lesion such as a polyp or Meckel's diverticulum may be missed.

5. Higher rate of recurrence.

6. Enteric intussusceptions cannot be reduced by hydrostatic methods.

Operative Reduction (Fig. 103).—If the infant is dehydrated or collapsed resuscitative measures are adopted. In a warm theatre the patient is anæsthetised and a stomach tube is passed and left *in situ*. The abdomen is opened through the lower right rectus (except in the case of an obvious left colic intus-

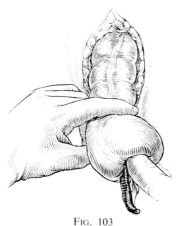

FIG. 103
Operative reduction of
intussusception.

susception). Speed and gentleness are essential. The mass is located and the major part of the reduction performed with two fingers inside the abdomen. It may be difficult to coax the mass round the splenic flexure, and if it should slip from between the fingers it is possible to continue " reduction " in the wrong direction! When the mass reaches the cæcum or ascending colon it is gently delivered and final reduction accomplished under direct vision (Fig. 104). Only experience can dictate the amount of pressure required to complete reduction. Packs wrung out of hot saline keep the bowel warm and help to reduce œdema. Small tears in the peritoneal coat serve as a warning that the bowel may tear if further pressure is exerted. If reduction is accomplished the peritoneal tears are rapidly closed with one or two catgut stitches. The experienced surgeon should know within a very few minutes if reduction will be possible. If he decides that the intussusception is irreducible the anæsthetist is warned and a careful but speedy resection or lateral anastomosis is performed. Long-continued attempts at reduction may so exhaust the infant that there is little prospect of success whatever further operative procedures are carried out. The infant may

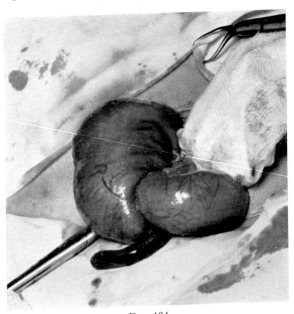

Fig. 104

Final reduction of intussusception under direct vision.
Note dark colour of the appendix.

die of shock following *forcible reduction.* Autopsy in fatal cases has shown that the reduced portion of bowel may remain inert even when the bowel is not gangrenous. A localised peritonitis is often found in such cases. Forcible reduction may reveal gangrenous bowel which must be resected. Although the recuperative powers of an infant can be little short of miraculous, post-operative collapse may be equally dramatic and saline or plasma may be required before the patient leaves the theatre. In some cases the superior ileocæcal fold appears to encourage re-entry of the ileum into the cæcum and it may appear advisable to cut this band. After reduction of the intussusception the appendix may be a dark plum colour (Fig. 104), but all those examined histologically after appendicectomy were still viable. It adds little to the operating time to remove the appendix routinely if reduction was easily accomplished, but it is unwise to open the alimentary tract unnecessarily and thus risk infection of a portion of bowel whose vitality has been lowered.

Unintentional heat loss is a formidable risk in surgery of infancy. The peritoneal cavity should not remain open longer than is absolutely necessary. Operative procedures should be minimal, and the sooner the infant is back in a warm bed the better. Almost invariably there is a post-operative rise in temperature (100° to 102° F.), but this returns to normal the day after operation.

IRREDUCIBLE INTUSSUSCEPTION

Resection and primary anastomosis is the best form of therapy *provided that the surgeon has extensive experience of intestinal surgery in children.* If the condition of the patient is poor, or if the surgeon is only occasionally dealing with intestinal problems in young children, there are two alternative forms of treatment :—

1. *Mikulicz Resection.*—The intussuscepted mass is exteriorised and the wound closed around it before the affected portion of bowel is cut away. The proximal ileum remains as an ileostomy and this must be closed within a week as the child will not tolerate prolonged loss of small bowel contents. If the infant is very ill it may be wiser to perform an ileostomy and simply exteriorise the irreducible mass. Resection and anastomosis can be performed when the patient's condition is sufficiently improved—usually thirty-six or forty-eight hours later.

2. *Simple side-to-side Anastomosis.*—The bowel above and below the mass is anastomosed (usually an ileotransverse colostomy), the intussusception being left *in situ*. If the viability of the ensheathing layer is doubtful the mass is exteriorised and if necessary resected later.

When the intussusception is irreducible the infant is usually very ill, and before operation an hour or two can be usefully spent in improving his condition with intravenous fluids, oxygen and antibiotics.   After operation the infant is nursed in an incubator or oxygen tent, and if an ileostomy has been performed the intravenous drip is continued and suction drainage applied to the ileostomy tube until continuity of the bowel has been restored.

CHRONIC INTUSSUSCEPTION

Subacute or chronic intussusception is arbitrarily defined as intussusception in which the symptoms have persisted from five days to two weeks or more.   An intussusception of this type has no complete obstruction to the intestinal lumen, and bowel movements may continue during the illness.   There may even be diarrhœa.

There is irregular or intermittent vomiting, slight or moderate abdominal pain and only occasionally passage of small amounts of blood in the stool.   Repeated examinations may be necessary before the mass is palpated, and a barium enema examination may be the deciding factor in establishing the diagnosis.   In these patients the prognosis is usually good, but it should be remembered that even this type of intussusception may suddenly become irreducible.

RECURRENT INTUSSUSCEPTION

Recurrence of the invagination is found in about 2 per cent. of patients with intussusception.   The interval between the intussusceptions varies from twenty-four hours to several years. In our series the condition has recurred on three occasions in one patient.   No surgical procedures are effective in preventing recurrence, but if a child has had more than three recurrences of ileocæcal or ileocolic intussusception it is justifiable to resect the terminal ileum and cæcum and perform an end-to-end anastomosis.   Many people have rediscovered and remarked upon Jonathan Hutchinson's observation of pigmentation of the buccal mucosa associated with polyps of the small intestine. These patients may have repeated intussusceptions and are apt to suffer from anæmia and occasional bloody stools.

INTUSSUSCEPTION DUE TO MECKEL'S DIVERTICULUM

A Meckel's diverticulum may form the apex of an intussusception, either by inverting itself or remaining uninverted, when its base forms the apex of the intussusception. Most patients are over a year old, and in almost half the intussusception is found to be irreducible at operation. The symptoms have usually lasted several days before admission to hospital and vomiting is a marked feature. Such cases form about 2 per cent. of all patients with intussusception.

Even if the intussusception can be reduced the small bowel in the region of the apex is particularly vulnerable and may not survive manipulation. It may be necessary to resect the bowel two or three inches on either side of the diverticulum and to perform an immediate anastomosis.

RECTAL BLEEDING IN INFANTS AND CHILDREN

The passage of blood from the rectum is surprisingly common in pædiatric practice, and in the out-patient department of a large children's hospital about 300 infants and children with this complaint are seen each year. In most cases the diagnosis is straightforward and quite obvious, but in a few the cause of bleeding is never found after full investigation and even laparotomy.

Mild Bleeding.—Most children seen in the out-patient department with rectal bleeding pass only small quantities of blood— usually from such minor conditions as anal fissure, rectal prolapse, proctitis and stercoral ulcer.

Moderate or Extensive Bleeding.—Each year about twenty patients in whom rectal bleeding is the principal or only symptom are admitted to the surgical wards of the hospital. One or two require blood transfusion. The most common lesions are rectal polyp, enteritis or enterocolitis, intussusception, Meckel's diverticulum, volvulus, duplication of the alimentary tract, systemic hæmorrhagic disease and hæmorrhagic disease of the newborn. In one patient the bleeding was caused by a sharp foreign body in the rectum.

Digital rectal examination, proctoscopy, sigmoidoscopy or barium enema may show a lesion (like a polyp) which can be treated quickly and effectively. Only too often sigmoidoscopy, barium enema and hæmatological studies reveal no abnormalities and laparotomy may be called for as the only means of detecting such conditions as Meckel's diverticulum, duplication of the bowel or intestinal polyp.

CONDITIONS DIAGNOSED AND TREATED IN
OUT-PATIENT DEPARTMENT

Acute Anal Fissure is the most common cause of rectal bleeding. There is a history of constipation and generally pain on defæcation. The bleeding is usually small in amount, bright red, streaked on the outside of the stool and occurs during or just after defæcation. The fissure is usually in the midline posteriorly. Multiple radiating fissures of varying depth are not uncommon. In the infant such fissures are often associated with gastro-enteritis or ammoniacal dermatitis. Most fissures are easily seen and digital rectal examination, which is very painful, is usually unnecessary and should be avoided.

Treatment.—The stool is softened with a mixture of milk of magnesia and liquid paraffin, and in the infant it is only rarely that further treatment is needed. In older children the fissure is anæsthetised by the application of 1 per cent. amethocaine ointment, and digital dilatation performed twice a day may help to relieve the spasm. Very occasionally sphincterotomy is required to cure the lesion.

Proctitis.—On proctoscopy the mucosa is injected and bleeds readily. The patient is given a low residue diet and small daily doses of milk of magnesia and liquid paraffin. Suppositories of 2 per cent. mercurochrome appear to alleviate the condition in some patients.

Rectal Prolapse.—Prolapse may be partial when the mucous membrane only is prolapsed, or complete when there is pro-trusion of the entire rectal wall (Fig. 105). The former is common and occurs in flabby overweight children with chronic constipation and is usually initiated by prolonged straining on the " pot." The complete prolapse occurs in debilitated or ill-nourished children and often follows an illness which has confined the child to bed. It is also seen in children with meningo-myelocele. The parents usually refer to the condition as " something coming down." Usually the prolapse has been reduced before the doctor sees the patient, but on rectal examina-tion the sphincter is felt to be lax and the withdrawn finger is often followed by redundant folds of rectal mucosa.

Treatment.—If the prolapse remains exteriorised it may be reduced merely by elevating the foot of the cot or raising the buttocks on a pillow. Gentle pressure with cotton wool moistened with warm water is probably preferable to lubricants such as vaseline. After reduction the buttocks are strapped together and the child given the liquid paraffin mixture daily. This may be all that is required. If the prolapse recurs the child should cease to use the " pot " and should be taught to defæcate lying on his side, or if old enough should use the adult

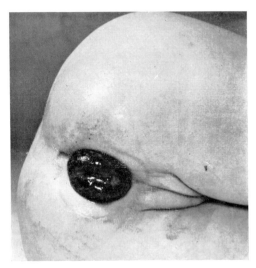

Fig. 105
Rectal prolapse.

toilet. The squatting position should be resumed as soon as possible lest the child develop a habit which may be difficult to eradicate. Rectal prolapse in children is usually a self-curing condition.

In a few cases it may be necessary to inject a small quantity of 5 per cent. phenol in olive oil into the submucosa to bring about fibrosis. The buttocks are strapped together after the sclerosing agent is injected. To the lay public a prolapse is rather terrifying and it is important that the anxious parents should be reassured.

CONDITIONS DIAGNOSED OR TREATED IN HOSPITAL

1. **Benign Intestinal Polyp.**—The single polyp of the rectum is a common cause of bleeding from the rectum. In the empty

rectum a low polyp is easily felt on digital examination. No attempt should be made to exteriorise it unless one is prepared to deal with an alarming hæmorrhage which may follow its tearing off. The polypus is a simple adenoma of the mucous membrane which becomes pedunculated by peristalsis and it may protrude at the anus as a pink mulberry-like object. Polyps high in the rectum and in the lower colon require sigmoidoscopy under general anæsthesia for proper visualisation. Treatment is by local excision. Polyps above the rectosigmoid can sometimes be demonstrated by contrast barium enema, and a transabdominal approach will be required for their removal. Polypoid adenomatosis of the small intestine may lead to bleeding and anæmia. This uncommon condition is discussed briefly under " Recurrent Intussusception " (p. 188).

Diffuse polyposis of the colon is rare, but as it is a precancerous lesion its presence must be excluded by barium enema and sigmoidoscopy.

2. **Enteritis and Enterocolitis.**—The history of bleeding is usually short and bleeding is accompanied by diarrhœa. Pus cells will be found in the motions and dysentery bacilli may be cultured. The treatment is medical.

3. **Ulcerative Colitis.**—This condition is uncommon in childhood and the patients are rarely admitted to the surgical wards. The bleeding may be of months' duration and there may be excess of mucus in the stools. The diagnosis is made by sigmoidoscopy and may be confirmed by X-ray. The treatment in childhood is medical and colectomy is rarely performed before puberty.

4. **Volvulus.**—In malrotation the symptoms are commonly those of obstruction of the duodenum or of intestinal obstruction, but in volvulus associated with vitelline remnants the obstructive symptoms may be overshadowed by the discharge of dark or altered blood. The diagnosis is confirmed at laparotomy.

5. **Meckel's Diverticulum.**—Hæmorrhage arises from a peptic ulcer in the diverticulum or adjoining ileum. Investigations by barium enema, barium meal and sigmoidoscopy are negative. At laparotomy the diverticulum is excised. Histology reveals aberrant gastric or pancreatic tissue.

6. **Intestinal Duplication.**—A large diverticulum may be

demonstrated by a barium meal but the diagnosis is usually made at laparotomy.

7. **Intussusception.**—In acute intussusception the diagnosis is not long in doubt, but in recurring or chronic intussusception there may be repeated episodes of bleeding without severe abdominal pain. The mass may be palpated or the diagnosis may be made by barium enema or barium meal and confirmed at laparotomy.

8. **Systemic Hæmorrhagic Disease.**—Anaphylactoid (Henoch-Schönlein) purpura, thrombocytopenic purpura and leukæmia may all present with bleeding from the rectum.

9. **Hæmorrhagic Disease of the Newborn.**—All patients in this group are under two weeks old. Bleeding usually stops six to twelve hours after treatment with vitamin K. Transfusion with fresh blood is occasionally required.

10. **Rectal Bleeding of Unknown Ætiology.**—In 20 per cent. of patients admitted to hospital no cause for the bleeding is discovered. Following sigmoidoscopy, barium enema and barium meal, complete blood studies are carried out with negative results. Even laparotomy fails to provide an answer. The majority of these patients recover spontaneously, but a few continue to pass small quantities of blood on infrequent occasions.

FOREIGN BODIES IN THE ALIMENTARY TRACT

Infants and children place in their mouths an unbelievable variety of indigestible objects, and in the first four years of life these objects are not infrequently swallowed. Commonly swallowed foreign bodies are coins, safety-pins, " Kirby-grips," pins, tacks, nails, buttons, brooches and small toys. In our experience 95 per cent. of these objects—sharp and blunt—move along the alimentary tract without becoming impacted or injuring the mucous membrane. Most foreign bodies which pass safely down the œsophagus will eventually come out through the anus. They start on their way with little more than a gulp or a cough and many are swallowed without the slightest difficulty. Only the disappearance of the object with which the child has been playing leads to parental suspicion of the accident. Most swallowed foreign bodies pass into the stomach, and there they rarely give rise to symptoms. Their final evacuation may be missed if all stools are not kept and carefully searched. Perforation of the intestine is rare and usually occurs so slowly that the opening is sealed and peritonitis is rare.

Occasionally a foreign body may become impacted in the œsophagus and give rise to choking, difficulty in swallowing and local discomfort. If left too long there may be reaction in the trachea, and a sharp object may occasionally perforate the œsophagus and cause mediastinitis or puncture the aorta, pericardium or pleura.

During the taking of a rectal temperature in a restless child a thermometer may very occasionally break in the rectum. The broken fragment is almost invariably passed along with the first or second bowel movement after the accident.

Radiography.—Even if one suspects that the child is romancing in saying that a foreign body has been swallowed, X-ray examination of the alimentary tract should never be omitted. Fortunately most foreign bodies are opaque to X-rays and their progress (or lack of progress) can be followed.

Treatment—(1) *Œsophageal Foreign Bodies.*—Because of large size or sharpness, foreign bodies may lodge in the œsophagus and must be removed. The higher the impaction the greater is the urgency for removal because of the risk of respiratory complications. Removal is done under direct vision by endoscopy.

(2) *Gastro-intestinal Foreign Bodies.*—With conservative treatment the child is kept on normal diet and purgation is avoided. All stools are collected in a suitable container and thoroughly examined. Most objects will be evacuated within a few days, but occasionally elimination may take several weeks. Mere size is not a deterrent to passage through the canal, so long as the object is smooth and rigid. In children under the age of 2 years a large " Kirby-grip " may have difficulty in passing round the duodenal bend. Sharp objects such as pins, needles, open safety-pins and broken glass must be regarded with some concern, and progress should be checked frequently by X-ray. If a sharp object remains in the one position for more than two or three days surgical removal should be considered. Children who have swallowed foreign

bodies are referred to the hospital daily, yet in one surgical unit during a five-year period laparotomy was required only on six occasions. The objects were a mucus extractor with rubber tubing attached, two darning needles, an open safety-pin, a " Kirby-grip " and a large fish bone perforating a Meckel's diverticulum.

Trichobezoar is discussed in Chapter VIII.

Foreign Bodies in the Air-Passages.—A foreign body in the larynx may cause local pain, spasms of coughing and pain on swallowing. Irritation may lead to laryngeal œdema. The object should be removed by direct laryngoscopy. In the trachea there may be no symptoms after the initial choking as, apart from a toy balloon, foreign bodies which pass the cricoid will not completely obstruct the trachea. Sharp objects and organic material will, however, cause tracheitis early and lead to dyspnœa. Radiography is of value if the object is radio-opaque. The foreign body should be removed by bronchoscope, but where facilities for bronchoscopy do not exist a tracheotomy may be necessary to save life. Foreign bodies in the bronchi cause local pain and cough and, if large enough, lead to dyspnœa, emphysema or, where there is complete obstruction, atelectasis and possible lung abscess. Organic bodies produce early inflammation. Radiography may give accurate localisation of radio-opaque objects, but if the presence of a foreign body is suspected early bronchoscopy should be performed.

Foreign Bodies in the Ear.—The common foreign bodies inserted into the ear are peas and beads and occasionally a small insect is found. The intruder may be hidden by the curve of the meatal floor. Removal can usually be effected by syringing with *warm* water. Although peas and other animal and vegetable matter may swell, they become soft and can be broken up in a day or two if syringing is unsuccessful. If syringing fails to dislodge a bead or a small pebble it may be removed with a small blunt hook.

Foreign Bodies in the Nose.—Peas, pebbles, buttons, etc., are frequently inserted up the nose. They may be removed with a small blunt hook or aural dressing forceps. The removal of foreign bodies from the ear or nose is unpleasant and few children are able to remain still during the procedure. Sudden movement by the child may result in displacement of the object farther in or injury to the meatus. A general anæsthetic is usually advisable.

Foreign bodies in soft tissues, bladder and vagina are considered in appropriate chapters.

CONSTIPATION

In infancy constipation is judged by the consistency of the stools rather than by their frequency. Hard dry stools are commonly due to *underfeeding, inadequate fluid intake* and *change from breast to artificial feeding.* If the stools are hard and streaked with blood there is probably an *anal fissure*, and pain on defæcation tends to perpetuate constipation. A mixture of milk of magnesia and liquid paraffin softens the motions and allows the fissure to heal. If healing does not take place, daily digital dilatation is carried out following the local application of 1 per cent. amethocaine ointment. Very occasionally the anus is stretched under general anæsthesia. Severe constipation in infancy may be due to anal stenosis or Hirschsprung's disease.

In childhood constipation is frequently due to habitual neglect from laziness or preoccupation with other activities. The rectum becomes insensitive and does not answer the call to defæcation. A vicious circle is often established by the regular exhibition of purgatives. The cure lies with the parents, who are instructed in regulation of the child's bowel habit. If necessary the bowel is cleared by saline washouts and re-educative measures instituted. The child is aroused in the morning in plenty of time to go to the lavatory and should not be allowed to take along books or comic papers. The diet is adjusted and mixed fruit, wholemeal bread, All-bran and copious fluids are given. For some years we have used a standardised preparation of senna (Senokot) in the treatment of children with stubborn constipation. The usual dose is one teaspoonful nightly and this is gradually reduced and eventually discontinued. There has been no evidence of habit formation.

MEGACOLON

In 1887 Harald Hirschsprung of Copenhagen described the condition which still bears his name. From the early weeks of life there is stubborn constipation and the colon becomes distended and filled with gas and fæcal material. Since Hirschsprung's time there have been many conflicting theories on the ætiology of the condition, but there is now almost universal agreement as to the causal factors. Cases of megacolon may be divided into three main groups :—

1. *Organic Megacolon.*—This may occur at any age. In infancy it is most commonly due to anal stenosis; in adult life it may be caused by stricture or tumour.

2. *Hirschsprung's Disease* (congenital megacolon) is due to

diminution or absence of ganglion cells in the myenteric plexus of the distal colon. Constipation is present from early life.

3. *Idiopathic Megacolon* (colonic inertia).—In this condition there is no constant ætiological factor. Constipation is not present from birth and the onset is usually slow and insidious. Faulty bowel habits and an elongated sigmoid with excessive water absorption are contributing factors. The colon is dilated all the way down to the anus.

HIRSCHSPRUNG'S DISEASE

CONGENITAL MEGACOLON

In this disease there is obstruction without any obvious mechanical cause. The proximal colon is greatly hypertrophied and dilated and there may be mucosal ulceration. The rectum and rectosigmoid have a normal calibre but appear to be relatively narrow. The narrower (or unexpanded) segment may be short or long. The megacolon may be confined to the sigmoid loop, but the enlargement may extend to the splenic flexure or transverse colon. In advanced cases the entire colon from the rectosigmoid upwards is grossly distended and the distension may extend into the ileum. The obstruction is caused by a neuromuscular defect and the peristaltic waves cannot pass through the affected segment. On histological examination there is complete absence of *parasympathetic ganglion cells* in the intramural myenteric plexus of Auerbach throughout the unexpanded segment. Proximally the ganglion cells are normal, but they become scanty at the transitional area (Fig. 106).

Clinical Features.—Although the child appears to be healthy at birth, constipation and progressive abdominal distension appear in the first few days or weeks of life. Eighty per cent. of the patients are male. *In the newborn infant* the disease may present with abdominal distension and vomiting (Fig. 107). X-ray reveals dilated coils of bowel (Fig. 108), and clinically and radiologically the condition may simulate other forms of neonatal obstruction (Chap. IX). On insertion of the little finger into the rectum gas and yellow liquid fæces may be evacuated and the distension reduced. (In gastro-enteritis there may be vomiting, abdominal distension and frequent motions,

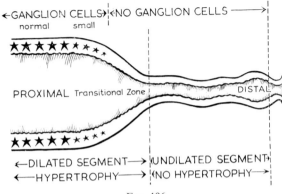

FIG. 106

Diagrammatic representation of histopathology in
Hirschsprung's disease.

(By permission of Dr M. Bodian and " Lancet.")

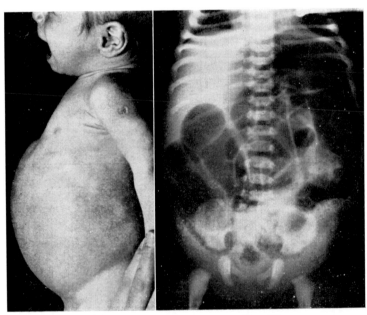

FIG. 107   FIG. 108

Fig. 107.—Abdominal distension in neonatal Hirschsprung's disease.
Fig. 108.—Radiographic appearances in neonatal Hirschsprung's disease.

and the response to rectal examination may be similar to that in neonatal Hirschsprung's disease.) If the loose motions continue in neonatal Hirschsprung's disease it is suggestive of *ulcerating colitis* and may be an indication for early surgical relief of the obstruction. Barium enema may show an unexpanded rectosigmoid with proximal dilatation but it is unusual for this " typical " appearance to present until the infant is 3 weeks old. The classical radiographic picture may not develop for three months. Unless the condition is carefully handled in hospital, the outlook in neonatal Hirschsprung's disease is grave and until recently three-quarters of the patients died in the first year of life. When the disease presents as a neonatal obstruction the gut may be deflated by a finger or tube passed into the rectum. If obstruction persists in spite of daily saline washouts and a diagnosis cannot be made following a barium enema, the abdomen is opened and the diagnosis confirmed by demonstration of the unexpanded distal colon and proximal distension. A colostomy is performed in the dilated bowel and a piece of colon is taken from its margin for biopsy to confirm the presence of parasympathetic ganglion cells. A rectosigmoidectomy of the aganglionic bowel is performed when the child's condition permits, but rarely before the age of 6 months.

Some patients show less well defined clinical signs. There may be intermittent constipation and abdominal distension in the neonatal period, but these are controlled by conservative measures and may be so controlled for many years. Constipation becomes more stubborn and there is marked enlargement of the abdomen (Fig. 109). The abdominal skin may become thin, tense and shiny, and dilated veins may course over the wall. Peristaltic waves may be seen to pass along the dilated and hypertrophied colon. Fæcal masses are usually palpable through the abdominal wall. Digital rectal examination may reveal an empty rectum with fæces at its upper limit or palpable in the sigmoid colon through the rectal wall ; less commonly the rectum contains much fæcal material. Constipation may be masked by fæcal incontinence (*encopresis*) or spurious diarrhœa, and soiling of the underclothes is common. Growth is usually retarded and puberty may be delayed in untreated children ; the child is often sallow and listless. The abdominal distension is often intermittent and may be relieved by the passage of quantities of foul-smelling fæces, particularly at night. Acute obstruction may occur at any time and there may be ulceration of the mucosa and occasionally perforation of a stercoral ulcer.

Radiography.—Plain radiography of the abdomen is the

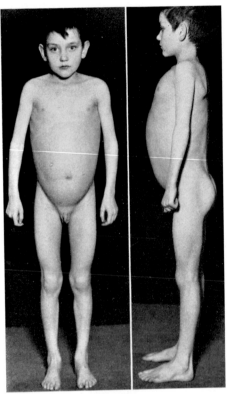

FIG. 109
Hirschsprung's disease in a boy of 10 years.

most useful investigation. Dilated large bowel and fæcal masses suggest the correct diagnosis. If the haustrations are taken up by distension, even a skilled pædiatric radiologist cannot always differentiate large and small bowel distension and it may be impossible to differentiate Hirschsprung's disease from other forms of obstruction. Examination with a barium enema should be carried out with great caution. The bowel can hold enormous quantities of barium which the child is unable to expel, and death may occur from shock. Small quantities of barium are instilled (infants must first be sedated) and the patient is examined in the anteroposterior, lateral and oblique positions

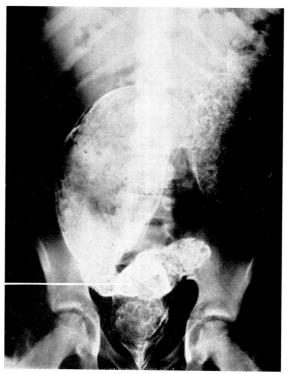

FIG. 110

Unexpanded rectosigmoid segment outlined by barium enema in Hirschsprung's disease.

until the unexpanded aganglionic segment is demonstrated distal to the dilated region (Fig. 110).

If the clinical diagnosis is not confirmed by radiography, rectal biopsy is a most useful diagnostic measure. The diagnosis is based on the state of the submucous or myenteric parasympathetic plexus.

Treatment.—Hirschsprung's disease varies in severity and it is not necessary to operate on patients with the milder forms of the disease. With supervised diet, laxatives, saline washouts and olive oil enemata, some patients can be carried along for lengthy periods. They usually require periodic admission to hospital when fæcal impaction becomes troublesome. If a soap and water enema made with tap water is given, severe shock may arise from " *water intoxication.*" There is rapid diffusion of water into the circulation from the greatly dilated bowel. Enemata and washouts are therefore made up with saline and all fluid is recovered.

The accepted surgical method of treatment of confirmed Hirschsprung's disease is removal of the obstructing aganglionic segment of bowel. After pre-operative preparation of the bowel by colonic lavage and chemotherapy or antibiotic, a *recto-sigmoidectomy* is performed by a pull-through technique ; this may be accomplished by a one-stage, two-stage or three-stage procedure. In the two-stage and three-stage operations, recto-sigmoidectomy is preceded by a colostomy. After careful pre-operative preparation the aganglionic segment is mobilised down to the anal sphincter and the distended sigmoid loop excised. (In the two-stage procedure the colostomy is resected along with the aganglionic bowel.) The rectum is then everted upon itself and pulled out through the anus. The proximal colon is drawn through the rectum, the excess rectum cut away and an anastomosis performed just outside the anus. When the bowel is inverted into its normal position the line of anastomosis is less than an inch above the anus. Intravenous glucose saline and blood are necessary during and after this operation. (In the three-stage procedure the transverse colostomy is closed two weeks after the rectosigmoidectomy.)

Following abdominoperineal rectosigmoidectomy most patients have normal sphincter control, take a normal diet and require no laxatives.

IDIOPATHIC MEGACOLON

In this condition there is simple dilatation of the colon forming a pear-shaped terminal reservoir above the anus. Constipation usually starts after the second year of life. The abdomen may become distended and fæcal masses may be palpable through the abdominal wall. On digital rectal examination there are fæcal masses in a dilated rectum.   There may be encopresis.

The radiographic appearances may be typical of the *terminal reservoir* type of megacolon (Fig. 111), or the left colon may be

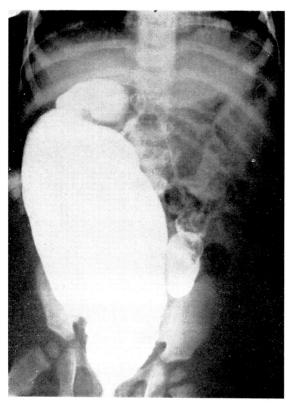

Fig. 111
" Terminal reservoir " demonstrated by barium enema.

dilated and redundant (dolicho-colon).   If the radiographic appearances are equivocal rectal biopsy is performed.   In idiopathic megacolon ganglion cells will be present.

Treatment.—There is no satisfactory radical treatment for this condition, but if the patient is carried along with medical measures as already described the constipation is usually relieved spontaneously between the ages of 8 and 12 years.   It may be necessary to perform a rectal biopsy to exclude the presence of Hirschsprung's disease. Dramatic cures sometimes follow the internal anal sphincterotomy which can be performed during the biopsy.

CONGENITAL MALFORMATIONS OF THE RECTUM AND ANUS

Embryology.—In the five-week embryo the urogenital sinus and hind-gut empty into a common cavity—the *cloaca*—separated from the exterior by the cloacal membrane (Fig. 112, A). By the downgrowth of a mesodermic fold (urorectal septum) the separation of the urogenital tract from the rectum is normally completed by the seventh week (Fig. 112, C). For a time there is a small opening between the rectum and the urogenital tract known as the *cloacal duct* (Fig. 112, B). The urorectal septum also divides the cloacal membrane into the *urogenital membrane* anteriorly and the *anal membrane* posteriorly (Fig. 112, C), and these acquire external openings. A small invagination—the *proctodeum*—develops in the region of the future anus, and the proctodeum and rectum join by rupture of the anal membrane during the eighth week (Fig. 112, D). Rectal and anal anomalies and associated malformations are due to arrests in development in the seventh and eighth weeks of fœtal life.

Congenital anal stenosis may occur at the anus or at a level of 1 to 3 cm. above the anus. This partial obstruction is caused by incomplete rupture of the anal membrane. Rectal stenosis is due to incomplete development of the rectum. Persistence of the anal membrane leads to membranous imperforate anus. Most commonly the rectum ends blindly at some distance above the imperforate anus, due to a deficiency in the lower posterior part of the cloaca.

Fistulæ between the rectum and urogenital tract are established if the urorectal septum does not completely separate the rectum from the urogenital sinus. A rectoperineal fistula (Fig. 113, C) forms if the anterior portion of the cloacal duct is closed and the posterior portion remains open and is carried downwards by local growth. In the female, fistulæ between the rectum and the vagina occur as the Müllerian ducts descend along the posterior wall of the urogenital sinus (Fig. 113, G).

The external anal sphincter muscle develops from the regional mesenchyme and is not dependent upon the presence of the

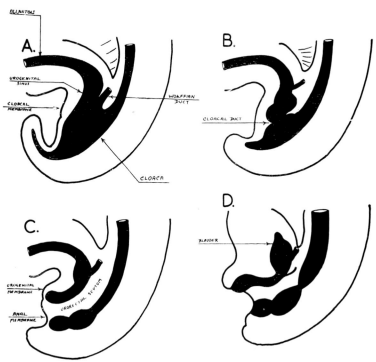

FIG. 112

Normal development of anus and rectum from 7·5 to 42 mm. stage.

terminal bowel.   The sphincter is usually fairly well developed in all types of imperforate anus.

CLASSIFICATION

The abnormalities have been classified according to the methods of treatment required.

Type I.—Here the anus and rectum though patent show some degree of stenosis.   The stenosis may be at the anus or 1 to 3 cm. above the anus (Fig. 113, A).

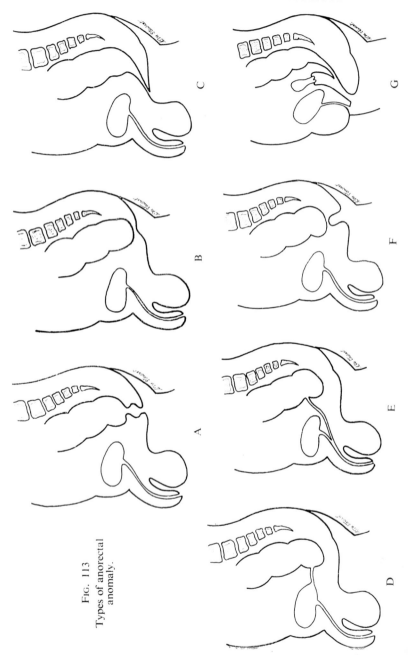

Fig. 113
Types of anorectal
anomaly.

Type II.—" Imperforate anus " with only a membranous obstruction (Fig. 113, B).

Type III.—*Rectoperineal fistula,* most commonly opening at the perineoscrotal angle (Fig. 113, C).

Type IV.—The rectal pouch ends some distance above the imperforate anus. This type is commonly associated with a fistula between the bowel and the genito-urinary tract (Fig. 113, D and E).

Type V.—The anus is apparently normal but the rectal pouch ends in the hollow of the sacrum separated by a variable distance from the anal pouch (Fig. 113, F).

Type VI.—*Rectovaginal fistula*—ectopic vaginal anus. The fistula may open anywhere along the posterior vaginal wall (Fig. 113, G), but most commonly opens into the fossa navicularis.

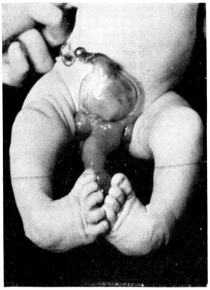

FIG. 114

Infant with imperforate anus and multiple developmental anomalies. The syndrome includes exomphalos, extroversion of the bladder, spina bifida and club feet. Ileum has intussuscepted through ileocæcal valve and has prolapsed through the transverse colon which opens on lower abdomen.

ASSOCIATED ANOMALIES.

There are other congenital anomalies in about one-third of the cases. Associated anomalies which may be directly responsible for death include hydrocephalus, œsophageal atresia, coarctation of the aorta, congenital heart disease, exomphalos, atresia of the small and large bowel, extroversion of the bladder and meningocele (Fig. 114).

CLINICAL FEATURES

Most of these patients suffer from intestinal obstruction from birth and are therefore usually seen in the first few days of life. They are brought to hospital, either because the doctor, nurse or parent observes that there is no anal opening, because the meconium comes from an abnormal orifice or on account of symptoms of acute intestinal obstruction. The abnormality may be overlooked for several days, particularly in the type with an apparently normal anus (Fig. 113, F).

Type I.—The complaint is difficulty in defæcation. The infant may pass ribbon-like stools—as though extruded from a toothpaste tube. If treatment is delayed the abdomen becomes distended but vomiting is a late feature. The stricture is felt on rectal examination.

Type II.—These patients are usually seen early because of the obvious abnormality. The napkin is not stained with meconium and the perineum may be seen to bulge when the infant cries or strains. After thirty-six hours the abdomen becomes distended and the other signs of obstruction develop.

Type III.—The absence of the anus is obvious but the perineal fistula may not be noticed. The fistula is usually too narrow to allow adequate evacuation of meconium. The passage of a probe may give information as to the position of the rectal pouch, and gentle dilatation of the fistula may allow postponement of the radical operation for twenty-four to forty-eight hours.

Type IV.—There is no bulging of the perineum on crying or straining. The presenting features are otherwise as in Type II. There is usually a dimple where the anus should be, and the skin is puckered when the sphincter contracts.

Type V.—The presence of a normal-looking anus will usually lead to delay in diagnosis. It is surprising how rarely the attending physician carries out a rectal examination. The condition is usually overlooked until the infant presents with signs of intestinal obstruction.

Type VI.—The fistulous opening in the vagina or fossa navicularis may be large enough to support life for a considerable time and the anomaly may not be noticed for weeks or even months. More commonly, stubborn constipation or even intestinal obstruction cause the patient to be brought to hospital early.

Recto-urinary Fistulæ.—A fistula connecting the rectum and bladder rarely manifests itself in the early period of life.

Presumably the fistula is plugged with inspissated meconium or by a flap of mucous membrane. The recto-urethral fistula is occasionally short and wide and fæces may be mixed with the urine at an early stage. Calculus formation may also follow.

RADIOGRAPHIC APPEARANCES

The infant is X-rayed in the head-down position with a metal marker fixed at the site of the anal dimple. The gas in the bowel rises and outlines the distal extent of the blind rectal

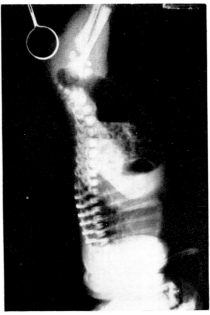

FIG. 115

Radiographic appearance in an infant aged 20 hours with imperforate anus. Inverted position allows gas to outline blind pouch. Metal marker indicates position of anal dimple.

pouch, indicating its position in relation to the anal membrane (Fig. 115). The infant is X-rayed in the anteroposterior and lateral positions and the information gained is of great value in deciding whether the perineal or abdominoperineal operation should be used. It is important to remember that the radiographic appearances may be misinterpreted in the first few hours of life. It may take fifteen to twenty hours for the gas to pass through the sticky meconium to the terminal gut, and only after this time do radiographic appearances provide an accurate picture of the position of the rectal pouch. It may be necessary to hold the infant in the inverted position for five to ten minutes to prevent a fallacious elongation of the distance between the blind segment and the perineum.

Rectovaginal and rectoperineal fistulæ can be outlined and the level of the rectal pouch determined by instilling viscous radio-opaque fluid into the tract.

As in other forms of intestinal obstruction in the newborn, barium by mouth is not used because of the danger of aspiration of barium that has been vomited.

TREATMENT

Type I—Anal or Rectal Stenosis.—On many occasions an infant with signs of acute intestinal obstruction has been cured by a simple rectal examination! (Neonatal Hirschsprung's disease may closely simulate stenosis in this respect, but here the " cure " is usually short-lived.) More commonly repeated dilatation with Hegar's dilators is necessary. The size of the dilators is gradually increased until the little finger can be inserted. It may be necessary to instruct the parent to continue digital dilatation for several months. Rarely some form of anoplasty may be necessary.

Type II — Membranous Obstruction.—This condition is treated by suitable incision followed by repeated dilatation.

Type III — Rectoperineal Fistula.—The fistulous tract is excised and the rectal pouch brought down and sutured to the skin as described in the perineal operation below. Dilatation of this type of fistula is rarely satisfactory and delay in operation may lead to stercoral ulceration and fatal peritonitis.

Type IV.—When the rectal pouch ends some distance above the imperforate anus, the operative approach depends on the position of the pouch as assessed by local and radiographic findings. If the pouch ends more than 2 cm. from the anal pit the final result following perineal operation alone is not likely to be satisfactory.

Perineal Operation.—A small rubber catheter is passed into the stomach and the infant anæsthetised. With the patient in the lithotomy position on a special table (Fig. 116), an antero-posterior incision is made in the midline of the perineum from the scrotum or vagina to the tip of the coccyx. The external anal sphincter is split and blunt dissection carried up through the levator ani keeping close to the hollow of the sacrum to avoid injury to the genito-urinary tract. When the pouch is identified it is freed widely. Traction sutures are inserted and

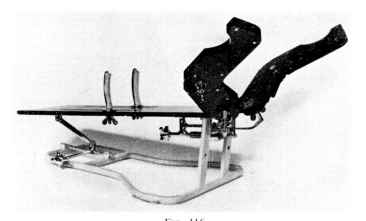

Fig. 116

Miniature operating table which is placed on top of operating table—used in perineal and abdominoperineal approach to anorectal anomalies.

the bowel pulled down so that it lies in the perineal wound without tension. The bowel is stitched to the levators (with silk sutures passed through the outer layer of the bowel in the four quadrants) and only then is the rectal pouch opened and the edges sutured to the skin with silk or fine catgut. Earlier opening of the bowel allows flooding of the operation field with meconium. Ten days after operation the stitches are removed and the anus gently dilated. Dilatation is repeated at increasing intervals, often for several months.

Treatment of associated vesical or urethral fistula by this route is difficult and may be impossible, and the combined abdominoperineal approach is preferable.

Abdominoperineal Operation.—A stomach tube is passed and the infant anæsthetised. An intravenous drip into the saphenous vein at the medial malleolus allows easy access for intravenous medication. A small urethral catheter is passed to localise the urethra and the abdomen is opened through a midline incision. The peritoneal cavity is opened and the grossly distended hind-gut full of green-black meconium is displayed and freed down into the pelvis. A urinary fistula, if present, is clamped and divided and a suprapubic cystostomy performed. With the infant in the lithotomy position a midline perineal incision is made as in the perineal approach already described and the freed rectum is seized and brought down. The abdomen is closed with a small drain in the space of Retzius for twenty-four hours. The bowel is fixed in position with fine silk stitches and then opened up. After operation the infant is nursed in an incubator for twenty-four hours. The de Pezzer catheter is left in the bladder for eight days. On the tenth day anal dilatation is commenced.

Type VI—Rectovaginal Fistula.—If the fistula is low down in the posterior vaginal wall or in the fossa navicularis (ectopic vaginal anus) repair should be carried out in the neonatal period by the perineal approach. The blind rectum is exposed through a midline perineal incision and the fistula displayed. The fistula is doubly ligated and divided and the operation concluded as described in the perineal operation.

Less commonly the fistula is high in the vagina and radical cure may be postponed until the parts are large enough to permit satisfactory dissection—about the age of 3 or 4 years. The fistula may be sufficiently large to permit defæcation or it may be dilated enough to allow defæcation. Excessive dilatation is not desirable as it enlarges an abnormal opening. Usually, silting of the colon makes colostomy necessary in the first year of life. Radical cure should be completed before the child goes to school.

CHAPTER XII

The Umbilicus

EXOMPHALOS (OMPHALOCELE)

IN this condition there is a herniation of abdominal viscera into the base of the umbilical cord. The covering is thin and translucent and consists of peritoneum and amniotic membrane.

Embryology.—Between the sixth and tenth weeks of fœtal life the alimentary tube grows so rapidly that the mid-gut

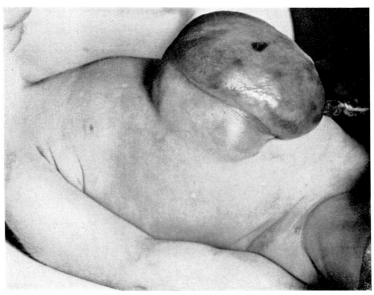

FIG. 117
Omphalocele.

herniates into the base of the umbilical cord. After the tenth week the abdomen enlarges at an accelerated pace and the mid-gut is withdrawn into it. If the development of the anterior abdominal wall is retarded the intestine or a portion of the liver may remain in the base of the umbilical cord.

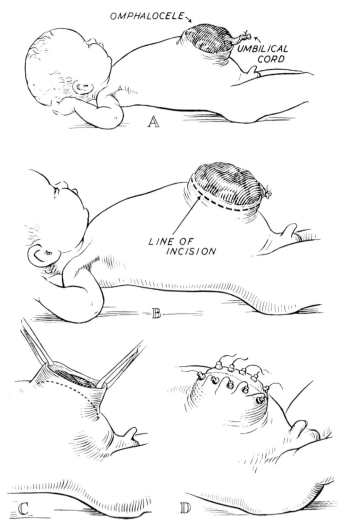

FIG. 118

Two-stage repair of large omphalocele. A, Omphalocele covered with transparent sac. B, Umbilical cord cut away : skin separated from sac. C, Skin freed and undermined from pubis, up on to chest and into both flanks, then pulled up over intact sac. D, Skin closed with interrupted double-stop sutures. At a second operation, six to twenty-four months later, the ventral hernia is repaired in layers.

Clinical Features.—Through the thin-walled sac the intestines, liver or other abdominal organs are exposed to view. The sac varies from a few centimetres in diameter to a swelling the size of a large grapefruit (Fig. 117). The umbilical cord arises from the apex of the sac. The defect in the abdominal wall varies from 2 to 8 cm. During the first day of life the sac wall is moist and pliable. After this it becomes dry, friable and more opaque, and may rupture and allow evisceration. Surgical

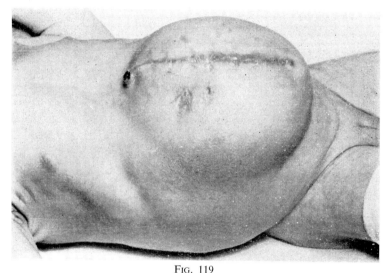

Fig. 119

Appearance of ventral hernia one month after first-stage operation for large omphalocele.

correction of the anomaly is therefore urgent. For the first twenty-four hours the baby suffers no pain and shows no evidence of obstruction or respiratory difficulty. There may be associated developmental anomalies.

Treatment.—Early operation is required to prevent rupture of the sac or spreading infection of the abdominal wall. If the exomphalos is small the sac is excised along with a narrow rim of adjacent skin, carefully ligating the two umbilical arteries and the umbilical vein. The muscle and fascial layers are freed and the abdomen closed in layers with fine silk. Large omphaloceles constitute a serious surgical problem. If the operation is carried out in one stage the diaphragm is displaced upwards with serious respiratory disturbance, the vena cava is compressed with circulatory collapse and pressure may lead to intestinal obstruction.   If the sac is more than 6 cm. in diameter operation should be performed in two stages (Fig. 118).   In the first stage the sac is thoroughly cleansed and the cord ligated at its base and divided.   A circular incision is made in the skin round the base of the sac and the skin freed well into both flanks and down to the pubis.   The skin is then pulled up over the intact sac and closed using double-stop sutures (Fig. 118).   This leaves the child with a large ventral hernia (Fig. 119).   The hernia is repaired in layers several months later.

UMBILICAL HERNIA

Umbilical hernia is common in infants and young children. It is due to a defect in the abdominal wall where it has been

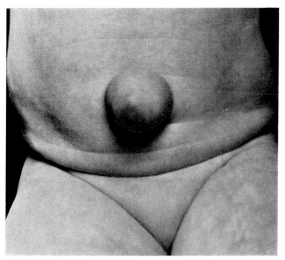

Fig. 120
Umbilical hernia.

pierced by the vessels of the umbilical cord.   The peritoneal sac is covered only with the subcutaneous tissue and skin of the umbilicus (Fig. 120).   The hernial ring has a firm edge and is usually confined to the peri-umbilical region, but there may be

divarication of the recti as far as the ensiform process.
Umbilical hernia is more common in girls than boys.

The hernia varies from a tiny protuberance to a bulge 3 cm.
in diameter which becomes larger and more tense when the
patient cries or strains. The sac may contain omentum or a

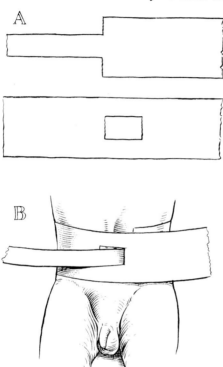

FIG. 121
Strapping for umbilical hernia.
A, Method of cutting adhesive tape.
B, Strapping applied.

knuckle of bowel. The hernia rarely disturbs the patient, but
the appearance is a constant source of worry to the parents.

Treatment.—Most umbilical herniæ are spontaneously cured
before the child goes to school. If the tip of the little finger can
be inserted through the fascial ring at the umbilicus when the
child is a year old surgical intervention may be required. If
the ring will not admit the finger tip at a year the sac will

probably be obliterated as the child grows. The practice of strapping a coin over the umbilicus probably interferes with the shrinkage of the hernial ring, although many herniæ are spontaneously obliterated in spite of this archaic method of treatment. During the first year proper strapping may expedite closure of the ring; it certainly helps to soothe anxious parents. Two pieces of 2-inch adhesive tape are cut as in Figure 121, A, one with a hole and one with a tongue. The straps are placed on either side of the abdomen and the tongue threaded through the hole and the free ends pulled tight, producing longitudinal wrinkles in the skin (Fig. 121, B).

Operative repair in the child should always retain the umbilical cicatrix. A small curved incision is made above the umbilicus, the sac is dissected free from the under surface of the navel and the peritoneum closed with fine silk. The sheaths are brought together in the midline and the skin wound closed with the normal umbilical appearance.

UMBILICAL DISCHARGE

Serious inflammation around the umbilicus (*omphalitis*) is now rare. Omphalitis in the newborn was once a serious condition and carried a grave risk of spreading cellulitis of the abdominal wall and even peritonitis. The umbilical arteries and vein may remain patent for the first few weeks of life and infection can reach the blood stream and give rise to septic foci anywhere in the body (*vide* " Sepsis in the Newborn ").

Discharge from the umbilicus in infants is frequently associated with granulation tissue which persists after the cord has fallen away. The granulations will disappear if treated with dusting powder. If the discharge persists one must look for some underlying cause. The persistence of remnants of the vitelline duct (sinus, cyst or fistula) has been discussed in Chapter XI. Urachal remnants may also lead to umbilical discharge.

Patent Urachus and Urachal Cyst.

The urachus is derived from the upper part of the allantois. The lumen is normally obliterated and a fibrous cord connects the apex of the bladder to the umbilicus. If the lumen of the urachus persists, the urinary bladder retains an opening at the umbilicus in post-natal life (Fig. 122). If only a segment of the tract remains, a cyst lined with transitional epithelium lies anterior to the peritoneum—a *urachal cyst*.

In *patent urachus* there is intermittent discharge of urine from the umbilicus. The condition must be differentiated from granulating umbilicus and vitello-intestinal fistula. Instillation of lipiodol will show whether the connection is with the intestine

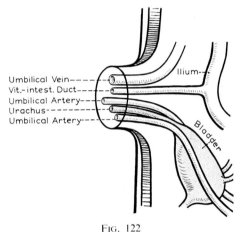

FIG. 122

Umbilical region showing embryological structures transmitted by umbilical cord.

or bladder. After ascertaining the presence of a normal urethra the fistula is excised through a midline incision below the umbilicus. The recti are separated and the tract peeled off from the peritoneum and ligated at the upper pole of the bladder.

A *urachal cyst* presents as a midline swelling below the umbilicus. If the cyst becomes infected it forms an abscess of the lower abdominal wall and may even simulate an appendix abscess. Before infection the cyst is easily excised. If an abscess forms it is incised and drained and the cyst removed at a later date.

CHAPTER XIII

Testis and Epididymis

Descent of the Testis.

The testis is developed from the germinal ridge, and in the embryo it lies on the inner side of the mesonephros (Wolffian

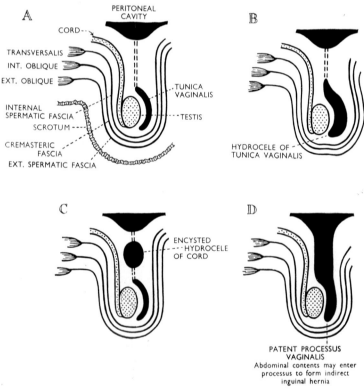

FIG. 123
Fate of processus vaginalis.

body) in front of the kidney in the lumbar region. Normal spermatogenesis cannot occur in the human testis retained in the abdominal cavity, and under hormonal control the testis should descend through the abdominal wall to its position in the cooler scrotum by the eighth month of intra-uterine life. From the lower pole of the testis a fibromuscular band (the *gubernaculum*) passes down to the subcutaneous tissues of the scrotal swelling. Additional strands extend to the root of the penis, to the saphenous opening, to the perineum or to a superficial inguinal position above and lateral to the external inguinal ring. In its descent the testis is accompanied by the degenerating mesonephros and its duct which form the epididymis and vas deferens. In front of the testis the peritoneum herniates as the *processus vaginalis*, passing through the muscle layers of the abdominal wall. The lower portion of the processus vaginalis persists as the *tunica vaginalis* testis. The upper part is normally obliterated shortly after birth, but may persist in varying degrees (Fig. 123), giving rise to hernia or hydrocele (Chap. XIV).

The testis may be retained within the abdomen, it may remain within the inguinal canal or it may lie at the external inguinal ring—*cryptorchidism* or *undescended testis*.

On the other hand the testis may descend but instead of passing into the scrotum it comes to occupy an abnormal position—usually superficial to the inguinal canal—*ectopic* or *misplaced testis*.

UNDESCENDED TESTIS

The cause of defective descent of the testis is unknown. Undescended testes are always small and it is probable that the imperfect development of the testis interferes with descent, and not that the imperfect descent interferes with development. (Ectopic testes are usually well developed.)

Unless the testis is retained within the abdomen a hernial sac is usually present. The scrotum is imperfectly developed because it has never been opened up by the processus vaginalis or by the testis. The term cryptorchidism should only be applied when the testis lies in the canal or is retained within the abdomen and cannot be palpated.

CLINICAL FEATURES

Undescended testis must be distinguished from *retractile testis*. In the young the strong cremasteric reflex can draw the testis into the upper scrotum or into the superficial inguinal pouch. This retraction is particularly marked if the child is examined in a cold room or with a cold hand. By gentle traction the retractile testis can be brought partially or completely into the scrotum. The condition is not pathological and the parents can be reassured that descent will eventually occur spontaneously. These patients constitute about 80 per cent. of the cases of " undescended testis " sent for surgical opinion. An undescended testis cannot be palpated while it remains in the inguinal canal. It may be " milked " out at the external inguinal ring, but it cannot be pushed over the pubic brim into the scrotum or laterally into the superficial inguinal pouch as the spermatic cord is too short. The scrotum on the affected side is small. The condition is commonly right-sided and is bilateral in less than a quarter of those affected. The diagnosis may be difficult in cases of early male obesity where there is excessive fat and tiny gonads. It is important that the testes should be in the scrotum before puberty—if possible before the twelfth birthday. If the diagnosis of retractile testis cannot be made confidently from bilateral cryptorchidism, particularly in a fat boy, the advice of an endocrinologist should be sought before the child reaches puberty.

COMPLICATIONS

The mal-descended testis is more exposed to trauma and torsion is not uncommon ; chronic discomfort may interfere with the playing of games. An abdominal or inguinal testis has diminished spermatogenic activity. The undescended testis is frequently associated with indirect inguinal hernia. There is statistical evidence that malignant change is more common in the undescended or ectopic testis.

Fertility.

    (a) *Bilateral Cryptorchidism.*—Abdominal or inguinal testes do not produce spermatozoa, and if the defect persists after puberty the patient is irrevocably sterile.

(*b*) *Unilateral Cryptorchidism.*—Fertility is identical in treated and untreated cases and unilateral retention of the testis does not in itself call for any treatment.

The frequency of testicular atrophy is high after surgical intervention, and this must be borne in mind when considering the future of a cryptorchid from the point of view of fertility.

TREATMENT

Spontaneous Descent.—Eight out of ten cases diagnosed in childhood as suffering from undescended testis have merely delayed but normal development. The remaining 20 per cent. suffer from either cryptorchidism or ectopia. Although the testes should be in the scrotum at birth the descent process may be delayed and continue during childhood years.

Hormone Treatment.—The mechanism of descent which is accelerated by androgenic or chorionic gonadotrophic hormones is poorly understood. Stimulation of the endocrine system has harmful potentialities and may result in glandular imbalance.

Hormone therapy should be used only in bilateral cryptorchidism in the boy who is fat and who has underdeveloped genitalia (Frölich adiposogenital syndrome). *Pregnyl* (chorionic gonadotrophic hormone) is injected in a dose of 500 units at weekly intervals for six weeks. The patient is examined before each injection for evidence of hypertrophy of the phallus or painful enlargement of the testes. If one testis is normally descended there is no point in endocrine therapy and operation will probably be required.

Orchidopexy.—The optimal age for therapeutic placement of the testis in the scrotum is between the ninth and twelfth years. If an associated hernia is troublesome herniorrhaphy may be required earlier and orchidopexy should be attempted at the same time. It may not be possible to replace the testis in the scrotum without tension on the spermatic vessels, and it is essential that the parents are interviewed before the operation and are warned that it may be necessary to sacrifice the testis.

Operation.—The inguinal canal is opened, the testis freed and a hernial sac if present is dissected up to the neck, transfixed and the excess removed. The testis and cord are freed by sharp and blunt dissection and the freeing of the testicular vessels is continued upwards behind the peritoneum until the testis can be placed in the scrotum without tension. An adequate bed for the testis is made by stretching the under-developed scrotum with two fingers passed through the inguinal wound. If the testis cannot be placed in its bed at this stage no trans-septal orchidopexy or Keetly-Torek procedure (in which the testis is brought through the base of the scrotum and embedded in the thigh) will fix it there without inducing testicular atrophy. Even if the cord is freed sufficiently to allow replacement without tension, an unattached testis tends to retract to a high position where it will become adherent. The operation is therefore concluded by passing a stitch through the gubernaculum and tying it over gauze on the outer aspect of the scrotum. An alternative method is to pass the testis through two slits in the pubic fascia (Browne's modification of Bevan's operation). This strap ensures retention of the testis in the scrotum. The tunica albuginea is incised to diminish the consequences of reactionary œdema of the testis. If the vas and vessels are too short to allow the testis to be placed in the scrotum without tension, the testis is brought down as far as possible and allowed to remain there for a year or more. Complete mobilisation is again carried out, and it may be possible to place the testis in the scrotum without tension by this two-stage procedure.

Results

Judged by size, consistency and final position of the testis, the results are satisfactory in about 70 per cent. of cases in which the testis has been placed in the scrotum. Unfortunately replacement is possible in only about half the patients who come to operation. In the others the testis is small and atrophic, or sufficient lengthening of the cord cannot be obtained and orchidectomy or a two-stage operation is performed.

The results with regard to sexual recovery are difficult to assess. In unilateral cryptorchidism treated by orchidopexy, fertility is normal or only slightly reduced. Unfortunately our own figures can offer no *proof* of fertility following orchidopexy in a bilateral cryptorchid. Undoubtedly a man with bilateral *ectopia* can father children after orchidopexy, and it is possible that claims of successful function following orchidopexy apply to ectopia and not to true cryptorchidism. On the other hand, some of the " undescended " testes which have been successfully brought down before puberty might have descended spontaneously if the surgeon had dared to wait a little longer.

ECTOPIA TESTIS

In this condition the testis descends but instead of passing into the scrotum it comes to lie in some adjacent region (Fig. 124), most commonly superficial to the external oblique fascia in the inguinal region. It is difficult or impossible to palpate an undescended testis lying in the inguinal canal, and a testis in the region of the canal that is easily palpated is usually

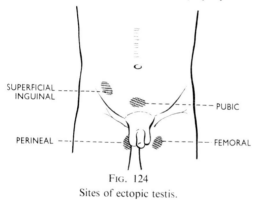

SUPERFICIAL INGUINAL

PERINEAL

PUBIC

FEMORAL

FIG. 124
Sites of ectopic testis.

ectopic (Fig. 125). By gently but firmly pressing the testis laterally along the line of the inguinal canal the undescended organ will disappear into the abdomen while an inguinal ectopic testis will become more prominent. The ectopic testis cannot be made to enter the scrotum. Less commonly an ectopic testis is found in the perineum, at the root of the penis or at the saphenous opening. As with incompletely descended organs the testis and epididymis may be atrophic and are sometimes completely separate. A hernial sac may accompany the testis.

TREATMENT

The only treatment of an ectopic testis is surgical. Not only is hormonal treatment futile, but it may cause degenerative changes in the mechanically retained testis.   Spontaneous descent will never occur.

In the occasional patient with perineal ectopia, operation is performed at an early age to prevent discomfort or even serious damage to the misplaced organ.   Where the ectopic testis is in

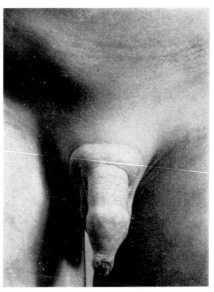

Fig. 125
Right inguinal ectopic testis.

the inguinal region operation may be performed at any age, but unless there is local pain or discomfort or the associated hernia is giving trouble, surgical treatment is not carried out until the child is 9 or 10 years old.   Through an inguinal incision the testis is freed from its abnormal position and placed within the scrotum.   The cord is usually long enough to allow replacement without extensive dissection.   If a hernia is present radical repair is carried out at the same time.

TORSION OF THE SPERMATIC CORD
(TORSION OF THE TESTIS)

Torsion of the testis is a misnomer ; it is the spermatic cord that undergoes torsion.   The condition is less frequent in infancy and childhood than in adult life. Imperfect descent of the testis is a predisposing cause; the testis is unduly mobile and it may be suspended from the epididymis by a mesentery-like attachment. In childhood, torsion may occur in the fully descended organ due to a sharp blow or to some sudden movement as in swimming.

CLINICAL FEATURES

There is sudden severe local pain and tenderness. The testis becomes swollen and hard and œdema may extend up the cord. A hydrocele develops in the tunica vaginalis. If mechanical relief is delayed, necrosis of the testis and epididymis supervenes and the scrotum becomes discoloured and œdematous.

Differential Diagnosis.—This may be difficult and torsion may be confused with incarcerated hernia or with acute orchitis. The diagnosis is frequently made only at operation.

TREATMENT

The treatment is immediate operation. A delay of a few hours may lead to irreparable infarction. In the adult it may be possible to reduce the torsion by manipulation through the scrotum, but this procedure is very rarely successful in childhood. Spontaneous reduction of the twist may occur, and certain cases diagnosed as orchitis in infants are probably examples of partial torsion.

At operation the cord is exposed and the testis dislocated from the scrotum. Reduction of the torsion may permit a return of circulation if the injury is of short duration. In most cases necrosis has already occurred and the testis must be removed.

TORSION OF THE APPENDIX TESTIS

The appendix testis or hydatid of Morgagni on the superior aspect of the testis occasionally becomes twisted on its pedicle and the resulting symptoms are similar to those of torsion of the spermatic cord. The condition occurs most commonly between 5 and 15 years of age.

Treatment.—At operation œdema and vascular engorgement

without an obvious twist of the cord should arouse suspicion. The tunica vaginalis is opened, the twisted pedicle ligated and the appendix testis removed. If the tunica is not opened in all cases of torsion, testes may be removed unnecessarily.

DISEASES OF THE TESTIS AND EPIDIDYMIS

Acute Orchitis and Epididymitis.

Infection of the testis and epididymis is rare before puberty and nowadays even tuberculosis of the epididymis is seldom seen in a children's hospital. Acute orchitis arises during mumps, but this is rare before the age of 12. Orchitis may appear during the course of many bacterial infections such as osteitis or diffuse peritonitis. Swelling and œdema after torsion or trauma may closely simulate orchitis.

Treatment.—Having excluded torsion, treatment consists of bed rest, elevation of the scrotum and antibiotic treatment of any associated systemic infection.

Tuberculous Epididymitis.

Hæmatogenous infection of the epididymis occurs occasionally in infants and young children who have a primary focus of tuberculosis elsewhere. The disease may extend from the epididymis into the body of the testis and may be first noticed when the testis and epididymis form a tumour mass. The scrotal wall may become involved in a cold abscess. The vas deferens is usually thickened and nodular.

Spontaneous healing may occur, and conservative treatment should be adopted in most cases. Streptomycin, P.A.S. and isoniazid are given.

Tumours of the Testis.

Benign tumours of the testis are practically unknown in children, although a teratoma may occasionally remain benign. There are numerous varieties of testicular neoplasm, and the nomenclature is simplified for the convenience of the surgeon and radiotherapist if two groups are distinguished.

1. TERATOMA.—The tumour may be found at birth and varies greatly in size. There may be a long history and the tumour

progresses slowly by direct extension and metastasises late. Microscopically teratomata show their tridermal origin and there may be cartilage, bone, muscle, lung tissue, hair, nerve or even a typical carcinoma.

2. SEMINOMA.—These tumours are highly malignant in childhood and are composed of large round or polyhedral cells of embryonic type.

Metastases.—Malignant testicular tumours metastasise widely, spreading first to the iliac and lower lumbar glands. Invasion of the vessels allows metastases to liver, brain, lungs and bone.

Clinical Features.—Pain does not appear until late, and the earliest sign is the difference in size of the two testes. A small nodule may be followed in a short time by a large metastatic abdominal mass. An overlying hydrocele may make early diagnosis difficult.

Prognosis.—The prognosis is always bad. The mortality of simple castration is negligible, but with this treatment alone 95 per cent. of cases end fatally within five years.

TREATMENT.—Unless there are demonstrable metastases in the abdomen or lungs, immediate orchidectomy is the treatment of choice. The cord is severed as high as possible before mobilising the tumour. A course of deep X-ray therapy follows operation.

CHAPTER XIV

Hernia and Hydrocele

INGUINAL HERNIA

INGUINAL hernia in childhood is almost invariably of the indirect type and represents a persistence of the processus vaginalis described in the paragraph on descent of the testicle in Chapter XIII (Fig. 123, D). In the female the peritoneal pocket develops in a similar manner and, descending with the round ligament, forms the canal of Nuck; it may persist into post-natal life. The right testis descends at a later date than does the left, and accordingly the processus vaginalis is closed off later on the right side. This probably accounts for the greater frequency of congenital inguinal hernia on the right side. Inguinal hernia is rare in the young female and constitutes about 5 per cent. of inguinal herniæ in infancy and childhood.

Percentage Distribution of Inguinal Hernia in Childhood

Right-sided	.	.	. 60 per cent.
Left-sided	.	.	. 20 per cent.
Double .	.	.	. 20 per cent.

Surgical Anatomy.—An indirect inguinal hernia traverses the inguinal canal and appears on the surface through the external inguinal ring. It is invested by the coverings of the spermatic cord (Fig. 123):—

1. External spermatic fascia from the external oblique.
2. Cremasteric fascia from the internal oblique.
3. Internal spermatic fascia from the fascia transversalis.

The sac lies in the middle of the cord surrounded by these coverings. The pampiniform plexus of veins is on its antero-lateral aspect and the vas deferens and its artery lie on the postero-medial surface. The individual coverings are fairly easily distinguished. The cremasteric layer usually has well-developed muscular fibres. The internal spermatic fascia is often extremely thin and not easily recognised by the in-experienced operator.

CLINICAL FEATURES

A hernia may be discovered at or shortly after birth, and very large scrotal herniæ may appear during the first few weeks of life. Most commonly the hernia is first noticed during the second or third month and may follow a period of crying or straining. The hernia usually disappears spontaneously when the child ceases to cry or strain. If this does not occur it can

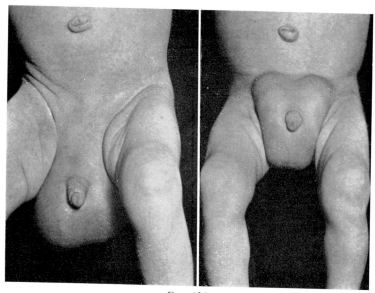

FIG. 126

On reader's left—bilateral hydrocele; on right—bilateral inguinal hernia.

usually be reduced with ease. The hernia may be small and appear at the internal ring, or it may be elongated and extend through the entire canal. Less frequently the mass may fill the scrotum on the affected side (Fig. 126). In a progressive case the hernia gradually increases in size, the walls of the sac stretch, and more and more viscera enter it. Many small herniæ appear to regress during childhood, though they may reappear in adult life. Most children are little disturbed by the presence of the hernia, but the swelling is often blamed for fretfulness, loss of appetite and failure to gain weight. In some cases there are bladder symptoms such as frequency of micturition or incontinence. Usually the hernia distresses the parents more than the child.

The examination of a child for inguinal hernia is quite different from that employed in the adult. As in all examinations of children one must first attempt to gain the confidence and co-operation of the patient. Before the child is touched the parts are inspected and the appearance and disappearance of the swelling during coughing or straining may be all that is required to make the diagnosis. If the child wishes to stand he should be allowed to do so as the erect position may induce the hernia to bulge. If a mass is present gentle pressure is exerted on it from below upwards to see if it can be reduced. The testes are then palpated to see if these organs are fully descended and in their proper position. If a hydrocele is present its relationship to the testis and cord is defined. In infancy both hernia and hydrocele can be transilluminated.

There may be a good history of a recurrent swelling, but often no inguinal swelling is found during the examination. The middle finger is placed on the spermatic cord and by rolling the cord from side to side one can, with practice, estimate the thickness of the structures within the canal. If the hernia is unilateral the cord will be found to be slightly thicker on the affected side even although the hernial sac is empty. If the cord is picked up gently between the finger and thumb and the constituent parts allowed to slip through the examining fingers a similar comparison between the two sides can be made. With practice the examiner learns to recognise the abnormal thickness of the cord. This is important in bilateral hernia where there is no normal cord for comparison. Invagination of the scrotum and palpation of the external ring rarely give any helpful information, and no attempt should be made to introduce a finger into the canal.

Incarcerated Hernia.

Although strangulation of the contents of an inguinal hernia is rare in childhood, incarceration is not uncommon and occurs in approximately 5 per cent. In a third of these cases the hernia has not been recognised prior to the time of incarceration and the incarceration occurs in a small sac through a narrow external ring. The local swelling is usually painful and the infant or child may show evidence of great discomfort or even agony. Even if intestine is present in the sac there may be no signs of obstruction, but *reflex vomiting* is not uncommon. Incarceration is most common in the first six months of life and is relatively rare in older children.

THE DIAGNOSIS OF INGUINAL HERNIA IN THE MALE

There is rarely much difficulty in making the diagnosis; a reducible swelling which passes from above downwards and makes its appearance through the external inguinal ring is unlikely to be anything other than a hernia. The chief difficulty arises in those cases in which the contents are not present in the sac at the time of the examination. Attention must be paid to the history, but too much importance should not be attributed to it. In the lay mind any swelling in the inguinal regions ranks as a " rupture." Thickening of the cord suggests the presence of a hernial sac, and if comparison is possible with a normal cord on the opposite side the observation is particularly valuable.

Certain conditions may sometimes be mistaken for inguinal hernia.

1. **Hydrocele of the Tunica Vaginalis.**—Usually there is little difficulty in differentiating a hydrocele from a hernia (Fig. 126), but occasionally there may be certain difficulties. Hernia and hydrocele may co-exist. A hernia with a narrow neck may be very difficult to reduce and may contain fluid and can be mistaken for a hydrocele. Intermittent hydrocele is not common, but in this condition, although the patency of the processus vaginalis is too small to permit of herniation, fluid may pass from the abdominal cavity into the tunica vaginalis. Although a thickening of the cord is demonstrable, its girth is never increased by the presence of contents passing into it from above.

2. **Encysted Hydrocele of the Cord.**—There is a localised swelling of the spermatic cord, incorporated with the cord and irreducible. This condition is frequently mistaken for an incarcerated hernia although there are none of the symptoms which are associated with an irreducible hernia. It is usually

possible to palpate a normal cord above the upper limit of the swelling. Occasionally the hydrocele extends upwards through the external ring and the differential diagnosis can be very difficult. An encysted hydrocele of the cord is movable both in the long axis and across the cord, fluctuation may be detected, and the swelling shows no expansile impulse on coughing.

3. **Undescended Testis.**—An undescended or ectopic testis may be mistaken for a hernia and is not uncommonly complicated by the presence of a hernia. The swelling of a simple hernia is elastic and painless on pressure, while that of an undescended or ectopic testis is firm and tender.

TREATMENT

Spontaneous Cure.—Obliteration of the processus vaginalis should be completed in late fœtal life, but occasionally obliteration continues into the first few months of post-natal existence. Natural closure after birth is rare and at operation one can often demonstrate that an attempt at natural closure has proceeded up to a certain point. There is an area of thickened tissue which surrounds the sac as a dense white ring.

Parents often inquire about the possibility of a spontaneous cure. It should be made clear to them that natural closure of the sac is only likely during the first three months of life, that such closure is rare, and that although the condition may appear to be cured the sac may reopen in later life. When the hernia is detected at birth, natural closure may be encouraged by avoiding constipation, crying, coughing or any condition which may increase intra-abdominal pressure and thereby open up the sac. In some centres a truss of wool is applied with the object of giving light pressure over the inguinal region. The essential aim of these measures is to keep the sac collapsed so that its walls can coalesce. If a hernia is still present after three months natural cure will not occur.

Conservative Treatment.—Conservative treatment is advisable in the first three months of life and in feeble and diminutive infants. In the first year of life the cord and hernial sac are delicate and the dissection requires some degree of skill and patience. There is no place for the injection treatment of herniæ in childhood. It is difficult to inject sclerosing fluid without extensive and possibly permanent injury to the delicate spermatic vessels and vas deferens.

Operative Treatment.—The operative treatment of hernia in infants and children is safe, can be performed at any time and the results are highly satisfactory. Operation should be carried out any time after the infant has passed the age of 3 months. The operative procedure differs from that which is carried out in adults. In infants and children a preformed sac is the cause of the hernia and there is no weakness in the musculature of the inguinal canal. The length of the canal is so short that it is possible to bring the internal ring into view and thus perform a radical cure without opening the inguinal canal (Mitchell-Banks operation). In the hands of experienced pædiatric surgeons this operation has given excellent results over many years. It is not an operation for the beginner, who can readily lose his way in the depths of a small incision. In the United States most surgeons use a modification of the Ferguson operation which entails splitting the aponeurosis of the external oblique from the external to the internal ring. Some British surgeons consider that the external abdominal ring should not be divided (Chiene) and perform the operation through an incision in the line of the inguinal canal just above the external ring. The same operations are performed in the female in whom the external ring can be closed tightly around the round ligament.

Post-operative Care.—The healing process is rapid and in the first year of life the patients remain in hospital only for a few hours. Older children remain in hospital for one or two days; they are then allowed to go home, where they are encouraged to stay in bed for a week.

Results of Treatment.—The operation for repair of inguinal hernia in infancy and childhood is one of the most satisfactory in surgery. There should be no operative mortality, and if the sac is properly isolated and secured recurrence is practically unknown.

TREATMENT OF INCARCERATED INGUINAL HERNIA

Although strangulation of an inguinal hernia is rare irreducibility is common, particularly in the first six months of life. It occurs in two varieties of hernia : (1) the small hernia which is appearing through a narrow external ring in a young infant; (2) the large old-standing hernia with a considerable quantity of omentum or intestine in an extensive sac.

Conservative Measures.—An incarcerated hernia in the child should always have a sufficient trial of conservative therapy before operative procedures are adopted. If light pressure will not reduce the mass no forceful efforts should be made to accomplish reduction. Attempts at reduction in a crying and struggling child are useless and may damage the contents of the sac.

The infant should be given an adequate dose of syrup of chloral (in the older child opoidine or some such morphine derivative is used) to abolish pain, to induce sleep and to relax the abdominal wall. The patient is then placed on his back with the foot of the cot or bed elevated to an angle of about 20 degrees to the horizontal, or a pillow is placed under the buttocks. When this position has been maintained for an hour or two the intestines usually return spontaneously to the abdomen or will do so when the mass is gently pressed by the fingers. Almost 90 per cent. of incarcerated herniæ in infancy are reduced by conservative measures.

Conservative treatment should not be continued for longer than three or four hours because of the danger of strangulation of the incarcerated bowel, but one must remember that surgical reduction may be a difficult procedure in infants and young children. The landmarks are obscured by œdema, and even when the hernia has been reduced satisfactorily, repair of the thin, friable and œdematous sac may be difficult or almost impossible. When the patient is anæsthetised and before the incision is made, a last gentle attempt at reduction is made. If this is successful the child is returned to bed. After conservative reduction it is better to wait for two or three days until the œdema subsides before proceeding with operative repair.

Operation.—Under general anæsthesia and with a tube in the stomach, an oblique incision is made exposing the œdematous coverings of the sac. The external ring is incised and external oblique fascia is slit upwards and outwards. The constricting ring may be difficult to identify; it may be the external ring or the constriction may be a fibrous ring in the sac wall itself. After opening the sac and evacuating some fluid (often blood-stained) the ring is stretched or divided from within the sac lumen. The intestine must not be allowed to slip back into the abdominal cavity until it has been examined and the operator is satisfied as to its viability.

Fortunately strangulation is rare, and in infancy bowel that the inexperienced operator may consider to be of doubtful viability has remarkable powers of recovery when replaced in the peritoneal cavity.

INGUINAL HERNIA IN THE FEMALE

Inguinal hernia is relatively uncommon in the female child. The ovary is an intra-abdominal organ and the processus is poorly developed and seldom descends along the canal of Nuck with the round ligament. When a hernial sac is present it is pear-shaped and seldom attains any great size. The ovary is commonly present in the sac. Incarceration is rare.

The differential diagnosis is from hydrocele of the canal of Nuck, femoral hernia and enlargement of the inguinal glands.

As in the male, treatment is by operation and the principles are as already described. At the neck of the sac the branch of the uterine artery which accompanies the round ligament may be injured and the ensuing hæmorrhage may be difficult to control.

FEMORAL HERNIA

Femoral hernia is rare in childhood and we have never seen the condition in a male child. The anatomy is the same as in the adult and the sac usually contains omentum.

Clinical Features.—In a thin child the swelling is easily palpated and the neck of the sac lies below and to the outer side of the spine of the pubis. Pain is a common feature of femoral hernia in childhood and the condition may cause the child to limp. The differential diagnosis is from enlarged inguinal glands.

Treatment.—The sac is best approached by an inguinal incision and the sac dislocated from the thigh into the wound. After ascertaining that the sac is empty the neck is ligated flush

with the peritoneum and the excess sac cut away. It is unnecessary to close the medial part of the femoral ring.

HYDROCELE

The development of the *processus vaginalis* has already been
described (p. 221), and the degrees of persistence are illustrated
in Figure 123. Accumulation of fluid within any portion of this
tract constitutes a hydrocele. Most commonly the fluid
accumulates within the tunica vaginalis—*hydrocele of the tunica
vaginalis*. If the upper part of the processus persists and is
closed off from the peritoneum and from the tunica vaginalis,
accumulation of fluid in this space constitutes an *encysted
hydrocele of the cord* (or in the female a hydrocele of the canal
of Nuck).

Clinical Features.

Hydroceles are common in infants and young children. They
are rounded or oval, cystic and rather soft and give rise to few
symptoms other than mild local discomfort. They are commonly
found around the testis; less frequently they appear along the
spermatic cord or in the canal of Nuck. Hydroceles of the
tunica vaginalis can distend the scrotum on the affected side
(Fig. 126), while hydroceles of the spermatic cord or of the canal
of Nuck are rarely more than 1 cm. in diameter and 2 cm. long.

A *hydrocele of the cord* or of the canal of Nuck may be
confused with an incarcerated inguinal hernia. Although
irreducible it is mobile in all directions, is usually painless and
is known to have been present for a considerable period of time.
These lesions seldom transmit light as they are covered by the
external oblique fascia.

Hydrocele of the tunica vaginalis seldom causes any difficulty
in diagnosis. It is a soft non-tender mass enveloping the testis
anteriorly. The upper pole can be palpated at or just below the
external ring. The testis may be faintly outlined by trans-
illumination. The hydrocele is occasionally accompanied by an
indirect inguinal hernia although this diagnosis may not be
confirmed until operation is performed.

A secondary hydrocele of the tunica vaginalis may arise in
association with disease of the testis or epididymis.

Treatment.

A hydrocele of the tunica vaginalis rarely requires operation in the first year of life. Many disappear spontaneously and treatment is only undertaken in infants if the mass is large enough to cause discomfort. Should the hydrocele persist after the first year, treatment will probably be required as the condition seldom regresses spontaneously after this time.

Hydrocele of the spermatic cord or of the canal of Nuck usually disappears spontaneously in the first few months of life, but those that appear after the first year usually persist and require surgical removal.

A hydrocele in a child should never be aspirated. Recurrence invariably takes place and in hydrocele of the cord the spermatic vein may be punctured with formation of a hæmatoma. The injection of sclerosing fluids is dangerous and may lead to increase in size of the hydrocele and damage to the testis or spermatic cord. It is wiser to expose the swelling and to remove the sac by dissection.

HÆMATOCELE

Hæmatocele may result from crushing injury to the testis or may follow operation for hernia or hydrocele where hæmostasis has been imperfect. Absorption of blood from the tunica vaginalis usually occurs more rapidly and certainly in childhood than in adult life. Occasionally it is advisable to evacuate the blood clot to expedite recovery.

CHAPTER XV

Liver and Spleen

LIVER AND BILIARY PASSAGES

Jaundice in Infancy.

Jaundice in the early months of life may arise from several causes. Physiological jaundice has always disappeared by the end of the first month. There is no bile in the urine and the stools are pigmented. *Jaundice due to sepsis* is associated with staphylococcal or streptococcal septicæmia. There is a profound toxæmia, fever, leucocytosis and a positive blood culture. This type of jaundice may be seen in neonatal osteitis. *Erythroblastosis fœtalis* (icterus gravis) may present a picture resembling biliary obstruction. The jaundice may be intense and the liver and spleen enlarged. The jaundice is due to rapid breakdown of Rhesus-positive red cells by antibodies transferred from the Rhesus-negative mother. Plugging of the bile ducts by pigment debris ensues. The jaundice may be mild and self-limited, but if the plasma bilirubin level remains high the baby is treated by *exchange transfusion*. *Hepatitis* is not uncommon in young babies. The ætiology is obscure but it is presumed to be a transmitted virus infection. *Obstructive jaundice* may arise from *obstruction of the biliary passages from inspissated mucus or bile*. The stools are pale and urine deeply pigmented. The jaundice may change in intensity from time to time, and this change may be the only means of differentiating the condition from atresia of the bile ducts. In **congenital atresia of the bile ducts** the block may be in the liver or in the hepatic or common bile duct. Jaundice is present at or soon after birth and is persistent and progressive. The stools are pale from birth and the urine contains bile pigments. The abdomen is distended by enlargement of the liver and later by ascitic fluid. In a few patients it may be possible to alleviate the condition by surgery. The ducts may only be blocked by inspissated material and can be cleared by saline irrigation through the gall-bladder. Where there is true atresia of the common duct it may be alleviated by anastomosing the gall-bladder or the common duct to the duodenum. Few patients survive.

Idiopathic Dilatation of the Common Bile Duct.—*Choledochal cysts* are rare in childhood. They present with intermittent *abdominal swelling, pain and jaundice*, and the diagnosis is rarely made before operation. Treatment is surgical and consists in anastomosing either the gall-bladder or the cyst itself to the duodenum.

Cholecystitis.—Cholecystitis is uncommon in childhood and rarely presents as an acute emergency. In adults acute chole-cystitis is usually associated with calculus, but in childhood it is a bacterial inflammation unaccompanied by stones and may resolve without surgical intervention.

Cholelithiasis is rather more common and presents with recurrent upper abdominal pain, nausea and vomiting. It may be associated with congenital hæmolytic anæmia. There may be jaundice from duct obstruction. The diagnosis is confirmed by radiography. At operation the ducts are explored and calculi removed. If the gall-bladder is thickened it is removed ; if the wall is not thickened cholecystostomy is performed. If there is a hæmolytic anæmia splenectomy is performed later.

Acute Distension of the Gall-bladder presents with upper abdominal pain and nausea or vomiting not associated with jaundice. It is probably due to blockage of the cystic duct by an enlarged cystic lymph node—part of a non-specific mesenteric adenitis. The pre-operative diagnosis is usually appendicitis or intussusception. The symptoms are relieved by simple aspiration of the gall-bladder.

Rupture of the Gall-bladder is rare except in association with severe abdominal injuries. It may, however, be caused by a direct blow over the right hypochondrium. The extravasation of sterile bile into the peritoneal cavity causes remarkably little discomfort or pain and there may be considerable delay before the diagnosis is made. Treatment is by cholecystostomy or, if the laceration is extensive, by cholecystectomy.

Hepatic Tumours.

Neoplasms of the liver are rare. Primary liver-cell *carcinoma* is the most common malignant tumour. It grows rapidly and metastasises widely. *Hæmangiomata* usually do not give rise to symptoms and are found accidentally at operation or autopsy. If large there may be a palpable mass and the tumour may rupture and cause intraperitoneal hæmorrhage. Multiple hæmangiomata are treated by deep X-ray therapy. *Hamartomata* are rare, but surgical removal is possible and the prognosis is good.

THE SPLEEN

There are many pathological states of the spleen related to abnormalities of the blood and circulation, and some of these disorders can be cured or alleviated by surgical measures.

Congenital Hæmolytic Anæmia (Acholuric Jaundice).

This condition is characterised by chronic or recurring anæmia, hæmolytic crises and by characteristic abnormalities in the blood picture. The anæmia may be discovered at any age. It is typical of the disease to have periods of exacerbation and remission. The *hæmolytic crisis* is associated with fever, abdominal pain, pallor and jaundice, but a mild degree of jaundice may be present most of the time. The crisis may be so severe that blood transfusion is required. The spleen is enlarged and there may be retardation of growth. There is a familial incidence in about 70 per cent. of cases. The erythrocytes tend to be globular—so-called *spherocytosis*. *Reticulocytes* appear in the peripheral blood and counts of 20 or 30 per cent. are common, due to hæmolysis of red cells. Normal red cells begin to hæmolyse in a solution of about 0·45 per cent. sodium chloride and hæmolysis is complete in concentrations of about 0·20 per cent. In congenital hæmolytic anæmia the cells begin to disintegrate in much higher concentrations and hæmolysis is usually complete in concentrations of 0·40 per cent. *Urobilinogen* is excreted in the urine and stools in many times the normal amount. Increased excretion of blood pigments may lead to development of *gall-stones*.

Treatment.—Splenectomy is specific and gives rapid and permanent relief. Although the erythrocytes retain their increased fragility, abnormal destruction of red cells ceases.

Acquired Hæmolytic Anæmia.

This disease is rare before adolescence. The results of splenectomy are disappointing.

Idiopathic Thrombocytopenic Purpura.

In this disease there is a bleeding tendency due to a diminished number of circulating platelets. The platelet count is decreased from the normal 200,000 per c.mm. usually down to 75,000, occasionally down to zero. Clotting time is normal, but bleeding tends to be prolonged and clot retraction is delayed and poor. The disease may appear at any age but is most common between 3 and 7 years. There is spontaneous oozing from mucous membranes, and ecchymoses are induced by the slightest trauma. In the *tourniquet test* the application of a sphygmomanometer band or a tourniquet around the arm produces petechial hæmorrhages within a matter of minutes. The spleen may be enlarged.

Treatment.—There may be spontaneous remissions and the patient should first be treated with rest, sedation and, if necessary, transfusion of fresh blood. If the symptoms are severe and have recurred over a long period *splenectomy* is curative in a high percentage of cases.

Portal Hypertension (Banti's Syndrome).

Hypertension in the portal system can be caused by obstruction of the portal veins (developmental or from thrombosis following trauma or infection), or by obstruction in the liver secondary to cirrhosis. Rise in the portal blood-pressure leads to splenomegaly and the development of œsophageal varices.

Clinical Features.—The clinical picture may include *hæmorrhage from the œsophagus and stomach, enlargement of the spleen* and *liver failure*. Bleeding from œsophageal varices is apt to be severe, persistent and exhausting to the point of shock. There is vomiting of blood and tarry stools. The enlarged spleen may diminish markedly in size during or after a bout of bleeding. There are usually prominent veins on the upper abdomen and lower thorax, and the liver may or may not be enlarged depending on the site of portal obstruction. Hepatic failure is manifested by lassitude, malnutrition, anorexia, jaundice or ascites. Œsophageal varices may be demonstrated by radiography following a barium swallow or by very careful œsophagoscopy.

Treatment.—Non-surgical measures have comparatively little to offer and there is little that can be done beyond repeated blood transfusions. Before surgery is undertaken the liver function should be assessed. Anæmia is corrected by blood transfusion and a high protein, high carbohydrate diet, supplemented by vitamins B_{12} and K, and by such food factors as *choline* and *methionine*. When the portal block is secondary to cirrhosis of the liver the outlook is poor. The object of treatment is to establish a large and permanent fistula between the portal and caval venous systems to reduce the portal hypertension and its complications. Shunts can be *porto-caval* or *lieno-renal*. In childhood the only indication for porto-caval anastomosis is for children who have previously been subjected to splenectomy and who still have œsophageal bleeding. Above the age of 3 years there are no particular difficulties in performing a lieno-renal anastomosis. The spleen is removed and an end-to-side anastomosis performed between the splenic and renal veins, preserving the left kidney.

Traumatic Rupture of the Spleen.

Rupture of the spleen is generally caused by a crush or run-over injury, but may result from a blow on the abdomen or a fall from a height.

Clinical Features.—When the spleen is damaged the most important sign is that of intraperitoneal hæmorrhage. It may be difficult to decide whether the local pain and tenderness are due to trauma of the abdominal wall or injury to viscera. A rising pulse, falling blood-pressure, pallor, thirst, air hunger and a falling red-cell count are indications for laparotomy. " Silent " rupture of the spleen is rare in childhood, and the signs and symptoms are seldom delayed as they may be in an adult with a subcapsular hæmatoma.

Treatment.—The blood is typed and a cannula is inserted into the saphenous vein at the ankle so that blood may be given promptly during splenectomy if this should be necessary. The abdomen is opened through a transverse incision, blood and clot are removed from the peritoneal cavity and further hæmorrhage is prevented by digital compression of the vessels of the splenic pedicle. The spleen is then removed.

Cysts of the Spleen.

Small cysts of the spleen are sometimes found at autopsy, but a large *serous cyst* of the spleen may present with painless abdominal swelling. It may be possible to remove the cyst, but it may be simpler to remove the entire organ. Sarcoma and hæmangioma of the spleen have been described, but the authors have never encountered a tumour of the spleen during life.

CHAPTER XVI

Genito-urinary System

DISORDERS OF MICTURITION

THE clinical features of urinary disorders in infancy and childhood are similar to those of adult life, but the interpretation of these features is modified by certain physiological and pathological problems peculiar to the young. Before discussing the regional problems of the genito-urinary system it is appropriate to consider certain disorders of micturition, the correct interpretation of which may lead to early recognition of urinary anomaly or disease.

In infancy micturition has a sharp beginning, quick voiding and a decisive ending. Even in the youngest infant there should be dry periods and there should be no straining and no dribbling (see *posterior urethral obstruction*, p. 257). When the infant is wearing napkins and wetting himself frequently it is only too easy to overlook straining and dribbling.

Increased Frequency.

Increased frequency persisting beyond infancy or returning after micturition has become normal is usually caused by local irritation—either external (*ammoniacal dermatitis, vaginitis, threadworm infestation* or *anal fissure*); or internal (*urethral* or *vesical calculus* or *cystitis*). Polyuria will cause increased frequency and the fluid intake and output should always be measured when frequency persists.

Dysuria.

The most common cause of dysuria is *ammonia dermatitis*, leading to *meatal erosion* in the male and *ammonia burns of the vulva* in the female. *Cystitis* and *bladder calculus* are less common causes. Pain on micturition often leads to urinary retention as the child will tolerate a greatly distended bladder rather than suffer the pain of passing urine.

Retention of Urine.

ACUTE RETENTION is commonly due to pain and spasm caused by local irritation of the urethra or bladder. It may be mechanical from impaction of a small stone or sulphonamide crystals in the urethra. A pelvic appendix abscess irritating the bladder wall will also cause a reflex retention.

CHRONIC RETENTION presenting with dribbling overflow may be due to a partial urethral obstruction caused by *urethral valves, congenital bladder neck obstruction*, congenital or post-traumatic *urethral stricture* ; it also accompanies the " *neurogenic bladder* " associated with developmental anomalies of the spine and spinal cord such as spina bifida (p. 261). Infants with agenesis of the abdominal muscles almost invariably suffer from chronic urinary retention (p. 260).

Incontinence of Urine.

Many patients with urinary incontinence appear first with a diagnosis of enuresis. On examination, they fall roughly into three groups :—

1. *Dribbling Incontinence.*—Continuous dribbling, or in the tiny infant squirts of urine every few minutes, indicates chronic retention. This type of incontinence is found with posterior urethral obstruction and also in the neurogenic bladder.

2. *Involuntary Voiding.*—The involuntary voiding of large quantities of urine (several ounces) at intervals occurs with severe cystitis and is also found in the neurogenic bladder.

3. *Vertical Incontinence.*—If there is urinary leak when the child is upright but not when in bed it is usually diagnostic of *ectopic ureter* (p. 256).

Pyuria.

Cloudiness of urine is commonly due to phosphatic deposit and indicates lack of fluid intake and alkalinity. Turbidity which persists when the urine is warmed and acidified is due to albumen and indicates the need for microscopic examination of the deposit. The common causes of pyuria are shown in Figure 127. Pyuria is common in children with dilatation of parts of the urinary tract. A male child with pyuria should always be thoroughly investigated. The short urethra allows

PYURIA

Obstruction → Stasis → Infection

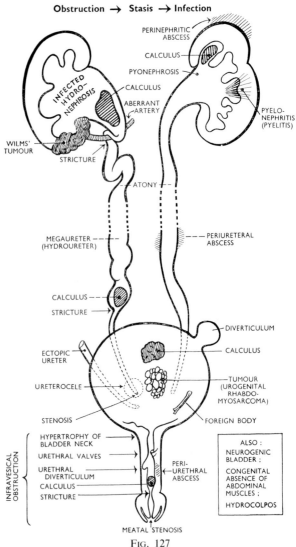

FIG. 127

Obstruction of urinary tract.

an ascending infection to occur more readily in the female. In the male infant a specimen of urine can be obtained by strapping a sterile test-tube over the cleansed penis; in the female, sterile specimens must be obtained by catheterisation.

Hæmaturia.

Unless there is an obvious lesion of the prepuce or meatus, hæmaturia is almost always of serious significance. One must exclude bleeding from the bowel or from the vagina. Red urine may be due to eating beetroot or dyed boiled sweets. Fear on the part of the mother usually leads to early investigation of hæmaturia.

In little boys, bleeding from a meatal ulcer is the most common cause and this lesion is almost always accompanied by pain. The meatus is scabbed over and the child is miserable. Hæmaturia may also be accompanied by pain when due to passage of a clot, crystals or a calculus. Painless hæmaturia may be a presenting feature of Wilms' tumour. Recurrent bouts of slighter bleeding are common in hydronephrosis and may be an early sign in renal tuberculosis. Trauma may produce frank blood in the urine. Finally, hæmaturia can occur in such general diseases as purpura, leukæmia and endocarditis. The most important differential diagnosis is from acute hæmorrhagic nephritis; casts in the urine confirm the diagnosis. The common causes of hæmaturia are illustrated in Figure 128.

METHODS OF INVESTIGATION

An accurate history is important and in infants and young children this can only be obtained from the parents. General examination of the patient and of the urine, together with renal function tests when indicated, are carried out as in the adult. In infants *excretion urography* may be technically difficult and the results are often unsatisfactory. A vein may be difficult to find, but with practice it should always be possible to inject the dye into a scalp vein. Diodone (50 per cent.) solutions can be injected subcutaneously or intramuscularly, 1 ml. of hyaluronidase being added to expedite absorption. With either method of administration concentration of the dye by the infant's kidneys may be poor. In the infant it may be almost impossible

HAEMATURIA

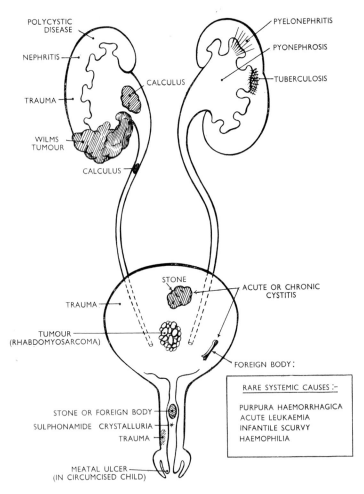

COMMONEST CAUSES OF HAEMATURIA IN CHILDHOOD :— NEPHRITIS ; PYELONEPHRITIS ;
SULPHONAMIDE CRYSTALLURIA ;
TUBERCULOSIS ; CALCULUS .

FIG. 128
Causes of hæmaturia

to eliminate intestinal gas, but clarification of the renal areas can be assisted by giving a drink of aerated water. The resulting gaseous distension of the stomach will give a good view of at least the left kidney. *Catheterisation* seldom presents any serious difficulties. A well-lubricated size 5E catheter can usually be passed in small male children. It may be difficult to see the urethral orifice in female infants. *Cystoscopy.*—In girls a single catheterising cystoscope can be passed almost from the time of birth so that retrograde pyelograms can be obtained during the early weeks of life. The male urethra varies considerably and it is rarely possible to pass an examining cystoscope through the urethra under the age of 6 months; a double-catheterising instrument cannot be used until the age of 2 years or more. A general anæsthetic is always required. If endoscopy is really essential a cystoscope can be passed through a perineal urethrostomy. *Retrograde pyelography* is usually simple in childhood. One millilitre of dye is injected into the renal pelvis for each year of life up to the age of 5 or 6 years. The patient is then screened and more dye is injected if necessary. *Cysto-urethrography.*—The bladder is filled with 35 per cent. diodone and the child is X-rayed while voiding urine. *Cine-radiography* is necessary to give really accurate information. When posterior urethral valves are present there is dilatation of the posterior urethra, and very occasionally the valve may be visualised. It may be necessary to examine the posterior urethra with a *urethroscope*. Occasionally *cystometry* may give helpful information in difficult cases.

ENURESIS

Enuresis strictly refers to " making water in the bed," but the term is applied to urinary " incontinence " for which no organic cause can be found. *The term should only be used for lack of control after the age of 4 years.* Involuntary micturition is physiological in infancy and only becomes significant after the age at which bladder control is normally established. An intelligent child receiving adequate but not excessive attention usually acquires control by day during his second year and ceases to wet the bed at night towards the end of the third year. Normal children may intermittently wet their beds during the fourth year and even later following minor illness or sudden change of temperature, or even such psychological upsets as the birth of another child and the deprivation of a certain amount of parental attention.

In most patients referred to hospital with a diagnosis of enuresis no organic abnormality is found. But as organic disease may be responsible for the symptoms, a careful history is taken and a thorough examination of the child and the urine is made. The history may bring forth symptoms which suggest disease of the urogenital system—frequency, urgency, dysuria or pain—and appropriate investigations are then made. Watching the act of micturition may show difficulty in starting, an obstructed flow or dribbling incontinence. The history may indicate that large amounts of urine are passed and this will be accompanied by evidence of excessive drinking or thirst. The habit of drinking large quantities of fluid shortly before going to bed is not in itself likely to provoke enuresis in an otherwise normal child. If there is no other evidence of organic disease endoscopic examination should be avoided, but if the condition fails to respond to conservative measures after a period of some months, it is advisable to review the case fully to make certain that some organic cause has not been overlooked.

Treatment.—Enuresis may be regarded as a symptom of a wide variety of emotional disturbances and each case must be considered individually. Although the home circumstances may be highly unsuitable it is usually necessary to treat the child in his own home. The prognosis will often depend on the degree of co-operation obtained from the parents and on the clinician's success in gaining the child's confidence. Patients who are sent to a urological clinic tend to be those who have failed to respond to simple measures or who have become the despair of a child-guidance clinic.

The parents should be instructed to adopt towards the child an attitude of kindly but firm discipline. All patients over the age of 5 should be told by the doctor that they must really help themselves in the treatment. The child is given a calendar on which the dry nights are marked with a star, a dry week being rewarded by some special treat or by a gift. Emphasis is placed on encouragement and not on disapproval or punishment. Success is gained with such a variety of treatments that the importance of suggestion hardly needs emphasis. Drugs which have been used successfully include belladonna, phenobarbitone, probanthine, ephedrine, methyl ephedrin and amphetamine, and various combinations of these, but the varying mode of action casts doubt upon their role in cures.

It is usually advisable to lay down a routine of treatment. The last drink is taken at a fixed hour, possibly two hours before bedtime. The mother rouses the child to pass urine at a certain hour, before enuresis has occurred, probably about the time at which she herself is going to bed. If necessary the child may be roused again by an alarm clock about 4 a.m. Deep sleep may be an ætiological factor, and the hardness of the bed, scantiness of bedclothes and an avoidance of over-fatigue during the day are all factors which lighten the level of sleep. The most simple and effective way of ensuring that the fullest use is made of the sensation of bladder distension causing the child to awake is to use sleep-lightening drugs, of which dextroamphetamine seems to be among the most effective. Over the age of 5 years this drug is given in a dose of 2·5 mg. at bedtime, and if the child is dry when lifted at 11 p.m. the dose may be repeated at this time and increased by 2·5 mg. at a time until the maximum tolerated dose is reached. Symptoms of overdose are restlessness, nightmares and a feeling of intense fatigue the following day. The alarm bell which rings when the sheets are wet is a much quoted method of treatment, but the apparatus is not mechanically perfect and is rarely satisfactory in the young child.

In the treatment of day symptoms the co-operation of the school authorities must be obtained. Starting at home the child is sent to pass urine at hourly or even half-hourly intervals. At school he does not ask to go out but is sent out hourly by the clock. During week-ends at home the interval can be slowly extended until the child empties his bladder two-hourly. After four or five weeks of progressive time-training during the day the nocturnal enuresis may also be cured.

A difficult decision in treating enuresis is when to make a full urological investigation. If after three months' treatment along the lines suggested above, enuresis is not materially improved, a full urological investigation is justifiable. Any gross urological or genital anomaly will have been dealt with initially and only those patients with no obvious organic lesion or in whom such lesions have been eliminated must now be considered. Excretion pyelography is the first procedure. The residual urine, if any, is obtained by catheterisation and is measured and examined bacteriologically. Cystometry may be performed at this time and cystoscopy and urethroscopy can be carried out on the same occasion or left until the effect of the passage of the catheter has been noted. The discovery of a structural anomaly does not necessarily mean that the cause of the enuresis has been found, but any such abnormality should be corrected. Constipation with fæcal accumulation in the pelvis is often overlooked as a factor in maintaining functional urinary incontinence, particularly in the patient with the so-called terminal reservoir. Regulation of bowel function often leads to complete disappearance of the urinary symptoms.

DEVELOPMENTAL ANOMALIES OF THE UPPER URINARY TRACT

ANOMALIES OF THE KIDNEY (Fig. 129)

Renal Agenesis.—In the bilateral form the child is stillborn or dies soon after birth, but unilateral agenesis occurs with sufficient frequency to be of practical importance. As a rule the ureter is absent also, and that half of the bladder may be underdeveloped. There will be no shadow on intravenous pyelography and the normal kidney may show hypertrophy and its ureter may be dilated.

Renal Hypoplasia.—This is more common than agenesis. Renal dwarfism is found in bilateral renal hypoplasia. As in agenesis *it is important to recognise the unilateral type when contemplating major procedures on the opposite kidney*.

Ectopia.—Ectopic kidneys are usually misshapen and are commonly malrotated with the pelvis projecting from the anterior aspect. They are commonly found in the iliac fossa or in the pelvis, and if associated with pain may be mistaken for an appendix abscess or intussusception. Ectopic kidneys are particularly liable to hydronephrosis and infection.

Fused Kidneys.—The *horseshoe* type is the most common form of fusion. There may be vague abdominal pains and a mass may be palpable in the epigastrium in a thin child.   Like other renal anomalies fused kidneys are liable to hydronephrosis and infection.

Polycystic Kidney.—There are two forms of polycystic disease in childhood :—

1. The renal parenchyma of both kidneys is replaced by innumerable small cysts and the tubules attached to the cysts end blindly.   The infants are stillborn or die very soon of renal failure.   Occasionally the condition may be unilateral and present with a painless abdominal swelling.   There is often a

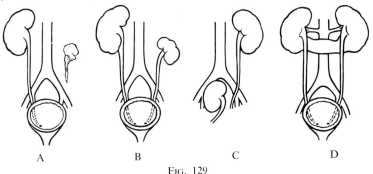

A   B   C   D

FIG. 129

Developmental anomalies of kidney. A, Agenesis. B, Hypoplasia.
C, Pelvic ectopic kidney. D, Horseshoe kidney.

family history of the anomaly, and siblings of the patient may also be affected.

2. The adult form of the disease is occasionally seen in later childhood.   In this type most of the cysts are formed in the course of patent and functioning tubules.   One kidney may enlarge before the other and if the enlargement is accompanied by hæmaturia the condition may simulate renal neoplasm.   In this form the disease usually progresses slowly and seldom causes renal failure in childhood.

ANOMALIES OF THE URETER

Duplication.—During investigation for urinary tract infection it is not uncommon to find duplication of the upper urinary tract. The anomaly may be unilateral or bilateral, and dilatation and infection are common complications.   The diagnosis is made by pyelography. Infection may be treated conservatively, but heminephrectomy may be required.

Ectopic Ureter.—The characteristic *vertical incontinence* is easily missed in early childhood and the patient is usually treated for enuresis. In the male the ureter may open into the posterior urethra and may be seen on urethroscopy. In the female the extravesical opening may be in the urethra, at the external meatus, in the vagina or even in the uterus. There is continual dribbling of urine despite micturition at normal intervals, but the child is usually dry when lying down. The rare deformity of double urethra may lead to difficulty in diagnosis. The diagnosis is sometimes confirmed by pyelography. In the female the dye test is useful. The bladder is filled with a 0·4 per cent. solution of indigo-carmine, a vulval pad is applied and the child kept up and about without micturating for an hour or two. If the pad is wet but not dyed the bladder is excluded as the source of incontinence. The symptoms may be relieved by simple ligation of the lower end of the ectopic ureter but heminephro-ureterectomy may be required.

Ureterocele.—A congenital pin-hole orifice may be responsible for cystic dilatation of the intravesical portion of the ureter. Megaureter follows and there may be infection and calculus formation. The cyst is excised by open operation through the bladder.

URINARY OBSTRUCTION (Fig. 127)

Retention (arrest) or *stasis* (retardation) of the urinary flow at various levels is common in the young. Obstruction is followed by dilatation of varying type and degree and is almost invariably complicated by infection. The outstanding dilatation may be local—in bladder (*vesical retention*), in a ureter (*megaureter*) or in the kidney pelvis (*hydronephrosis*), but generally the tract should be considered as a whole.

Vesical Retention.

Infravesical obstruction may be due to a variety of lesions, and these have already been enumerated. The bladder responds by muscular hypertrophy, but sooner or later vesical distension occurs. Back pressure affects the upper urinary tract, the ureters become dilated and tortuous and, as in the adult, hydronephrosis may develop. The onset of uræmia may be insidious.

In the neonate no urine may be passed in the first twenty-four hours or longer, but this need cause no alarm if the bladder is not markedly distended. Evidence of birth injury is sought and the external genitalia examined for an anomaly such as hypospadias with a narrow ectopic urethral orifice. The risk of introducing infection is great, but if retention is complete the bladder must be emptied using a No. 3E or 4E soft rubber catheter. When posterior urethral valves are suspected the tests described on page 259 are carried out.

In the older child *acute retention* is usually due to minor causes such as meatal erosion and crystalluria and should be relieved by immediate catheterisation. *Chronic retention* may also demand immediate drainage, but usually there is time for complete urological investigation. Urethral valves, bladder neck obstruction, vesical diverticula and urethral strictures may all be dealt with by various surgical procedures. The handling of a patient with neurogenic bladder requires all the co-operation of the child and the parents. Most patients are supplied with a portable urinal; others have been dealt with by making a sigmoid or ileal bladder.

Posterior Urethral Valves.—Posterior urethral obstruction is not uncommon but there is usually delay in diagnosis because of failure to suspect the condition. At this point it is appropriate to repeat the statement that in infancy micturition has a sharp beginning, quick voiding and a decisive ending. If micturition is not of this type a few simple tests should be performed to detect, if possible, posterior urethral obstruction. It is only too easy to overlook dribbling when an infant is wearing napkins and wets himself at frequent intervals.

Posterior urethral valves usually arise from the verumontanum (Fig. 130) and produce urinary obstruction and extensive damage to the kidneys. The kidneys excrete urine during the early months of fœtal life and urethral obstruction may cause severe renal damage even before birth (Fig. 131).

Clinical Features.—The infant has difficulty in voiding urine from the earliest days of life, and if he is observed during the

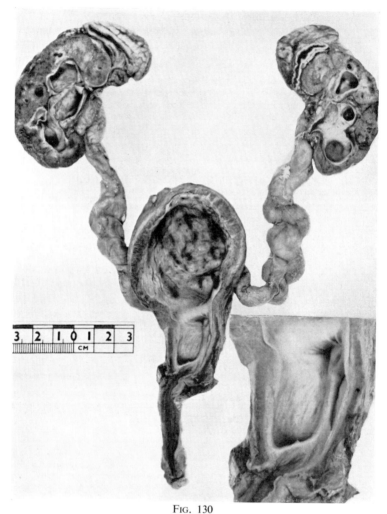

FIG. 130

Autopsy specimen from infant with posterior urethral valves, showing
hypertrophy of bladder and bilateral hydroureter and hydronephrosis.

act of micturition there will be diminution in the volume and force of the urinary stream : there may be only a gentle dribble from the meatus. Palpation of the abdomen usually reveals a distended bladder, but it may be necessary to confirm this by a bimanual examination with one finger in the rectum. The urine

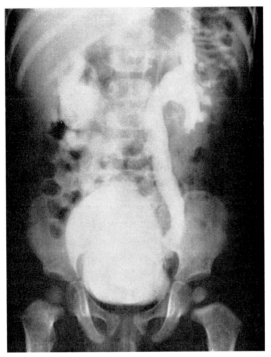

Fig. 131

Cystogram with reflux up dilated ureters in infant with posterior urethral valves.

is infected early and the infant may show signs of uræmia—drowsiness, vomiting and failure to thrive.

Treatment.—When posterior urethral obstruction is suspected a small rubber catheter is passed and the bladder partially decompressed. The blood urea or non-protein nitrogen is measured. Using 35 per cent. diodone or 12 per cent. sodium iodide, a voiding cysto-urethrogram is performed and this may confirm the diagnosis. If the kidneys are enlarged and tense,

bilateral nephrostomy is preferable to cystostomy. When the
infant's general condition has improved (this may take many

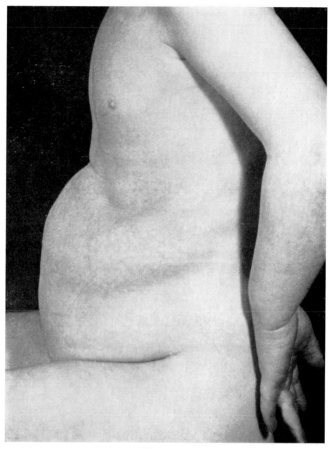

FIG. 132
Agenesis of anterior abdominal wall.

weeks), the urethral valves may be removed through a retropubic
or perineal approach.

Congenital Absence of Abdominal Muscles.—Agenesis of the
abdominal muscles is rare and almost invariably occurs in male
infants (Fig. 132). The muscles may be entirely absent or
reduced to a thin fibrous sheet. In patients with this anomaly

there is usually some dilatation of the urinary tract, but this may not be suspected until signs of renal failure develop. The dilatation usually extends down to the posterior urethra, but typical valves are rarely found. Some workers suggest that the dilatation of the urinary tract is secondary to the deficiency of the abdominal musculature; others consider that the vesical distension in fœtal life interferes with development of the abdominal muscles. Autopsy in one of our cases revealed diminution of the anterior horn cells of the spinal cord in the lower thoracic region. The muscle defect and the urinary tract dilatation may both be secondary to the cord defect; the vesical distension is possibly due to chronic retention in a neurogenic bladder.

Most infants with this anomaly die of renal failure in early life and gross dilatation of the urinary tract may be present at birth. In a few patients with a thin sheet of abdominal muscle, intensive physiotherapy and an abdominal support may prolong life for many years without serious deterioration in renal function.

Neurogenic Bladder.— Vesical retention of neurogenic origin may present as incontinence with retention or, very rarely, as continuous dribbling without retention. The neurogenic bladder is commonly associated with congenital deformities of the spine (Chap. XXI); it may also follow traumatic paraplegia.

Clinical Features.—When associated with spina bifida, dribbling incontinence is present from birth. The bladder is usually distended and urine can be expressed by manual pressure. Ammoniacal dermatitis and ulceration around the genitalia develop readily (Fig. 143). Some residual urine is present in most cases. The bladder is trabeculated and often sacculated, and vesico-ureteral reflux is a marked feature. Urinary infection eventually occurs in all cases with further deterioration in function and progressive damage to the renal parenchyma.

Treatment.—Operation on a meningocele or meningo-myelocele will never improve bladder function and may even make the situation worse.

Urinary infection is controlled by chemotherapy, and excessive leakage may be avoided by keeping the volume of urine in the bladder as small as possible. The mother, and later the child, is taught to empty the bladder at regular intervals by

16

manual pressure. By school age a boy can usually manage a portable urinal, but this apparatus is rarely successful in the female. In the female it may be justifiable to form an artificial bladder from a free ileal loop, but on a few occasions we have known girls gain reasonable urinary control when they reached puberty.

Dilated Ureter.

If the site of obstruction is at the *ureterovesical* level, the outstanding feature is dilatation of the ureter. Stagnation and infection follow, and back pressure and spread of infection lead to secondary effects on the kidney. *Megaureter* (hydroureter) may follow obstruction at the bladder neck or below and it is then bilateral (Fig. 131). It may also result from cystitis. Obstruction at the ureteric orifice from stricture, ureterocele or impacted calculus will lead to unilateral dilatation.

In some patients early relief of obstruction is called for ; in others expectant treatment is wiser, provided that infection can be controlled by chemotherapy.

Hydronephrosis.

Dilatation of the renal pelvis most commonly follows back pressure and is often bilateral. In " idiopathic " hydronephrosis the obstruction is at the pelvi-ureteric junction and has been ascribed to kinks and adhesions, to stricture, to aberrant vessels and to " achalasia." This lesion is usually unilateral. The dilatation chiefly affects the pelvis, but the calyces later dilate at the expense of the kidney substance. The kidney may be reduced to a thin shell of tissue upon a large hydronephrotic sac. If the hydronephrosis becomes infected renal function deteriorates rapidly and stone formation may complicate the problem of treatment. In infancy and childhood hydronephrosis may present as a symptomless tumour filling the loin or possibly the abdomen. If the swelling is large the differential diagnosis includes ovarian and mesenteric cyst, megacolon and renal tumour. A large hydronephrotic sac is usually translucent. A sterile hydronephrosis may give rise to periodic attacks of pain and vomiting, and during the attack the kidney may be palpably enlarged and tender. In infected cases an attempt should be made to sterilise the urine by chemotherapy before operation. At operation the kidney is inspected, its condition estimated and a decision made as to whether or not it is worth conserving. The obstruction may be relieved by division of adhesions, division of an aberrant vessel or by various plastic procedures on the pelvi-ureteric junction. In childhood the kidney can be preserved in a high percentage of patients with idiopathic hydronephrosis.

RUPTURE OF THE KIDNEY

The kidney is most commonly damaged in run-over accidents but rupture may follow a direct blow or a fall from a height. The injury varies from a small laceration to a complete tear across the kidney. There is severe pain in the abdomen and loin and severe shock. A perirenal hæmatoma may develop, with a tender swelling in the loin. Hæmaturia may be severe but usually subsides spontaneously in a few days. Each specimen of urine is kept for comparison so that diminution or increase in hæmorrhage may be assessed. Blood clots may cause renal colic, and in the bladder may cause retention. Treatment is almost always conservative. Only if severe hæmorrhage threatens life should operation be undertaken. Suture may be possible but nephrectomy is usually necessary.

UROLITHIASIS

Lithiasis is now a relatively rare disease in children in Britain. The calculi are almost invariably secondary to infection or urinary stasis associated with some defect in the urinary tract and are mainly phosphatic in structure. Less commonly the calculi occur in an otherwise normal urinary tract and are due to some disturbance in metabolism, acquired or congenital. These are formed of calcium oxalate, uric acid, ammonium urate or rarely of cystine or xanthine. Most stones, however, are of mixed composition with an outer covering of phosphates and contain a variable amount of organic material.

Renal Calculi are rarely observed in the first months of life unless there is a recto-urinary fistula (Chap. XI). Most children with urinary calculi have infected urine, and pyuria is usually apparent to the naked eye. Pain is a presenting symptom in a third of the patients, but renal colic is much less frequent in the child than in the adult, because the child's ureter dilates readily and allows stones to pass on to the bladder. Stones may form very quickly—within two or three months.

Staghorn Calculi.—This form is fairly common in patients with urolithiasis and is often preceded by "pyelitis," the organism commonly being a bacillus proteus. Renal function is usually well preserved in these patients.

Impacted Pelvic Stones.—Calculus hydronephrosis with impaction often leads to pain. There is a rapid deterioration in renal function with the formation of secondary stones.

Stones are prone to occur in anomalous kidneys due to urinary stasis.

Vesical Calculi.—These are usually associated with calculi in the upper urinary tract or with foreign bodies in the bladder (*e.g.*, "Kirby grip"). They may also follow untreated recto-urinary fistula associated with certain anorectal anomalies (Chap. XI). If they are small enough vesical calculi may be passed *per urethram.* They occasionally become impacted in the posterior urethra or the meatus, causing acute retention. The diagnosis is usually made from the history of the passage of a stone or following the investigation of pyuria, hæmaturia and recurrent urinary infection. The disease can seldom be diagnosed from a history of typical renal colic. Vesical calculi and calculi impacted at the lower end of the ureter may be palpated with a finger in the rectum in small children. Stones in the bladder may be seen on cystoscopy.

Treatment.—Treatment consists of : (1) removal of the stone ; (2) elimination of the stasis in the urinary tract ; (3) control of infection ; (4) elimination of stone-forming substances excreted in the urine ; and (5), very rarely, closure of congenital recto-urinary fistula.

URINARY TUBERCULOSIS

Urinary tuberculosis is not common in childhood, but the condition must always be remembered when investigating pyuria or hæmaturia. It is the same disease as in the adult.

Pathology.—The earliest lesions are small multiple cortical foci in the kidneys. There are no urinary symptoms at this stage, but albumen and tubercle bacilli may be found in the urine should it be examined by chance. Such early lesions can heal completely. A secondary lesion may be formed in one of the renal pyramids, usually in one kidney, and this lesion undergoes caseation and finally ulcerates into the calyx. Pus cells and tubercle bacilli are then found in the urine, and spread of infection to the urinary passages leads to increased frequency, hæmaturia and sometimes pain in the loin. Tubercles in the renal pelvis may obstruct the pelvi-ureteric junction, leading to hydronephrosis. This facilitates spread to the other calyces and finally leads to pyonephrosis. Calcification may occur early. The ureter becomes thickened and fibrosed and the bladder is first affected at the ureteric orifice, giving rise to the typical " golf-hole " ureter. Interstitial cystitis leads to severe contraction of the bladder.

Clinical Features.—The disease follows a primary focus elsewhere in the body. There are initially no urinary symptoms, and pus cells and tubercle bacilli may be found in the urine accidentally. Almost a quarter of the cases occur in sanatoria in patients suffering from bone and joint tuberculosis. The most common presenting sign may be hæmaturia or there may be frequency with burning pain on micturition. Very occasionally the kidney may be palpable. Older children may complain of a dull ache in the loin. There is no marked upset in the general condition of the patient. The urine is usually acid and without smell, but there may be secondary invasion by *B. coli* in the later stages. On cystoscopy the bladder is often normal but there may be grey tubercles on the mucosa and a " golf-hole " ureter may be apparent. Intravenous pyelography may show fluffiness of the calyces with dilatation or a filling defect. In retrograde pyelography there is danger of dissemination of the disease by catheterising the infected kidney, but the apparently healthy side should be catheterised to exclude bilateral disease. The first morning specimen of urine should be examined on repeated occasions until the organism is isolated by culture or guinea-pig inoculation.

Treatment.—If tubercle bacilli are found in the urine and there is no pyelographic deformity, treatment should be conservative and directed to the focus elsewhere in the body. When early lesions are found in a patient undergoing treatment for bone or joint disease, it is often wise to defer surgical treatment of the urological condition until orthopædic procedures are completed.   In advanced bilateral renal tuberculosis, surgery is rarely possible, and it is only with sanatorium regime and chemotherapy that any hope of improvement can be expected.   With these exceptions the treatment of renal tuberculosis is essentially surgical.   A course of chemotherapy is given for approximately three months before undertaking surgery.   This usually consists of streptomycin (45 mg. per kg. weight per day) with P.A.S. (250 mg. per kg.) plus isoniazid (10 mg. per kg.).   At the end of this period a total *nephro-ureterectomy* is performed.   Post-operatively streptomycin, P.A.S. and isoniazid are given for six to eight weeks.   In our own small series the prognosis has been good in early cases subjected to surgery, but from an extensive review of the literature it would appear that the prognosis is worse than in adults.

NEOPLASTIC DISEASE

TUMOURS OF THE BLADDER

Villous papillomata are never seen in childhood, and the only important tumour of the lower urinary tract is the rhabdomyosarcoma.

Rhabdomyosarcoma (Sarcoma Botryoides : Embryonic Sarcoma).

This is a rare mesenchymal tumour which may originate in the bladder as well as in the vagina.   The embryonic tumour cells can differentiate to form smooth and striped muscle, cartilage and bone.   Although a lethal tumour which grows rapidly and invades locally, it is characterised by delayed metastasis.   The tumour forms round gelatinous masses (like small white grapes) on a tough solid base.   The earliest clinical manifestations are those of a persisting infection with increased frequency, urgency and dribbling incontinence.   Severe spasmodic pain may make the child scream and strain.   Sooner or later the patient passes bright red blood with the urine.   On bimanual examination a solid tumour is felt to be filling the bladder.   The diagnosis is confirmed by cystoscopy.

Treatment.—The tumour is not radiosensitive and the only possibility of cure is by radical surgery. The ureters are transplanted into the sigmoid colon and a total cystectomy is performed. There are few recorded cures.

RENAL TUMOUR

The outstanding renal tumour of childhood is the nephroblastoma (Fig. 133).

Nephroblastoma (Embryoma, Wilms' tumour) is a tumour

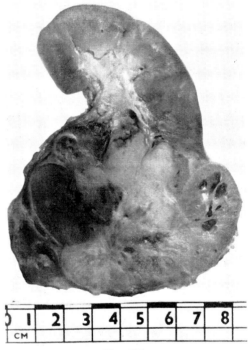

FIG. 133
Wilms' tumour (nephroblastoma).

of embryonic origin and contains mesenchymal and epithelial elements with every variety of differentiation—fibrous tissue, smooth and striped muscle, cartilage, bone, primitive glomeruli and tubules. The tumour outgrows its blood supply and shows areas of necrosis and hæmorrhage. Rarely it may be bilateral.

Growth is very rapid and the swelling soon becomes fixed to surrounding structures. The lymph glands around the pedicle are invaded early, but the dangerous spread is from growth into the renal vein.

Clinical Features.—The tumour is most commonly seen in the first year of life and is rare after the age of 3. The onset is insidious until an abdominal swelling is noticed. Occasionally hæmaturia may lead to early recognition, but the urine is usually normal. When nephroblastoma is suspected, *palpation should be as gentle and as brief as possible and should be performed only by the physician who first sees the patient and by the surgeon who is to operate.* Repeated palpation and demonstration of the tumour for teaching purposes will sign the child's death warrant. The swelling arises from the loin and passes forwards towards the midline. The mass is dull to percussion and does not trans-illuminate. Excretion pyelography usually reveals no shadow on the affected side, but some portion of the kidney may be secreting and a distorted pelvic shadow may be seen. Several authors have noted mild or moderate raising of the blood-pressure associated with Wilms' tumour, but hypertension has not been a significant feature of our cases.

Differential Diagnosis.—A large tense hydronephrosis may simulate a solid tumour, but it can usually be transilluminated. Neuroblastoma may be impossible to differentiate from nephro-blastoma, but here the pyelogram shows the outline of the pelvis and calyces and the shadow is displaced downwards and may be distorted. Retroperitoneal teratoma may simulate a renal or suprarenal tumour.

Treatment.—The lung fields are X-rayed to exclude gross metastasis. Pyelograms confirm the presence of a second kidney. The condition is regarded as a surgical emergency and should be operated on within a day or two of admission to hospital. Transperitoneal nephrectomy is followed by a course of radiotherapy. More than half the patients die within six to twelve months.

PARARENAL TUMOURS

It is appropriate to consider here tumours of the adrenal gland or in the sympathetic chain on the posterior abdominal wall.

Adrenal Cortical Tumours.

Tumours of the adrenal cortex are rare and may present with local swelling or with endocrine disturbance due to excess output of androgens. Endocrine disturbance may arise from a tumour too small to be clinically evident and it may be impossible to distinguish between tumour and simple hypertrophy of the gland. The adrenogenital syndrome has different effects in the male and female. In both sexes growth is abnormally rapid and centres of ossification appear early. In the male there is precocious development of the external genitalia with enlargement of the penis and growth of pubic hair, but the testes do not partake in the development. In girls the clitoris is enlarged, hair is of male distribution (Fig. 134) and feminine contours are lost. Pyelography may demonstrate displacement of the associated kidney and the outline of the adrenal may be shown radiographically following insufflation of oxygen into the perinephric space.

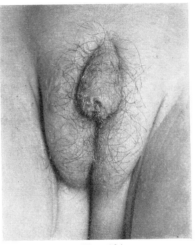

Fig. 134
Female pseudohermaphrodite.

Treatment.—If the tumour is malignant the prognosis is poor. In benign tumours and with hypertrophy, excision of the mass usually leads to a permanent cure with regression of the virilising changes.

Neuroblastoma (Sympathicoblastoma).

This is a malignant tumour arising from the autonomic ganglia or from the suprarenal medulla. The tumour may consist of small, round or polygonal undifferentiated cells or the cells may be arranged in characteristic rosettes. Areas of necrosis and hæmorrhage are common. The tumour grows rapidly and metastasises early. There may be massive involvement of the liver (*Pepper's syndrome*), but more commonly the secondary deposits occur in the skull and long bones, and in *Hutchison's syndrome* there are cranial and orbital deposits with exophthalmos.

Clinical Features.—The tumours occur in the same age group as the nephroblastomata. In the adrenal area the tumours are highly malignant and present with abdominal swelling. Lethargy, anorexia, pallor and wasting appear earlier than in renal tumours. Pyelography may show displacement of the renal pelvis. When the tumour arises from the lumbar sympathetic differentiation from renal tumour is usually easy.

Treatment.—Surgical excision should be attempted, but only too frequently local invasion or metastases render this impossible. In our experience all sympathicoblastomata arising within the adrenal have been fatal. Tumours arising from other parts of the sympathetic chain present a more hopeful picture. Following local excision and radiotherapy there have been a few five-year cures. A neuroblastoma may occasionally undergo spontaneous evolution to ganglioneuroma and this maturation may explain the cures which have apparently followed the administration of massive doses of vitamin B_{12}. We ourselves have seen no benefit arising from this form of therapy in tumours of the adrenal.

Phæochromocytoma (Paraganglionoma).

These adrenaline-secreting tumours which arise from the suprarenal medulla or sympathetic chain are rare in childhood. Although histologically benign their secretion induces hypertensive cardiovascular disease. There is progressive elevation of the blood-pressure with paroxysmal exacerbations of hypertension associated with headaches, palpitations, sweating, polydypsia and polyuria. There may be an excess of adrenaline in the blood. Intravenous injection of dibenamine hydrochloride induces a temporary fall in blood-pressure. The tumour may be demonstrated by pyelography or by injection of oxygen into the perirenal space, but laparotomy is necessary to demonstrate a lesion in the abdominal sympathetic. Operative removal of a phæochromocytoma is a risky procedure; there may be an excessive release of adrenaline or a dangerous fall in blood-pressure when the supply of adrenaline is cut off.

Other causes of hypertension in childhood are coarctation,

hypothalamic tumour, hyperthyroidism or renal hypertension caused by atrophic pyelonephritis or congenital hypoplasia of the kidney. Hypertension may occasionally be associated with Wilms' tumour; the mechanism is probably different from that found in the scarred kidney.

DEVELOPMENTAL ANOMALIES OF THE EXTERNAL GENITALIA

HYPOSPADIAS

Embryology (Fig. 135).—On the external aspect of the cloacal membrane, below the infra-umbilical aspect of the abdominal

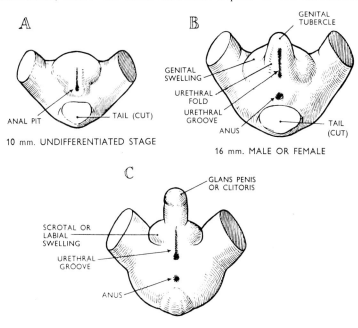

A

10 mm. UNDIFFERENTIATED STAGE

ANAL PIT — TAIL (CUT)

B

GENITAL TUBERCLE

GENITAL SWELLING

URETHRAL FOLD

URETHRAL GROOVE

ANUS

TAIL (CUT)

16 mm. MALE OR FEMALE

C

GLANS PENIS OR CLITORIS

SCROTAL OR LABIAL SWELLING

URETHRAL GROOVE

ANUS

21 mm. FAILURE OF DEVELOPMENT IN MALE LEADS TO PERINEAL HYPOSPADIAS

FIG. 135

Development of external genitalia.

wall, three protuberances appear. They are the *genital tubercle* and the *two genital swellings*. The urogenital orifice opens on the ventral aspect of the genital tubercle as the *urethral groove*. The groove is bounded on either side by the *urethral folds*. In the male the genital tubercle enlarges to form the phallus. In the female the tubercle is bent tailwards to form the clitoris.

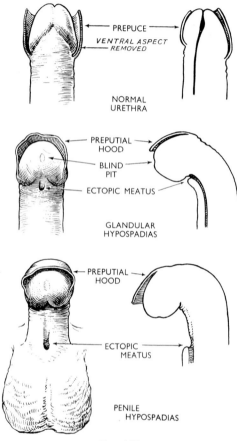

FIG. 136
Hypospadias.

The genital swellings form the scrotum in the male and the labia majora in the female. In the male at 45 mm. the urethral folds fuse over the urethral groove but the groove only extends to the coronary sulcus. The glandular urethra is formed from a cord of ectoderm which later becomes canalised. If the urethral groove fails to close, the deformity of hypospadias is found. In the female there is no closure of the urethral folds and the lips of the groove form the labia minora.

Clinical Features.—The terminal urethral orifice may open in the coronary sulcus, *glandular hypospadias*; at any point along the shaft of the penis, *penile hypospadias* (Fig. 136); or in the perineum, *perineal hypospadias* (Fig. 137). In perineal hypospadias the labioscrotal swellings fail to unite, and in extreme

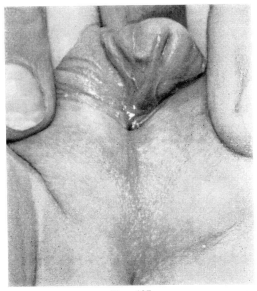

Fig. 137

Perineal hypospadias. The urinary " meatus " in the glans is a blind pit.

cases the presence of a pseudo-vagina may render sex determination difficult (p. 287). The prepuce has a characteristic hooded appearance due to a ventral defect caused by failure of closure of the urethral folds and this gives an appearance of partial circumcision. Some degree of ventral curvature of the penis (*chordee*) is present in all but the most minor degrees of the deformity. The chordee is caused by the short urethra and failure of development of the corpus spongiosum which is represented by a fibrous cord. The terminal meatus, particularly in glandular and penile hypospadias, is often minute and may be difficult to demonstrate and a blind pit in the glans may be mistaken for the urethral orifice (Fig. 137). The deformity is always distal to the urinary sphincters and there is rarely any defect in bladder control.

Treatment.—Three problems may present in infancy— *inadequacy of the urethral orifice, deformity of the penis* and, in perineal hypospadias, the *sex* of the child.

The infant may not pass urine after birth and a pin-hole meatus may require early relief by dilatation or *meatotomy*. In minor degrees of the deformity the penis is straight, and if the

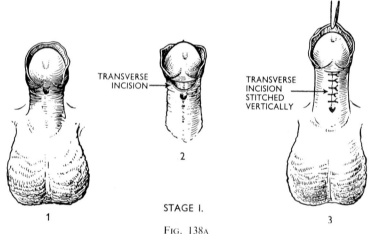

TRANSVERSE
INCISION

TRANSVERSE
INCISION
STITCHED
VERTICALLY

2

STAGE I.

1   3

FIG. 138A

Operation for hypospadias. Stage I—Repair of chordee and meatotomy.

orifice is adequate no treatment is required. In penile hypospadias, where chordee causes the urinary stream to be directed downwards, and in perineal hypospadias, surgical correction should be completed before the boy goes to school. The chordee is corrected and the penis straightened between 18 months and 2 years. Many ingenious operations have been devised for reconstruction of the urethral tube and the interested student should consult a textbook of operative surgery. We find the three-stage procedure of Denis Browne (Figs. 138A and 138B) is the most satisfactory operation. As in most recommended procedures the chordee is corrected and an adequate urethral outlet is constructed by meatotomy. The final stage of reconstruction of the urethra is, whenever possible, carried out before the boy goes to school (for obvious psychological reasons), but it may be postponed for a few years if the penis is not adequately developed. A perineal urethrostomy is performed to divert the urinary stream and the new urethra is

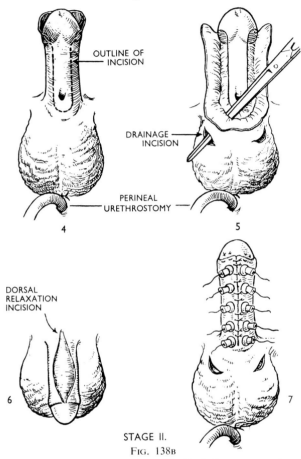

OUTLINE OF INCISION

DRAINAGE INCISION

PERINEAL URETHROSTOMY

DORSAL RELAXATION INCISION

4

5

6

7

STAGE II.

FIG. 138B

Operation for hypospadias. Stage II—Denis Browne operation—perineal urethrostomy and construction of urethra.

constructed from a simple ventral strap of penile skin. After extensive undermining the lateral flaps are approximated with double-stop sutures formed from a glass bead and a small section of soft aluminium tubing. The urethrostomy catheter is removed on the tenth day and the sinus closes spontaneously in three or four days.

ECTOPIA VESICÆ AND EPISPADIAS

Both deformities arise from deficiency in the midline of the infra-umbilical abdominal wall. In *ectopia vesicæ* (extroversion of bladder) the defect is complete, the anterior bladder wall is absent and the vesical mucosa prolapses through the defect in the abdominal wall. The umbilicus is lower than normal and is represented by a scar at the apex of the bladder. The trigone and the ureteric orifices lie exposed (Fig. 139). The pubic bones

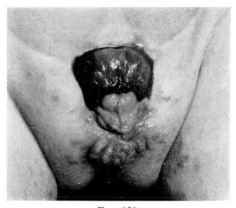

Fig. 139
Ectopia vesicæ.

are widely separated (Fig. 140). In the male the penis is short, thick-set and up-tilted. The urethra forms a groove on the dorsal surface of the penis and the prepuce is split dorsally (*epispadias*). The scrotum is normally fused but may be empty. In the female a vaginal orifice lies below the bladder, the clitoris is divided and lies below and posterior to the urethra. The urethral meatus is represented by a wide transverse slit.

In lesser degrees of the defect the umbilicus lies above the exposed posterior bladder wall. The bladder may be covered in, leaving only a defect of the sphincter and urethra—the common type of epispadias (Fig. 141). In still milder degrees the sphincters may be present and epispadias may be the sole anomaly.

Ectopia Vesicæ.

The exposed vesical mucosa is tender, and with the unmanageable urinary incontinence severe excoriation of the skin develops. There may be a waddling gait due to instability of the pelvis.

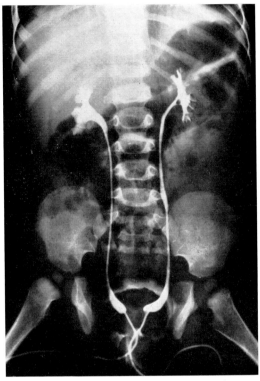

FIG. 140

Retrograde pyelogram in patient shown in Figure 139 shows no abnormality in upper urinary tract. Note wide separation of pubic bones.

Treatment.—Continence can almost always be obtained following transplantation of the ureters into the sigmoid colon. The operation is performed at the age of 18 months or 2 years —that is, when the period of physiological diuresis is over. During the waiting period constant attention is required to the raw bladder and the surrounding skin. Napkins are changed frequently, the skin is protected by vaseline or other emollient

17

and exposed to the air whenever possible. These patients sometimes suffer from recurrent rectal prolapse and this is treated
before ureteric transplantation is carried out. In patients with
bowel incontinence (*e.g.*, deficient perineal musculature and
rectal prolapse or meningocele associated with ectopia vesicæ),
transplantation of the ureters into the sigmoid should never be
carried out. It is necessary in such cases to use a free ileal loop
to make an " artificial bladder." The ureters are transplanted
into this artificial bladder which drains through an ileostomy

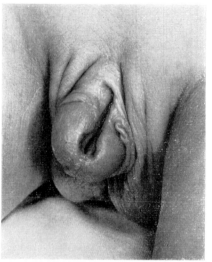

Fig. 141
Epispadias.

in the right anterior abdominal wall. The exposed vesical
mucosa is excised with diathermy when the child has achieved
full continence after transplantation. The raw area is covered
by lateral flaps and the penile deformity is repaired by an
adaptation of the Denis Browne procedure for hypospadias.

Epispadias (Fig. 141).

Most patients with epispadias are incontinent. Attempts
are made to build up the urinary sphincter before resorting to
ureteric transplantation. The urethra can be reconstructed by a
modified Denis Browne procedure.

THE PREPUCE AND CIRCUMCISION

Circumcision is one of the most common operations performed in this country. Before deciding whether a child's foreskin is to be removed or not the doctor should know something of the history of the operation and also something of the normal anatomy and function of the structure at different ages.

Ritual circumcision is practised over a wide area of the world by one-sixth of the world population. In some instances the procedure can be grouped with various forms of tribal marking by burning and incision and piercing of prominent folds such as the lips and ears. It may be performed to reduce sexual desire, to make a better warrior for a tribe and a more faithful husband and a less frequent disturber of the society in which the native warrior lives. Apart from ritual circumcision the procedure is common only in the English-speaking peoples. It is rare in Continental Europe and in Scandinavia. The earliest Egyptian mummies were circumcised and the practice was introduced into the Roman Empire with Christianity. There is no trace of the operation in medieval Europe, and apparently it was carried out only by adherents of the Jewish faith until the rise of surgery in the nineteenth century when the status changed from a religious rite to a common surgical procedure. The age at which circumcision is performed varies. In Mosaic practice it is carried out at the eighth day and in many Africans at puberty. Female circumcision as practised in the Sudan may include not only removal of the clitoris but often the major labia, the labia minora being stitched together.

Development of the Prepuce.—The mammalian penis serves the double purpose of urination and generation. The development of the penis and urethra have been discussed on page 271. The prepuce appears at the eighth week of intra-uterine life as a ring of epidermis at the base of the glans. It grows forward more rapidly on the upper surface. At twelve weeks the glandular urethra has not yet formed and arrest at this stage gives rise to the hooded prepuce of hypospadias. At sixteen weeks the prepuce covers the glans but there is as yet no preputial sac. The embryonic fusion between the prepuce and the glans gradually disappears due to the development of epithelial " pearls " that fuse until the preputial sac is complete.

At birth less than 5 per cent. of foreskins are completely retractable. In a little more than 50 per cent. the external meatus can be displayed, but in almost 40 per cent. of male infants even the tip of the glans cannot be uncovered. At the age of 6 months four out of five foreskins are still non-retractable. At a year 50 per cent., at 2 years 20 per cent. and at 3 years 10 per cent. are still non-retractable. The non-retractable state is due to congenital adhesions and rarely to a tight prepuce. The non-retractable prepuce can be regarded with equanimity up to the age of 3 years, but over 5 the smegma may become malodorous and steps should be taken to render the prepuce retractable and capable of being kept clean. Phimosis means stenosis of the preputial orifice. Acquired phimosis results from trauma. If the preputial ring is forcibly stretched, cracks appear and fibrotic contracture will occur later. Acquired phimosis may also follow inflammation of the prepuce associated with ammoniacal dermatitis. In the child the term phimosis should be confined to the acquired lesion.

Function of the Prepuce.—It is no accident that during the years when the child is incontinent, the glans is clothed by the prepuce. Deprived of this protection the glans is easily abraded by sodden clothes and napkins. Meatal ulceration is seen only in circumcised children but is almost unknown in Jewish babies circumcised in the first week of life when the urea concentration in urine is very low. For this reason it is advisable to perform circumcision within the first ten days or to wait until the infant is out of napkins.

Indications for Circumcision.

There are no convincing surgical grounds for circumcision in early infancy. If after six or twelve months the process of separation of the prepuce appears too dilatory, if there is any real risk of paraphimosis or in very rare instances ballooning of the preputial sac, the baby is anæsthetised and residual preputial adhesions gently separated with a probe. In severe acquired phimosis following ammoniacal dermatitis, the preputial opening may be enlarged by making an adequate dorsal slit with scissors. In older boys a non-retractable prepuce may give rise to such complications as balanoposthitis with a purulent discharge, or to recurrent paraphimosis, and these are undoubted indications for circumcision.

AMMONIACAL DERMATITIS (Napkin Rash)

A red erythematous rash covers the napkin area. There is œdema and desquamation and secondary infection may lead to ulceration. In the uncircumcised male the tip of the prepuce becomes œdematous and swollen (Fig. 142). In the circumcised

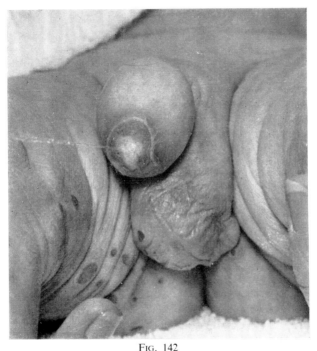

Fig. 142

Ammoniacal dermatitis with ulceration of prepuce and secondary phimosis leading to ballooning of preputial sac and thin urinary stream.

boy, blisters and ulcerated patches appear on the glans (Fig. 143). The meatus becomes reddened and everted or the seat of an ulcer or erosion. This meatal erosion causes the child great pain ; it scabs over and makes micturition difficult or impossible to start. When, with straining, micturition is finally started the tearing open of the crack causes severe pain, screaming, reflex stoppage of the urinary stream and sometimes the escape of a drop or two of bright red blood. Acute retention may occur.

The napkins smell strongly of ammonia.   In the breast-fed baby the condition is virtually unknown until weaning.   The condition is in fact an ammonia burn, the source of the ammonia being bacterial decomposition of the urea of the urine.   In the breast-fed infant the stools are acid in reaction and bacterial activity is inhibited, but bottle feeding changes the reaction of the stools to alkaline and this activates the fermentation process of the

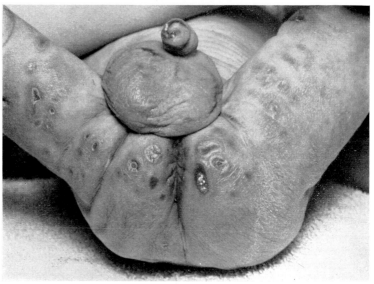

FIG. 143

Ammoniacal dermatitis with meatal erosion and ulceration
of buttocks and thighs.

ammonia liberated from the urine in the confined atmosphere of the soaked napkin.   In the female the urethra is protected by its position and urinary upset is minimal.

Treatment.—The mother is instructed in strict napkin drill. All traces of soap or detergent must be removed from the napkins by frequent hot rinsing after washing.   The liberal use of talcum or boracic acid powder will help to check fermentation. When the child is sleeping or likely to be wet for long periods no napkins at all are worn.   The clothing should be loose and requisite towelling and mackintosh are spread beneath him. Rubber or plastic protective pants are forbidden at all times.

Oral administration of either soya-bean flour or folic acid encourages the growth of lactobacilli, and this may inhibit the growth of ammonia-producing organisms in the stools. Soya-bean milk is made by adding 1½ oz. of soya flour to a pint of water and this is used to replace half the quantity of cow's milk normally taken. Folic acid is given in a dose of 10 mg. of the elixir daily.

Meatal Ulcer.—This lesion is almost never seen in the uncircumcised infant and preventive treatment is therefore the avoidance of circumcision. The treatment of the lesion is mainly that of the associated ammonia dermatitis. When the ulcer is covered by a scab the baby is helped by softening the scab in a bath or by gentle sponging. Local application of bland ointment is necessary and in older boys the glans must be protected from friction from the trousers. Untreated, scarring and contracture may lead to pin-hole meatus. Meatotomy may be necessary but this is never undertaken until all risk of re-ulceration from ammoniacal dermatitis has passed.

Paraphimosis.

In this condition a tight prepuce has been retracted and the resulting constriction causes swelling of the glans and mucous membrane distal to the constriction. If seen early a cold compress and gentle pressure reduces the œdema ; the retracted prepuce can then be drawn forward. If hyaluronidase is available, 0·5 to 1 ml. injected into the œdematous area quickly dissipates the swelling and reduction can be easily accomplished. If treatment has been delayed, a general anæsthetic is administered and a small vertical incision is made in the midline posteriorly through the constricting band ; the paraphimosis can then be reduced. If paraphimosis recurs the child should be circumcised.

Balanoposthitis.

Inflammation of the glans and under surface of the prepuce may be due to retained smegma, poor hygiene or may be associated with ammoniacal dermatitis (Fig. 142). There is redness, pain and swelling and a seropurulent discharge from under the prepuce. The condition usually subsides with sitz baths, but a dorsal slit may be required. If the child has attained voluntary bladder control circumcision may be performed after the inflammation has subsided.

FEMALE GENITAL TRACT

Adhesion of the Labia.

At birth the labia may appear to be fused and the infant may not pass urine (Fig. 144). The adhesion is rarely dense and separation can usually be accomplished with fingers or a swab. Oozing of blood is negligible.

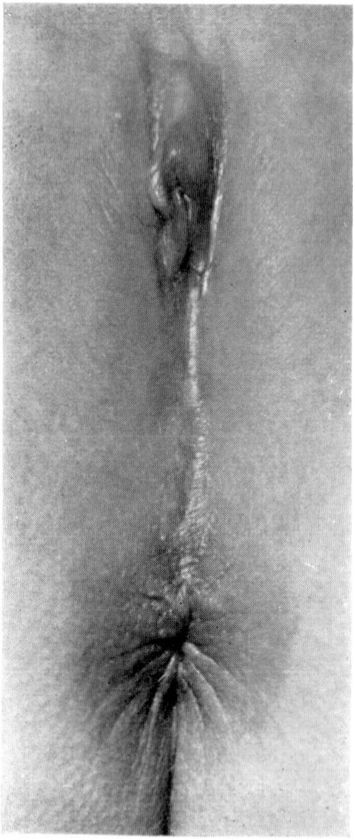

Vaginal Obstruction.

At birth the vagina may be completely occluded by an imperforate hymen or by atresia of its lower end. Maternal œstrogenic hormones may cause excess uterine or vaginal secretion and the vagina is greatly distended with accumulated fluid — *hydrocolpos*. Occasionally the cervical canal and uterine body may also be stretched —*hydrometrocolpos*. The cavity is filled with clear or mucoid fluid which tends to become purulent from bacterial invasion and gives rise to *pyocolpos*. The ballooned genital tract rises from the pelvic floor into the abdominal cavity and a midline lower abdominal swelling may be present at birth. The mass may lead to urinary obstruction, and enlargement of the bladder may prevent palpation of the vaginal tumour. On rectal

Fig. 144

Occlusion of vagina due to adhesion of labia.

examination the pelvis is filled with a mass projecting into the hollow of the sacrum.

The differential diagnosis is from ovarian cyst or tumour,

retroperitoneal tumour, urachal cyst, hydronephrosis or Wilms' tumour.

If the condition is due to an imperforate hymen or similar membrane, gentle separation of the labia will reveal the bulging membrane at or above the hymen. This bulge resembles a cystocele. The diagnosis is confirmed by inserting a needle through the membrane and aspirating the entrapped fluid. The membrane is nicked with a knife and the opening enlarged with sinus forceps, thus evacuating the fluid with consequent disappearance of the abdominal swelling.

When there is atresia of the lower vagina the distension may be gross and as well as urinary obstruction there may be rectal obstruction and respiratory embarrassment from upward displacement of the intestine. In this type there is no bulging membrane and the diagnosis is only confirmed at laparotomy. The unwary operator may attempt to excise the " cyst " only to find that he has removed most of the vagina along with the uterus, tubes and ovaries which are perched unobtrusively on the apex of the cystic swelling. Dense peritoneal adhesions may make demonstration of the exact state of affairs difficult. The cyst is carefully evacuated through its anterior wall. Before puberty an attempt is made to drain the vagina through the perineum and a new vagina is constructed.

At puberty an imperforate hymen leads to a collection of hæmorrhagic material within the vagina—*hæmatocolpos*. There may be abdominal or pelvic pain but rarely nausea or vomiting. There is tenderness on suprapubic pressure, and rectal examination reveals the tender swelling of the ballooned vagina. Hæmatocolpos should be suspected in a girl with pubic hair and enlargement of the breasts who has not yet menstruated.

As in the infant, incision of the bulging hymen gives immediate relief.

Vaginal Discharge.

Vaginitis may occur in young girls where personal hygiene has been poor, either from laziness or lack of adequate toilet facilities. The discharge ceases quickly with local cleanliness and sitz baths two or three times a day. Gonococcal vaginitis is rare in children, but if the diplococcus is recognised from a smear intensive penicillin therapy is instituted. Before puberty monilia and trichomonad vaginitis are also rare ; they are treated as in the adult.   If the discharge does not clear up quickly with local cleanliness and sitz baths, rectal examination may reveal a vaginal foreign body.   Purulent or hæmorrhagic discharge is often caused by a foreign body, and in such cases the vagina is examined with a small speculum.   Cotton wool may be introduced into the vagina, and such material cannot be palpated on rectal examination.   Very rarely a hæmorrhagic discharge may be caused by the highly malignant *rhabdomyo-sarcoma* (sarcoma botryoides) of the uterus or vagina.   Grape-like cystic masses are extruded from the vagina.   The tumour is highly malignant and is not radiosensitive.

Urethral Caruncle.

Dark red hæmangiomatous nodules may be seen on the urethral lips.   Unlike the adult caruncles these lesions are painless but may lead to local irritation and frequency of micturition.   The nodules are destroyed by a diathermy needle.

Prolapse of Urethral Mucosa.

The onset is sudden and the urethral mucosa rapidly becomes œdematous and very painful.   Unless epispadias is present the condition subsides with rest, local compresses and sitz baths.

OVARIAN CYSTS

Ovarian cysts are not uncommon before the age of puberty. They may present with lower abdominal discomfort or progressive enlargement of the abdomen.   Most commonly the first symptom is acute abdominal pain due to torsion of the pedicle.   The cysts are usually *dermoids* containing hair, sebaceous material, teeth and other ectodermal tissues.   Less commonly *simple unilocular cysts* are found.   The prognosis is excellent in both cases.

OVARIAN NEOPLASMS

Ovarian tumours in childhood are *teratoma, carcinoma* or, very rarely, *sarcoma*.   *Carcinoma* is the most common solid tumour of the ovary in childhood and may take the form of adenocarcinoma, *dysgerminoma* or *granulosa cell* tumour. In the granulosa cell tumour, production of œstrogens leads to *sexual precocity*—premature menstruation, development of breasts and pubic hair and advanced bone development. Solid ovarian tumours are usually painless unless there is torsion of the pedicle and present with an enlarging lower abdominal mass. If there is no radiographic evidence of metastases the tumour should be excised. In our limited experience ovarian neoplasms in childhood are less malignant than their histological appearances would lead one to expect.

HERMAPHRODITISM

Certain anomalies of the external genitalia may occasion difficulty in the determination of sex, and a brief review of the problem is given to assist the family doctor in the decision as to the upbringing of the child. It must be remembered that normally developed gonads and genitalia are not always accompanied by full masculinity or femininity of bodily form or psychology. In *intersex* the external genitalia are not fully characteristic of either male or female and this must be regarded as an extreme example of a common tendency. The " pragmatic " sex of an individual indicates the sex which the person feels himself or herself to be. If the sex is doubtful at birth the parents should be advised to have the child christened with some such name as Lesley, Francis or Evelyn, lest a change of sex should be necessary at a later date. The genetic sex may sometimes be established by the examination of the nuclei of a skin biopsy, from smears of oral mucosa or from polymorph nuclei using a blood film. (The nuclei of females contains a mass of sex chromatin which is inconspicuous in the nuclei of males.)

Female Pseudohermaphroditism.—The external genitalia of the female fœtus may be distorted by excess androgenic hormone from adrenal hypertrophy. Under normal ovarian influence the vagina, uterus and tubes are formed. The virilising adrenal cortex prevents the disappearance of the urogenital sinus and stimulates the growth of the phallus and labioscrotal folds. These patients have a single external orifice and the genitalia closely resembles the condition of perineal hypospadias in the male (p. 273). On endoscopy the cervix can be seen and salpingograms confirm the diagnosis. If adrenal hyperactivity continues after birth there will be evidence of continuing virilisation. Growth is rapid and ossification and epiphyseal effusion are in advance of normal. There is growth of pubic hair and prominent enlargement of the phallus (Fig. 134). Despite their female genetic sex these patients are often pragmatic males. Excessive amounts of 17-ketosteroids in the urine follow excretion of the androgenic hormone. Occasionally there is adrenal insufficiency with signs of Addison's disease. These infants present with anorexia, weakness and vomiting and there may be an adrenal crisis with a fall in serum sodium and a rise in serum potassium.

Treatment.—Treatment is difficult. A few patients can be cured by partial resection of the hypertrophied adrenal followed by amputation of the clitoris and plastic enlargement of the vagina. Most cases are happier as boys and the urethra is reconstructed by the Denis Browne procedure (p. 274). If the uterus and vagina are well developed they should be removed.

Male Pseudohermaphroditism.—Confusion of sex arises in children with perineal hypospadias and a small penis and undescended testes (Fig. 137). These patients are usually happier as males and the treatment is that of perineal hypospadias as already described.

True Hermaphroditism.—Individuals with both testicular and ovarian tissues are rare and a diagnosis is made only by histological examination of the gonads. Most patients have a hypospadiac type of penis and a vagina opening externally or into the urethra. There may be a testis on one side and an ovary on the other, or the gonads may contain characteristics of both —the *ovo-testis.*

Treatment.—Each case must be treated on its own merits. In patients brought up as males, hysterectomy may be necessary to prevent recurrent hæmorrhage. Interference with the gonads should be cautious as removal or damage to functional tissue may lead to eunuchoid changes.

CHAPTER XVII

The Thorax

MALFORMATIONS OF THE CHEST WALL

ABSENCE of the nipple (*athelia*) is usually associated with absence of the breast (*amazia*) and absence of the sternal portion of the pectoralis major, and is a rare anomaly. Congenital absence of the pectoralis major is more common

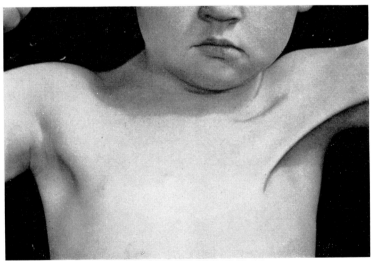

FIG. 145
Congenital absence of left pectoral muscles.

and there is remarkably little disability (Fig. 145). There may be an associated defect in the underlying ribs, but on the right side there is rarely any call for surgical intervention; on the left side, bone grafting may be required to protect the heart. Fortunately, all these defects are more common in the male.

Supernumerary nipples (*polythelia*) are common and are

usually symmetrical and situated below the normal nipple in the primitive mammary line. They are usually vestigial and may escape recognition until the areola becomes pigmented at puberty when excision may be performed.

Pectus Excavatum (Funnel Chest).

In this condition there is a depression of all or part of the sternum and adjacent cartilages (Fig. 146). The deformity may

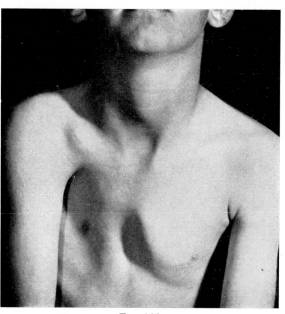

FIG. 146
Funnel chest.

be present at birth or may develop soon thereafter and often becomes progressively worse as the child grows. It is more common in males and is usually symmetrical. The cause is obscure, and although there is rarely evidence of rickets the bones are less rigid than normal.

Mild degrees of the deformity do not require treatment. If the deformity is severe an extensive operation is performed between the ages of 3 and 5 years. It consists of elevation of the sternum and costal cartilages after appropriate incisions.

Physiological Hypertrophy of Breast.

The breasts of many newborn babies of both sexes undergo some enlargement during the first week of life (Fig. 147), and this may be accompanied by the excretion of fluid which

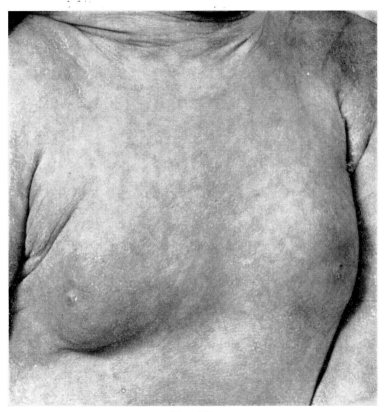

Fig. 147
Enlargement of breasts in the newborn.

resembles colostrum or milk. This condition is often erroneously referred to as mastitis neonatorum. It is only a response to maternal hormones which have crossed the placental barrier, the breast changes being precipitated by the withdrawal of maternal œstrogen with birth. The engorged breasts require no treatment and the swelling usually subsides within a few days.

Bacterial infection of the engorged breasts may lead to a true mastitis (p. 40).

Pain and swelling of the breast also occur in male and female children between the ages of 7 and 14 years. The condition is usually unilateral and there is a firm tender button-like swelling under the areola. There is no satisfactory

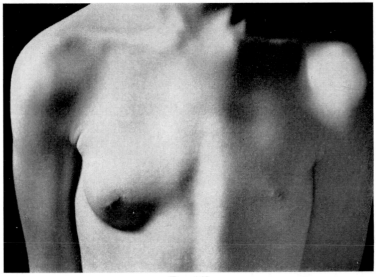

Fig. 148
Enlargement of one breast in boy of 9 years.

explanation for this condition and it subsides spontaneously within six to eighteen months. The tender part should be protected from friction and from the pressure of braces. (The condition is also seen in adolescent males, and young Service recruits may have to be excused the wearing of webbing equipment.) *Gynæcomazia* (hypertrophy of the male breast) may be unilateral (Fig. 148) or bilateral. For psychological reasons the breast should be excised.

INJURIES TO THE CHEST

Non-penetrating Injuries.

These vary from simple contusion of the chest wall to gross damage to the lung, heart and great vessels. In children, although the flexible chest wall permits severe visceral injuries without fracture, ribs may be fractured by a direct blow or in a crush injury. Although serious damage is rare, such injuries may be complicated by *subcutaneous emphysema* (Fig. 149), *pneumothorax* or *hæmothorax*. *Traumatic asphyxia* may follow compression of the thorax. There is sudden over-distension of the valveless veins with swelling and purple suffusion of the skin of the face, head, neck and shoulders. Subconjunctival and

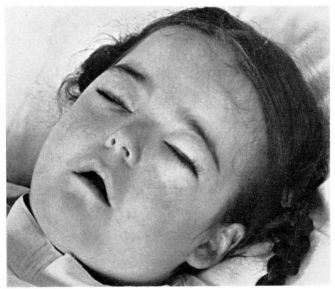

FIG. 149
Surgical emphysema in a girl of 5 years.

submucous hæmorrhage may occur. The swelling and discoloration pass off within a few days and no treatment is required.

Treatment.—The treatment of non-penetrating injuries of the chest is usually conservative. The child is propped up and a sedative such as opoidine is given to relieve pain. Oxygen may be required if the patient is cyanosed or if there is severe respiratory embarrassment. In patients with pneumothorax it may be necessary to evacuate excess air through a needle. The patient is X-rayed as soon as the general condition permits ; a portable apparatus is used. Operation may be required later

18

for hæmothorax or empyema. In a run-over accident there may be such complications as fractured spine, rupture of the diaphragm or injury to abdominal viscera.

Penetrating Wounds of the Chest.

These injuries are uncommon in childhood but may follow a spike wound or fall from a tree, when a branch may cause a penetrating injury. When the wound opens the pleural cavity, there is immediate danger to life. If the child survives, hæmo-thorax and empyema are late complications. When the wound involves the lung there are the added risks of valvular pneumo-thorax and severe hæmorrhage. Wounds of the heart and great vessels usually cause rapidly fatal hæmorrhage.

Treatment.—It may be difficult to distinguish a spike wound localised to the chest wall from a valvular penetrating wound which does not admit air to the pleural cavity. In all cases penicillin is given and the superficial wound is cleansed, explored and sutured. If an effusion develops it must be aspirated and penicillin is then instilled.

Large wounds of the chest wall are rare in childhood, but an open pneumothorax will present the same urgent problems of closure as in the adult.

Fracture of the Ribs.

Rib fractures are usually due to a crush injury; general treatment of the child is the first concern and the fractures may be initially disregarded. Fractures due to a direct blow are usually greenstick. Adhesive strapping causes more discomfort than the fracture and a cotton elastic bandage is the only support required. A shoulder strap prevents the bandage from slipping down.

Fracture of the Sternum.

Fracture of the sternum may occur in children without an associated fracture of the spine. If there is displacement, closed reduction can be carried out under general anæsthesia by placing the patient in hyperextension and applying head and foot traction and digital pressure. In an old fracture, closed reduction is impossible and there is no indication for open reduction.

DISEASE OF THE RIBS AND STERNUM

Hæmatogenous Osteitis of Rib.

Pyogenic infection of a rib is not common, but when it does occur it may present serious diagnostic problems in the early stages. It is rarely possible to find the bone focus until the pus ruptures through the periosteum, and in the early stages one can only treat the septicæmia. The principles of treatment are as in osteitis elsewhere (Chap. V).

Tuberculosis of Ribs.

The disease occurs most commonly at the costo-chondral junction, but may also occur in the body of a rib. The onset is insidious and painless and the patient usually presents with a cold abscess. The diagnosis is confirmed by isolation of the tubercle bacilli following aspiration of the abscess, and before operation the patient is started on a course of streptomycin, P.A.S. and isoniazid. The abscess is incised and at the costo-chondral junction the diseased bone and cartilage are removed with a sharp curette. When the disease affects the body of a rib the affected segment is excised, taking great care to avoid damage to the pleura. In both sites the wound is closed without drainage.

Tuberculosis of the Sternum.

The disease commonly starts in the mid-point of the front of the sternum and there is usually a smooth painless swelling when the child is first seen. Antibiotics and chemotherapy are given as for tuberculosis of the ribs, the abscess is incised and its walls curetted.

EMPYEMA

Pus in the pleural cavity is usually secondary to pneumonia and the disease is now rarely seen in the surgical wards of a children's hospital. With the modern treatment of pneumonia pneumococcal empyema is rare, and when it occurs it responds well to antibiotics and aspiration. Staphylococcal and streptococcal infections in infancy also respond to repeated aspiration and chemotherapy. Surgical drainage is never required during the acute phase of the illness.

LUNG ABSCESS

Solitary lung abscess is a rare sequel to pneumonia (Fig. 150). Multiple small abscesses are not uncommon in staphylococcal bronchopneumonia. An abscess may arise from infection round a foreign body such as a fragment of tooth or tonsil in a bronchus.

A localised abscess usually forms in the periphery of the

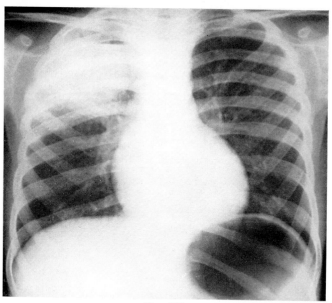

Fig. 150
Lung abscess in right upper lobe.

lung. At first it is a closed cavity, but it may rupture into a bronchus and pus is coughed up. If drainage is free the cavity may heal. When drainage is inadequate the abscess becomes chronic. Infection may leak into the pleural cavity with formation of empyema of a grave type.

Clinical Features.—There is a severe illness with high temperature, toxæmia and a troublesome cough. There may be localised dullness on clinical examination. The diagnosis is confirmed by radiography (Fig. 151, A and B).

Treatment.—When an inhaled foreign body is responsible,

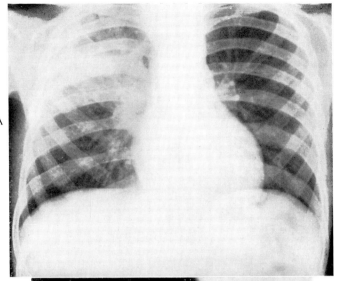

A

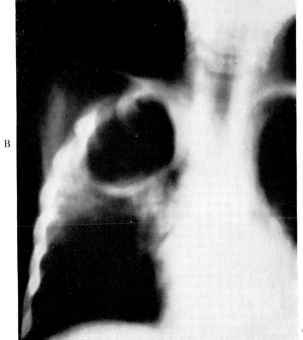

B

Fig. 151

A, Lung abscess after aspiration.
B, Confirmed by tomography

18 A

bronchoscopy and removal of the obstruction is undertaken. If free drainage can be established by way of the bronchi, most cases will recover spontaneously and completely with coincident antibiotic therapy. If the condition is of long standing, surgical drainage to the exterior or segmental resection of lung may be necessary.

BRONCHIECTASIS

The disease may be a sequel to bronchopneumonia compli-cating measles or whooping cough, it may follow virus infection

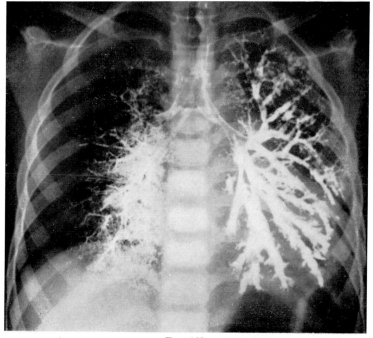

FIG. 152
Bronchiectasis.

of the bronchial lymphatic tissue, and it may occasionally follow inhalation of a foreign body into a bronchus. Inflam-matory destruction of the mucous membrane will lead to permanent bronchial dilatation.

The disease is chronic and the main features are attacks of

coughing followed by the expectoration of large quantities of foul-smelling pus. Clubbing of the fingers is only marked in patients with severe toxæmia and long-standing pulmonary suppuration. The diagnosis is confirmed by radiography following intratracheal instillation of lipiodol which outlines the dilated bronchi (Fig. 152), and indicates the lung segments involved.

Treatment.—Most cases are treated palliatively with good effect by postural drainage, physiotherapy and open-air treatment. Aerosol penicillin appears to help a few patients. In patients who are gravely handicapped in spite of conservative treatment, surgical procedures include *segmental resection, lobectomy* and *pneumonectomy,* to excise the permanently diseased lung tissue.

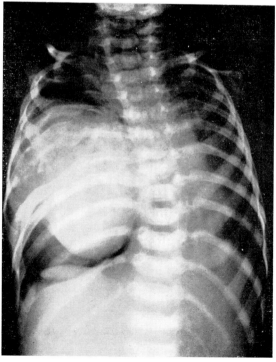

FIG. 153

Ganglioneuroma of right thorax, confirmed at operation.

CYSTS AND PRIMARY TUMOURS OF THE THORAX

Cysts and tumours of the thorax are not common in child-hood and in our limited experience the following have been encountered : *neuroblastoma, ganglioneuroma* (Fig. 153), *cystic hygroma, teratoma* and *duplication of the œsophagus*. Lesions reported from other children's hospitals include thymoma, bronchogenic cyst and neuro-enteric cyst. These conditions can be dealt with by thoracotomy.

The clinical features of thoracic cysts and tumours are various and include dyspnœa, cough and failure to gain weight. Radiographic examination reveals the intrathoracic mass, but the differential diagnosis may be difficult. Rarely there may be obstruction of the trachea or superior vena cava, and in one of our patients investigation of paraplegia led to the discovery of a thoracic neuroblastoma invading the spine.

CONGENITAL HERNIA OF THE DIAPHRAGM

Hernia of the diaphragm is not uncommon in the newborn. The diagnosis should be readily made by physical examination and can be confirmed by radiography. Most of these infants can be cured by early operation. If operation is not performed, 75 per cent. die before they are a month old.

Embryology.—The ventral diaphragm is formed from the *septum transversum* which separates the heart from the abdominal viscera. Mesoderm from the dorsal mesentery then bridges the cœlomic cavity from front to back, leaving openings in the postero-lateral parts of the diaphragm—*pleuroperitoneal canals*. These canals are closed by a double-layered membrane consisting of peritoneum below and pleura above. Striated muscle then develops between these serous layers. If arrest occurs in the early stage of this complicated developmental process there is free communication between the pleural cavity and the abdomen. If arrest in development occurs later, a thin hernial sac comprising both layers is present.

Congenital hernia may occur in several areas of the diaphragm :—

1. **Postero-lateral** (usually left)—that is, through the pleuro-peritoneal hiatus or foramen of Bochdalek.

2. **Œsophageal hiatus hernia.**
3. **Retrosternal hernia** (foramen of Morgagni).
4. **Antero-lateral**—a rare site for hernia.

Postero-lateral Hernia.—This is by far the most common type of diaphragmatic hernia which requires surgical repair in infancy and childhood. There is usually no hernial sac and the pleural cavity is filled to its apex with intestine and colon and, depending on the side involved, liver or stomach and spleen.

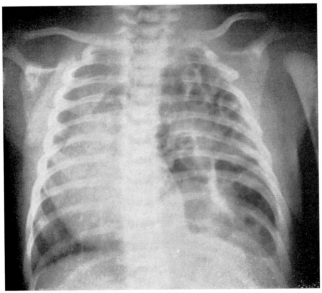

FIG. 154
Diaphragmatic hernia. Bowel in left thorax and heart displaced to right.

The lung on the affected side is collapsed and the heart is pushed to the opposite side.

Clinical Features.—The symptoms may be respiratory, circulatory or digestive. In a neonate with *cyanosis, dyspnœa* and *vomiting* the presence of diaphragmatic hernia must always be considered. Cyanosis may be improved by nursing the baby lying on the affected side in an incubator or oxygen tent. The pulse and respiration rates are increased, the affected side of the chest moves poorly and on percussion there may be dullness or tympanicity. On auscultation the breath sounds are diminished or absent. If gurgling is heard the diagnosis is obvious. The diagnosis is confirmed by radiography (Fig. 154). Administration of barium is dangerous and unnecessary.

Treatment.—Surgery should be undertaken within ten days

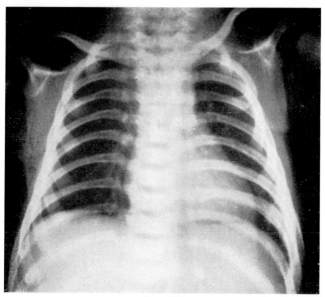

FIG. 155
Post-operative appearance in infant shown in Figure 154.

of birth, preferably within the first forty-eight hours, while the bowel is still empty of gas.

1. *Abdominal Approach.*—In the young infant it is easier to pull the viscera down from below. The edge of the ring is denuded and the aperture closed with silk. As in operation for a large exomphalos (Chap. XII) it may occasionally be advisable to adopt a two-stage closure of the abdominal wall (Fig. 155).

2. *Thoracic Approach.*— In older children there may be adhesions within the thoracic cavity and the operation may be more easily performed from above.

Retrosternal Hernia.—A hernial sac is present in 50 per cent. of retrosternal herniæ. Displacement of viscera is not so extensive as in the postero-lateral hernia. Symptoms are vague and are usually due to compression of some hollow viscus. The diagnosis is not usually made until the children are older, and radiography with a barium meal or even a barium enema may be necessary to confirm the diagnosis.

Treatment.—The hernia may be repaired through either a thoracic or abdominal approach.

Antero-lateral Hernia.—In this rare type of hernia symptomatology is similar to that of retrosternal hernia. Repair is most easily performed through the thorax.

Hiatus Hernia.

1. **Sliding hiatus hernia.**
2. **Para-œsophageal hernia.**

In both types of hiatus hernia in infancy there may be reflux of gastric contents with *œsophagitis, dysphagia, hæmatemasis* or *melæna*. It may be possible to differentiate the two types only by radiography following a barium swallow. In the sliding hiatus hernia a portion of the stomach is drawn upwards above the diaphragm by an œsophagus which appears to be shorter than normal (the so-called congenitally short œsophagus) (Fig. 156). In para-œsophageal hernia the œsophagus is of normal length and a portion of the fundus of the stomach is prolapsed alongside it. In both types of hiatus hernia a sac is always present. It may be possible to diagnose œsophagitis by radiography, and the diagnosis may be confirmed by œsophagoscopy.

Treatment.—Occasionally surgery may be called for in the early weeks of life owing to severe œsophagitis which may lead to stenosis and severe dysphagia. A gastrostomy may be necessary to put the lower œsophagus at rest and to save life. In most cases relief from symptoms can be obtained by feeding the baby in the sitting position as in cardio-œsophageal chalazia (Chap. VII). If the symptoms are severe operation is performed through a left thoracic approach. The results of operation in the para-œsophageal type of hernia are satisfactory, but a good result does not always follow repair of a sliding hiatus hernia

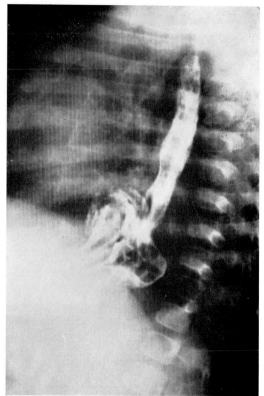

Fig. 156
Sliding hiatus hernia with œsophagitis.

in infancy. Of those patients who outgrow their symptoms without surgical intervention, some will probably require surgery in later adult life.

CONGENITAL LOBAR EMPHYSEMA

Breathlessness in a baby may be due to respiratory infection, diaphragmatic hernia, cardiac failure, vascular compression of the trachea (p. 309) and rarely, to *congenital emphysema of the lung*. In this syndrome the left upper lobe is most frequently affected. The condition is due to valvular obstruction, either from deficiency in the cartilaginous rings of the bronchi or caused by mucosal valves.

Clinical Features.—The usual symptoms are cough, stridor and difficulty in feeding due to breathlessness. Cyanosis is rare. Breath sounds are diminished, there is hyper-resonance on percussion and there is usually mediastinal displacement.

Radiography reveals downward displacement of the diaphragm and the distended lung herniates across the midline and shows increased translucency.

Treatment.—Paracentesis may occasionally bring about temporary relief but needling may lead to tension pneumothorax. Early thoracotomy should be performed and, when the chest is opened, the affected lobe does not collapse. The treatment is lobectomy.

HEART AND GREAT VESSELS

In recent years the surgery of congenital cardiovascular anomalies has excited widespread interest, and with the introduction of hypothermia and the artificial heart-lung machine the field has widened greatly. More then ever, precise methods of investigation are required to provide accurate anatomical and physiological information on the anomalies. The clinical findings of a skilled cardiologist are augmented by radiography, angiocardiography and cardiac catheterisation.

We shall consider here only the common and well-known deformities whose treatment is well established.

Patent Ductus Arteriosus.

During fœtal life the ductus arteriosus carries the greater part of the blood from the right ventricle direct to the descending aorta, by-passing the lungs. After birth the muscular ductus contracts as the lungs expand with the first breath and right ventricular blood is diverted to the pulmonary arteries. Expansion of the lungs leads to increased flow of oxygenated blood to the left atrium through the pulmonary veins.

When the ductus persists instead of fibrosing into the ligamentum arteriosum, high pressure in the aorta causes blood to flow from the aorta into the pulmonary artery. There is in fact an arteriovenous fistula and between 45 per cent. and 75 per cent. of the output of the left ventricle may be lost (Fig. 157). This leads to dilatation of the pulmonary artery and later to atherosclerosis. The right ventricle hypertrophies, as does the left ventricle, to compensate for the atrioventricular shunt.

The prognosis is not good. Physical development is usually retarded and most of the patients die before the age of 25 years from heart failure, infective endocarditis or occasionally from rupture of the ductus itself. There is no cyanosis in this type of anomaly. On auscultation the typical machinery murmur is heard, louder in systole. There is a low diastolic pressure with a high pulse pressure. On palpation a thrill is felt at the base of the heart. The radiographic appearances are variable, but there is sometimes fullness of the pulmonary artery. It is often impossible to hear a murmur in infancy because the aortic pressure is low and pulmonary pressure high and there is no appreciable flow through the ductus.

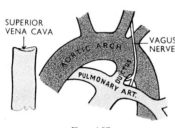

Fig. 157

Patent ductus arteriosus.

Treatment.—It is unusual for the diagnosis to be made in the first year or two of life, but a patent ductus may cause death from heart failure in the neonatal period and operation is occasionally called for in a small infant. After the age of 1 year there are no technical operative difficulties. Under general endotracheal anæsthesia the left chest is opened through either an antero-lateral or a posterior approach through the third interspace. The ductus is displayed by gentle dissection between the aortic arch and the pulmonary artery. After the ductus has been completely freed it is trebly ligated or divided and sutured.

Coarctation of the Aorta (Fig. 158).

Coarctation is a narrowing of the aorta and constrictions can occur anywhere from the midpoint of the arch down to the bifurcation of the vessel. In 98 per cent. the constriction is in the first part of the descending aorta.

The diagnosis of coarctation is rarely made in early

childhood, but the anomaly may present as cardiac failure in the neonatal period. The clinical picture, which includes breathlessness on sucking and choking attacks, may resemble that of mechanical feeding difficulty. In later life coarctation leads to serious complications or even death in most cases. Twenty-five per cent. live to a reasonable age; some die of bacterial endocarditis between the ages of 30 and 35 years; in others, sudden death occurs from rupture of the aorta between the ages of 20 and 30 years; in the remainder, death occurs from hypertension about the age of 40 years. The average age at death is 35 years. The condition is twice as common in males as in females. The diagnosis is made by the disparity in the pulse in the arms and legs. Blood-pressure is normally 20 to 40 mm. higher in the legs than in the arms, but in coarctation it is much lower in the legs. In children with coarctation, blood-pressure in the arm may be normal

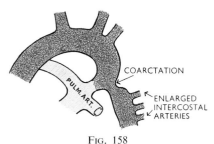

FIG. 158
Coarctation of aorta.

or only slightly elevated, but in older people there is usually hypertension. There is no characteristic cardiac murmur, but there is usually a systolic murmur over the præcordium. An electrocardiographic tracing does not help in the recognition of coarctation, but it may show evidence of myocardial strain. Radiography may show generalised cardiac enlargement, notching of the aorta and, after the age of 8 or 10, notching of the ribs from enlargement of the intercostal arteries. The exact position of the stricture and its length may be seen by angiocardiography using 70 per cent. Diodrast intravenously.

Treatment.—The optimum age for operation is during the first eighteen years of life before hypertension has caused irreversible changes in the arteries; operation is rarely of value after the age of 30 years. Coarctation of the aorta may present as cardiac failure in infancy. Following emergency medical treatment (digitalisation and salt-free milk feeds), successful resection has been performed in the neonatal period. The chest is opened through the fourth left interspace and the aorta and great vessels are mobilised. After clamping the aorta above and below, the narrow segment is excised and end-to-end anastomosis performed using very fine silk. If the gap is too great for end-to-end closure a graft is inserted.

Tetrad (Tetralogy) of Fallot.

In patients who survive infancy Fallot's tetrad is the most common of the anomalies of the heart and great vessels causing cyanosis. The tetrad consists of :—

1. *Pulmonary stenosis.* 2. *Intraventricular septal defect* (the aortic valve usually straddles this opening). 3. *Overriding of the aorta* (the aorta thus receives blood from both the right and left ventricles). 4. *Hypertrophy of the right ventricle.* There may be associated deformities such as patent ductus arteriosus, right-sided aorta and intra-auricular septal defect.

Clinical Features.—There is cyanosis from birth, increased by crying, straining or exercise. These children assume a squatting position but the reason for the assumption of this position is not understood. There may be spontaneous intra-vascular thrombosis due to sluggish circulation. The diagnosis is confirmed by radiography and cardiac catheterisation.

Treatment.—The optimum age for operation is between 4 and 14 years.

1. When the aorta is on the right side a Blalock operation is performed. The subclavian artery is anastomosed end to side to the pulmonary artery.

2. If the descending aorta is on the left a Pott's anastomosis is made between the aorta and the left pulmonary artery.

3. A direct attack may be made on the obstruction in the pulmonary valve or infundibulum by Brock's valvulotomy or infundibulectomy.

Double Aortic Arch.

Normally the aortic arch passes in front and to the left of the trachea and then proceeds as the descending aorta. In double aortic arch the ascending aorta bifurcates, one branch passing in front and to the left of the trachea ; the other to the right and posterior aspect of the œsophagus. Both then join to form the descending aorta (Fig. 159). Commonly the anterior arch is the smaller and can be safely divided.

Clinical Features.—There is difficulty in swallowing, crowing respirations and stridor. The baby tends to lie with the head extended. Radiography following a barium swallow shows indentation of the posterior wall of the œsophagus at the level of the third or fourth dorsal vertebra. Following instillation of lipiodol into the trachea a lateral view shows narrowing in the lower third.

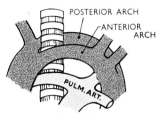

Fig. 159
Double aortic arch.

Treatment.—Through a left thoracotomy the thymus is removed and the great vessels exposed. The anterior arch is divided between the left common carotid and the left subclavian artery.

CHAPTER XVIII

The Head

Cephalic Meningocele.

A cephalic meningocele consists of a protrusion of meninges through a congenital defect in the skull. The most common situation is the occipital region (Fig. 160). There is a tense, rounded, pedunculated swelling present at birth. The swelling may be translucent and there may be an expansile impulse when the infant cries. A small occipital meningocele may lose its internal communication and it then resembles a dermoid cyst. Less commonly, a meningocele may present at the root of the nose or in connection with the anterior fontanelle. If a portion of the brain is included in the swelling it is called an *encephalocele* (Fig. 161), and should the protrusion contain part of a ventricle, it is known as a *hydrencephalocele*. In these more serious anomalies the child may be stillborn or may succumb at an early age. Should such a child survive, some degree of idiocy is almost inevitable.

Treatment.—The broad principles of treatment of meningocele are considered in Chapter XXI. Although the prognosis must always be guarded the results of surgical excision of simple cephalic meningocele are moderately good.

CIRCULATION OF CEREBROSPINAL FLUID

Cerebrospinal fluid is produced mainly by the choroid plexuses of the lateral ventricles. It circulates from the lateral ventricles through the foramen of Monro into the third ventricle in the posterior fossa. It passes thence into the subarachnoid space by way of the two lateral foramina (Luschka) and into the cisterna magna through the foramen of Magendie. The fluid is absorbed through the arachnoid villi and granulations —mainly in the skull but partly in the spinal canal. Some understanding of this circulation is important in hydrocephalus and in cerebral injury.

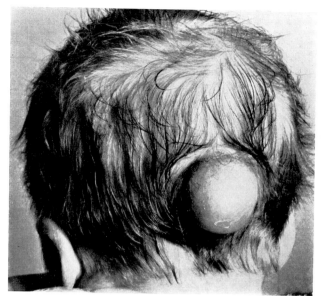

FIG. 160
Occipital meningocele.

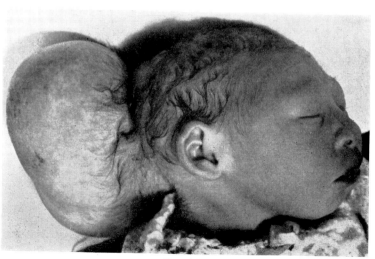

FIG. 161
Encephalocele.

Any obstruction in the main fluid pathways inside or outside the ventricular system may lead to hydrocephalus in which there is excess fluid within the ventricular system or over the surface of the brain.   Any increase in the volume of the brain, *e.g.* following trauma, may compress the subarachnoid spaces, impair circulation and absorption of cerebrospinal fluid and thus increase intra-ventricular pressure.

HYDROCEPHALUS

In *congenital internal hydrocephalus* there may be a defect in the aqueduct or in the foramina of the fourth ventricle (non-

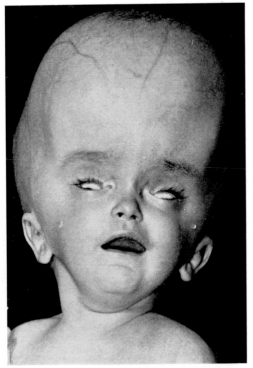

FIG. 162
Hydrocephalus.

communicating); or in the subarachnoid space or cisterna, when the fluid in the ventricles communicates with the lumbar fluid. Most cases of congenital hydrocephalus belong to the " communicating " type, and there is no agreement about the means by which the condition is produced.

Hydrocephalus may also occur in association with meningocele (Chap. XXI) and in such cases there is likely to be an associated malformation of the cerebellum and medulla. In this *Arnold-Chiari malformation* the cerebellum and medulla protrude through the foramen magnum with obstruction of the canal or subarachnoid space.

In later infancy and childhood hydrocephalus may be a sequel to meningitis. Inflammatory changes and adhesions interfere with the flow of cerebrospinal fluid.

Clinical Features. — Advanced hydrocephalus is easily recognised by the large skull, wide anterior fontanelle and separation of the sutures. The face looks very small, the eyes are displaced downwards and strabismus is common (Fig. 162). A variety of nervous signs and symptoms may be found— convulsions, mental deficiency, spastic paralysis, headache, optic atrophy, vomiting and nystagmus.

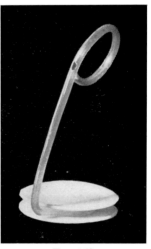

FIG. 163
Forrest plastic disc.

The *prognosis* varies with the cause of the hydrocephalus and with the severity of the condition. Severe and progressive primary hydrocephalus usually presents a hopeless problem, but some patients are relieved by early surgical intervention. Mild examples of the condition may remain stationary and the patient may reach adult life without gross mental or nervous disability. Established mental retardation and paralysis are not likely to benefit from surgical drainage.

Treatment.—The type of hydrocephalus is established by dye tests and by air encephalography. A ventriculogram shows the extent of ventricular dilatation.

In progressive cases the rate of enlargement may be temporarily diminished by repeated ventricular puncture. The operation of ventriculo-pharyngostomy has been abandoned and the present practice is to drain the cerebrospinal fluid from the lateral ventricle either into the subdural area by means of the Forrest plastic disc (Fig. 163) or into the peritoneal cavity through subcutaneous polythene tubing. Aqueduct blockage can be by-passed by a subcutaneous tube linking the lateral ventricles to the cisterna magna.

HEAD INJURIES

In the infant the suture lines of the skull are open and the cranium is to some extent elastic. This cushions the effect of a blow on the skull and thus protects the brain. In the older infant the sutures are closed, but ossification is incomplete and the skull is still elastic and the resilience provides some protection to the brain. In older children, after ossification is complete, the skull is rigid as in the adult and the effects of injury are very similar. In general, the presence of a cranial fracture in a child is of minor importance and there is often no evidence of the fracture apart from the X-ray films. A fracture assumes importance when it is compound or crosses an air sinus so that air or infection may be admitted into the cranial cavity or when it tears a blood vessel or nerve. The extent of the injury to the underlying brain is the governing factor in the management of all cranial injuries.

Birth injuries of the skull and brain are considered in Chapter III. Infants may fall from attendants' arms, from a high chair or from a bed. Head injuries are common in childhood from road accidents or following falls from a height.

Clinical Features.—The effects of head injury vary in severity with the stage of skull development and with the type of violence. There may be a period of unconsciousness (from seconds to hours) or there may be a lucid interval followed by delayed stupor or unconsciousness usually indicating subdural or extra-dural hæmorrhage. The duration of unconsciousness varies with the severity of the injury. Unconsciousness with pupillary changes, motor paralysis, changing blood-pressure, pulse and respiration indicate severe injury or hæmorrhage. A rising temperature follows brain-stem and hypothalamic injuries. Convulsions may indicate intracerebral or extracerebral hæmorrhage if there is no history of previous convulsions. Methods of localising cerebral lesions are the same as in the adult.

Treatment.—Observation of the state of consciousness is the key to management of closed head injuries. Treatment of shock improves extracerebral circulation. A free airway must be maintained to allow adequate oxygenation, and an oxygen tent may be required. Skeletal and visceral injuries must be recognised and treated; splinting of an injured limb, emptying of a distended bladder or application of a proper dressing may quieten a restless patient.

During the first twenty-four hours mild barbiturate sedatives may be necessary to calm an excited and restless patient. Pain is relieved by aspirin, and narcotics should rarely be used as they depress an already depressed brain. Pain from a fractured bone or other severe injury can usually be alleviated by codeine. Diagnostic lumbar puncture is rarely of practical value and any relief of intracranial pressure is only temporary and the procedure may promote further bleeding or result in a " pressure cone." Blood in the spinal fluid acts as a meningeal irritant and removal of blood-stained cerebrospinal fluid may be necessary but should be postponed for twenty-four hours. Intravenous hypertonic solutions are rarely used : although they may initially reduce intracranial pressure, the after effect is to increase pressure and brain volume above the original level. Food and fluid intake should meet physiological requirements and tube feeding may be required for the unconscious patient or parenteral fluid for those with excessive vomiting.

Many cases of head injury require some surgical treatment, varying from scalp suture to craniotomy. No scalp wound should be considered as trivial. The hair is clipped and the scalp widely shaved, and after thorough cleansing the wound is explored and repaired, under local anæsthesia if possible. Major elective surgical procedures are carried out in a neurosurgical unit. Subtemporal decompression should not be used indiscriminately for the relief of increased intracranial pressure and œdema. The brain herniates at the site of the decompression and additional brain damage may be caused. Defects in the skull following loss of bone in open or depressed fractures seldom need grafting in infants or children.

INTRACRANIAL SUPPURATION

As in the adult the various forms of intracranial suppuration described in this section are now rarely seen.

Extradural Abscess.—An abscess may form between the dura mater and the bone under a compound fracture. In this connection it should be remembered that fracture of the anterior fossa may involve the orbital plate and thus communicate with the nose. Extradural abscess is a rare complication of middle ear disease.

There are signs of toxæmia and there may be local pain. The infection may subside with antibiotic treatment, but it may be necessary to open the abscess.

Brain Abscess.—Abscess of the temporal lobe or cerebellum was once a dreaded complication of middle ear disease ; blood-borne brain abscess may follow such forms of intrathoracic suppuration as bronchiectasis and chronic empyema.

Such an abscess usually pursues a chronic course with impairment of cerebration but few localising signs. Treatment is by operation.

Sinus Phlebitis.—No infection of the lateral venous sinus or of the cavernous sinus has been encountered in the hospital since the introduction of antibiotics.

INTRACRANIAL TUMOURS

Intracranial tumours are not uncommon in infancy and childhood. They are mostly cerebellar and take the form of gliomata—cerebellar astrocytoma, medulloblastoma and ependymoblastoma. Rarely, craniopharyngioma, blood-vessel tumours and other varieties of glioma are found. The gliomata vary greatly in their malignancy—from the slow-growing astrocytoma to the vascular, rapidly growing medulloblastoma.

Clinical Features.—In infancy a tumour may attain large size before there is cerebral vomiting or papillœdema, as the open sutures delay the effect of increased pressure. In older children the sutures separate less readily and localising signs and evidence of increased intracranial pressure appear earlier. Early symptoms are headache and vomiting unrelated to feeding. Such features as hemiparesis or ataxia may be difficult to recognise or to interpret in the young child. Percussion of the skull may give a "cracked pot" sound. Radiography may reveal separation of sutures and ventriculography, air encephalography, cerebral angiography and electro-encephalography are all used to assist in diagnosis and localisation.

Treatment and prognosis depend on the nature and site of the tumour. The most favourable prognosis is in cerebellar astrocytoma : the prognosis is grave in medulloblastoma although cures have followed partial removal followed by radiotherapy.

RETINOBLASTOMA

This is the commonest orbital tumour in childhood. It is frequently bilateral and occurs within the first four years of life. Vision is interfered with, the pupil is dilated and the light reflex is bright yellow. There is marked proptosis and the tumour destroys the globe and grows back to involve the optic nerve. It is highly malignant. Early enucleation of the eye followed by radiation may save life, but the other eye may be subsequently affected.

CHAPTER XIX

Face, Mouth and Jaws

DEVELOPMENT OF THE FACE.—The face is formed from five processes which surround the stomodeum or future mouth : one fronto-nasal process, two maxillary processes and two mandibular processes (Fig. 164). The *fronto-nasal process* is divided into three by the olfactory pits : a *median nasal process* which forms the nasal septum, the philtrum of the upper lip and the premaxilla, and two *lateral nasal processes* which form the sides of the nose. The *maxillary processes* form the cheek and the entire upper lip apart from the central philtrum. The maxillary processes also form most of the

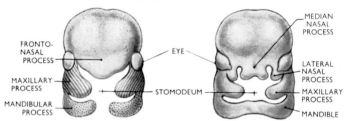

FIG. 164
Development of face.

upper jaw and the hard and soft palate apart from the premaxilla. The *mandibular processes* form the lower jaw. Defective fusion between the fronto-nasal process and the maxillary processes causes *cleft lip* and *cleft palate*. The very rare *median cleft lip* (true hare lip) is due to failure of fusion of the bulbous extremities of the median nasal process. Imperfect fusion of the maxillary and mandibular processes (usually unilateral) leads to *macrostoma* (Fig. 174) : excessive fusion of the processes causes *microstoma*.

Cleft lip may occasionally be associated with two small blind crypts in the lower lip (Fig. 165). The crypts are usually on the apices of nipple-like papillæ and they end blindly in the muscle of the lip. The walls are lined with squamous epithelium. Their ætiology is obscure and they are of no significance apart from their unsightly appearance, but these *inferior labial crypts*

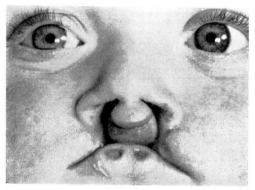

FIG. 165

Inferior labial crypts in an infant with bilateral cleft lip. Note wide separation of eyes (hypertelorism).

show a definite hereditary tendency. They should be excised before the child goes to school.

CLEFT LIP AND CLEFT PALATE

These anomalies occur in approximately 1 in 1,000 births and there is a family history of the deformity in 10 per cent. of patients. If one child is born with a cleft lip or palate the risk of a similar anomaly in future children of these parents is approximately 1 in 25.

The problems of cleft lip and cleft palate are so intimately connected that one condition cannot be discussed without the other. The deformities are usually divided into three groups :—

1. *Pre-alveolar cleft*, in which the lip or lip and nostril are involved.
2. *Alveolar cleft*, where the cleft involves lip, alveolar ridge and usually the palate.
3. *Post-alveolar cleft*, in which cleft is confined to the palate.

Pre-alveolar clefts may be complete or incomplete, and like alveolar clefts they may be unilateral or bilateral. Clefts are commonly accompanied by hypertelorism,

The aim of treatment is restoration of anatomical structure, correction of disfigurement, the provision of normal speech and improved function of deglutition and respiration.

Cleft Lip (Hare Lip).

The malformation may occur alone or in association with cleft palate. It varies from slight notching of the lip margin to right or left of the midline (Fig. 166), to a complete cleft running

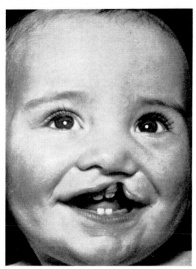

FIG. 166
Incomplete cleft lip.

up to the nostril. The alveolus may be cleft (Fig. 167) and the defect may extend back and communicate with a cleft palate. When the cleft is bilateral and complete the premaxilla is displaced forward (Fig. 168). In unilateral cases the nostril on the affected side is flattened (Fig. 167).

Treatment.—When the lip only is cleft, closure is carried out about the age of 3 months. There is rarely functional disability although feeding may be difficult at first and may call for the use of a large teat or spoon feeding. It is the disfigurement which requires early treatment as the parents are greatly distressed. Before operation is carried out a satisfactory feeding routine should be established and the infant should be

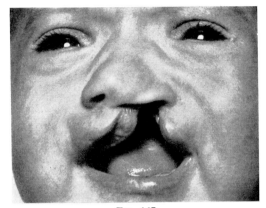

FIG. 167
Unilateral complete cleft lip showing
flattening of nostril.

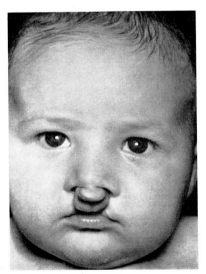

FIG. 168
Bilateral complete cleft lip.

in good condition, gaining weight and not anæmic.   Operation is always performed under antibiotic cover.   Tension on the suture line is relieved by the application of a modified Logan's

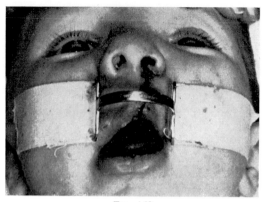

FIG. 169

Modified Logan's bow applied after closure of cleft lip.

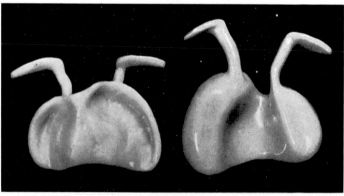

FIG. 170

One type of corrective prosthesis used to mould alveolus.

bow (Fig. 169), and light splints prevent exploring hands from reaching the wound.

Malalignment of the dental arch may be present at birth, and closure of a lip cleft over an arch thus deformed leads to an unsuccessful repair from both functional and æsthetic points of view. Lip closure may even produce further deformity, and this can take place very rapidly and during a few days following operation. Post-operative œdema may be sufficient to bring about further collapse of the already malformed dental arch. Early arch correction provides a sound foundation on which to close the lip and an æsthetically pleasing result follows the

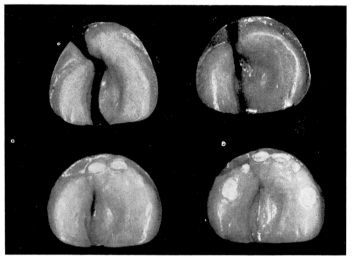

FIG. 171

Casts of palate and alveolus to show correction obtained by a series of corrective appliances.

primary operation. This treatment is conducted by a dental surgeon specialising in this problem, and dental supervision should begin when the baby is a few weeks old, using a series of intra-oral appliances (Fig. 170). These are constructed on models modified progressively towards the normal, and arch alignment is usually satisfactory by the time the infant is 3 months old (Fig. 171).

Cleft Palate.

The two halves of the palate fuse from before back and the last parts to fuse are the two halves of the uvula. Incomplete fusion may involve (1) the uvula only—*bifid uvula*; (2) soft palate only (Fig. 172, A); (3) the soft palate and hard palate (Fig. 172, B); (4) soft and hard palate with unilateral cleft of the alveolus—usually associated with unilateral cleft lip (Fig. 172, c) ; (5) soft and hard palate with bilateral cleft alveolus, usually associated with bilateral cleft lip (Fig. 172, d). Cleft palate unassociated with cleft lip shows a low familial incidence.

Clinical Features.—Both feeding and speech require an efficient nasopharyngeal mechanism. Regurgitation of feeds

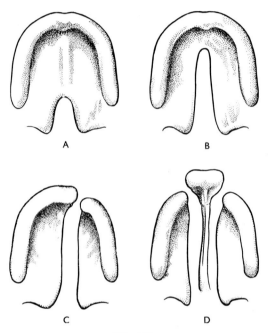

FIG. 172

Types of cleft palate. A, Cleft of soft palate (Veau I deformity). B, Cleft of soft and hard palate (Veau II). C, Cleft of soft and hard palate and alveolus (Veau III). D, Cleft palate and bilateral cleft of alveolus (Veau IV).

from the mouth into the nose interferes with feeding and may lead to malnutrition and nasopharyngeal infection. Later, the defect leads to difficulty in phonation and is responsible for the characteristic speech defect. Atrophic rhinitis is common and infection can readily enter the auditory tube and lead to deafness.

Treatment.—Operation is essential to provide a soft palate sufficiently long and mobile to meet the posterior pharyngeal wall, thus permitting closure of the sphincter between the nasopharynx and oropharynx. A mobile soft palate of adequate length must be provided before the child starts to talk, otherwise faulty speech habits may be acquired. Should such habits become well established they cannot always be corrected by speech therapy. Surgical closure of the palate is therefore performed about the age of 15 months. Early feeding difficulties are overcome by spoon feeding or by special flanged teats, and care is taken to avoid regurgitation or choking. Before operation a careful examination should be made for infection of the middle ear, antra, tonsils and teeth and appropriate treatment is given. Admission to hospital a day or two before operation is advised so that the child may become used to the nursing and feeding routine. Surgery is performed under antibiotic cover. After operation the arms are lightly splinted to prevent the child exploring his mouth. The post-operative diet consists of glucose drinks and soft foods and a drink of water is given after all food and drinks for ten days after operation. Hard sweets and hard foods are not allowed for two or three weeks.

If, after operation, speech is not satisfactory by the age of 3 years, suitable training is given by a speech therapist. Good speech demands more than an efficient mechanism, and a good surgical closure may yield disappointing speech results in an unintelligent child with unco-operative parents. On the other hand, it is astonishing how well a child may speak with an unrepaired or poorly repaired palate.

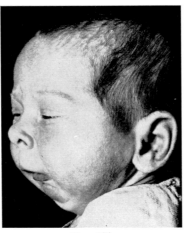

Fig. 173

Micrognathia. Baby has Veau II cleft palate—Pierre Robin syndrome.

Micrognathia.

Hypoplasia of the lower jaw (Fig. 173) is a not un-common cause of death from asphyxia in the early days or weeks of life. The anomaly may be associated with a wide cleft of the soft and hard palates and the poorly fixed tongue tends to fall back into the palatal gap and interfere with feeding and breathing (Pierre Robin syndrome). The infant should be nursed on his face and fed by means of a spoon or

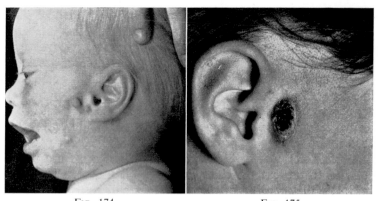

FIG. 174   FIG. 175

Fig. 174.—Accessory auricles and macrostoma.
Fig. 175.—Excoriation at opening of pre-auricular sinus.

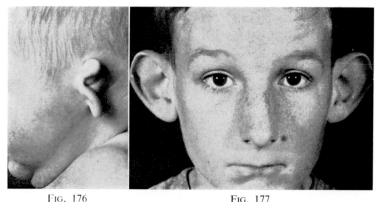

FIG. 176   FIG. 177

Fig. 176.—Maldevelopment of ear.
Fig. 177.—Bat ears.

naso-œsophageal tube. Should the baby survive for two months the disability becomes less, the shape of the mandible improves and the patient is usually fit for palate repair at the age of 15 months. For æsthetic reasons plastic operation to the mandible may occasionally be required in later life.

Supernumerary auricles are common (Fig. 174) and should be excised with their central core of cartilage. *Pre-auricular sinus* is less common. The opening is usually found at the root of the helix and a blind-ending tract runs downwards and slightly forwards. The sinus may become infected (Fig. 175) or, if its opening is occluded, a cyst may form. Treatment is excision of the sinus. *Under-development of one ear* is not uncommon. No satisfactory treatment can be carried out in early childhood (Fig. 176). *Bat Ears.*—Marked protrusion of the ears, particularly in a boy (Fig. 177), can lead to a life of misery at school. Plastic repair should be carried out before school age.

External Angular Dermoid. —Dermoid cysts may form in any of the fusion lines of the skull or face but the most common site is at the outer angle of the orbit (Fig. 178). This cyst may lie in a little depression in the skull. Secondary pyogenic infection may occur. The cyst should be excised any time after the age of 3 months.

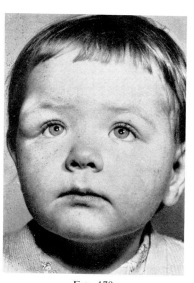

Fig. 178

Right external angular dermoid.

Tongue Tie.—A congenitally short frenulum of the tongue is not uncommon, but it rarely prevents a child from learning to speak normally. If the tongue cannot be protruded beyond the teeth the frenulum may be divided transversely under general anæsthesia. After adequate hæmostasis the wound is sutured longitudinally with chromic catgut. A snip with scissors without anæsthesia is both dangerous and ineffective.

Short Frenulum of the Upper Lip.—This deformity is invisible and rarely causes disability (Fig. 179). In later life it may lead to a wide gap between the central incisor teeth (Fig. 180). If the frenulum extends between the incisor teeth it should be excised completely under local or general anæsthesia.

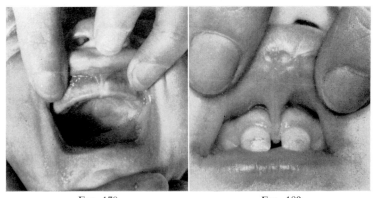

Fig. 179   Fig. 180

Fig. 179.—Frenulum of upper lip in infant.
Fig. 180.—Upper lip frenulum with gap between central incisors.

Ranula.—There is a soft translucent bluish swelling in the floor of the mouth, usually confined to one side of the frenulum of the tongue (Fig. 181). The condition must be distinguished

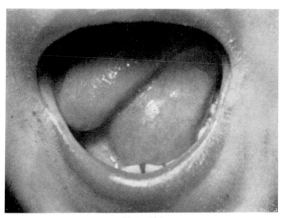

Fig. 181
Ranula.

from the firmer, opaque *sublingual dermoid*. Occasionally a ranula is subject to recurrent attacks of infection which makes the tongue protrude and leads to difficulty in swallowing. An attempt is made to dissect out the lining of the cyst but complete removal is difficult and recurrence is common.

Recurrent Swelling of the Parotid Gland.—Recurrent painful enlargement of a parotid gland is not uncommon in childhood. The condition is usually unilateral. It is never due to a calculus. The swelling may subside spontaneously in a day

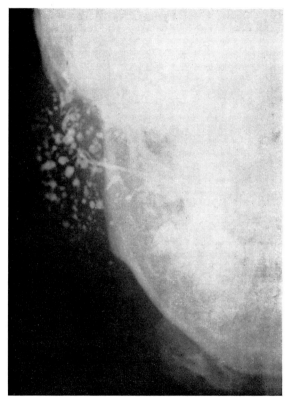

Fig. 182
Parotid sialogram showing sialectasis.

or two but it may persist for several weeks. Sometimes the orifice of the duct is congested and a little turbid fluid may be expressed. The condition may be relieved by canalising the duct with a fine cannula or it may subside after instilling penicillin into the duct. A sialogram may show obstruction of the duct or sialectasis (Fig. 182). If recurrence of the painful swelling persists after repeated attempts at canalisation, the

20

condition may be cured by treating the gland by deep X-ray therapy.

Recurrent enlargement of the submaxillary salivary gland is rare in childhood.

Osteitis of the Jaws.—The *maxilla* is the most common site for hæmatogenous osteitis in infancy (*vide* p. 44). There is swelling and redness under the eye and the lids may become

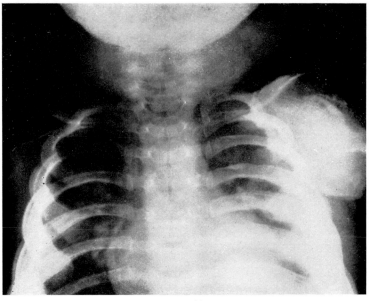

FIG. 183

Infantile cortical hyperostosis showing lesions in mandible, ribs and left scapula.

swollen so that the condition simulates orbital cellulitis. The organism is usually a staphylococcus resistant to penicillin, but the infection commonly responds to the administration of tetracycline. The abscess may point in the hard palate, at the alveolus or over the lower orbital ridge. There are no recognisable radiographic changes in the infant and there is no damage to the permanent teeth. Surgical intervention is rarely necessary. In older children an abscess may arise at the root of a canine tooth and simulate osteitis. This alveolar abscess may burrow posteriorly and point in the midline of the hard palate or it may rupture into the antrum and pus may discharge down the nose. In these older children the organism is usually sensitive to penicillin.

The mandible is an uncommon site for acute hæmatogenous osteitis. When it does occur the patient is usually gravely ill and requires intensive treatment with penicillin or one of the wide-spectrum antibiotics. Sequestra form slowly and several operations may be required for their removal. Even after extensive sequestrum formation there is satisfactory regeneration of new bone and deformity is slight.

Low-grade osteitis of the mandible may follow an alveolar abscess (gumboil). Extraction of the offending tooth may arrest the condition, but the abscess may point in the alveolar sulcus or below the jaw.

In infancy, osteitis of the mandible is very rare, and swelling of the lower jaw with radiographic bone change is more likely to be due to *infantile cortical hyperostosis* (Fig. 183). See Chapter V.

FACIO-MAXILLARY INJURIES

Abrasions and *lacerations* of the face are common following blows, falls and road accidents. *A general anæsthetic is essential* for effective cleansing. Ingrained dirt can be removed with a sterile toothbrush. Meticulous suturing of lacerations should be carried out; the rich vascularity allows primary closure even eighteen or twenty-four hours after injury. Fractures of the facial bones are uncommon in children, but in open face injuries it is best to treat underlying fractures at the same time as the soft tissue injury.

MALAR HÆMATOMA.—Following a blow on the face over the malar bone the child may develop a black eye. As the discoloration and diffuse swelling subsides there is often a firm residual hæmatoma over the malar. This lump may take many weeks to disappear, and not infrequently a linear depression appears during the second week giving rise to an unsightly blemish (Fig. 184). This lesion is caused by bursting of the small-meshed subcutaneous fat, the skin remaining intact. The parents can be reassured that the linear depression will eventually disappear spontaneously.

20 A

FRACTURES.—The most common bone injuries are to the nose, mandible, maxilla and malar bones. Fractures of the nose are reduced with a rubber-sheathed instrument in the nose and finger manipulation externally. Severely comminuted fractures require supportive splinting of light intranasal packing of vaseline gauze. Mandibular fractures are diagnosed by disturbances in occlusion, and ecchymoses under the mucosa

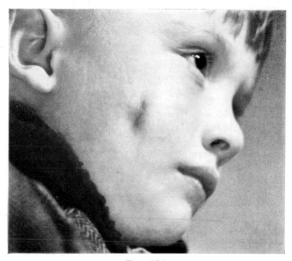

FIG. 184
Malar hæmatoma.

will point to the fracture site. Displacement of fragments is confirmed by radiography. Uncomplicated fractures of the body of the mandible are treated by manipulation and application of a barrel-type bandage and overlying plaster strips. More severe fractures are reduced under anæsthesia, and in older children the reduction is maintained by interdental loop wires at molar, canine and incisor positions. When only deciduous teeth are present, acrylic splints can be used. Mouth washes are used after feeding. Maxillary, malar and infraorbital fractures are treated as in the adult.

CHAPTER XX

The Neck

DEVELOPMENTAL ANOMALIES

PORTIONS of the branchial arches and branchial clefts may persist to give rise to several anomalies. The overgrown second branchial arch fuses with the fifth arch and the cervical sinus thus formed should disappear. If the sinus persists it will form a *branchial cyst*; should the second arch fail to fuse with the fifth, a *branchial fistula* will be formed.

The thyroglossal duct passes downwards exactly in the midline, from the foramen cæcum between the genioglossi to the upper border of the thyroid carti-lage. It then diverges to one or other side of the midline. At the hyoid bone the tract passes down in front of the bone then curves up behind the hyoid before con-tinuing down. The anomalies of persistence of the duct are *thyroglossal cyst* (Fig. 185), accessory and ectopic thyroid.

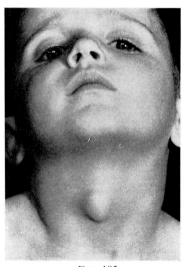

FIG. 185

Thyroglossal cyst.

Branchial Cyst is not com-monly seen in infancy but may become apparent during childhood. It usually lies beneath the upper third of the sternomastoid. The painless cystic swell-ing is difficult to differentiate from a tuberculous cervical gland. The cyst is removed through a transverse curvilinear incision.

Branchial Fistula.—The lesion is usually unilateral and the orifice may be found anywhere along the anterior border of the sternomastoid, usually in the lower third of the neck (Fig. 186). There may be irregular discharge of watery fluid and the tract may be demonstrated radiographically after instilling lipiodol (Fig. 187). The fistula should be excised before the child goes to school as it may be subject to recurrent infection. The operation constitutes an interesting anatomical exercise owing

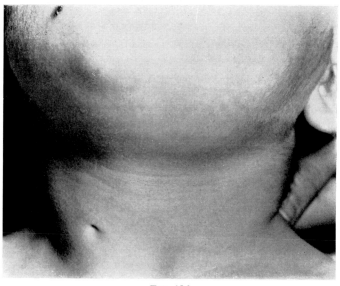

FIG. 186
Branchial fistula.

to the intimate relations of the tract to carotid vessels and the the glossopharyngeal and hypoglossal nerves as it ascends towards the tonsillar fossa.

Thyroglossal Cyst.—Cysts may occur anywhere in the line of the duct—above the thyroid cartilage, exactly central; below the thyroid cartilage, slightly to one side of the midline. They vary in size from a pea to a hazel-nut. They are subject to recurrent infection and may rupture spontaneously to form a *thyroglossal fistula* (Fig. 188). Thyroglossal fistula is never a developmental anomaly but follows rupture or incision of a thyroglossal cyst. The cyst moves up and down on deglutition or on protruding the tongue. Both cysts and fistulæ are removed

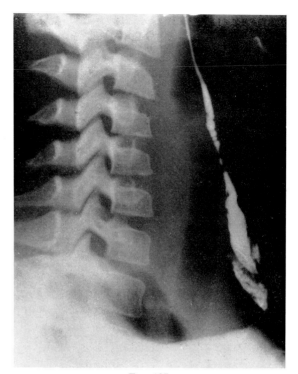

Fig. 187
Branchial fistula outlined with lipiodol.

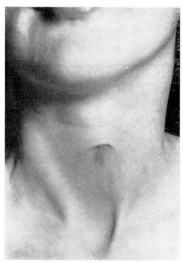

Fig. 188
Thyroglossal fistula.

through a collar incision, the central part of the hyoid bone being removed along with the tract which is excised as high as the foramen cæcum of the tongue.

Before removing a cyst some clinicians administer radio-active iodine and, using a Geiger counter, make sure that the

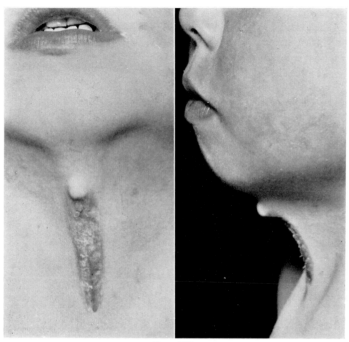

Fig. 189
Median cervical cleft.

swelling is not due to an ectopic thyroid which may be the only thyroid tissue present. This is not yet accepted surgical practice and the procedure is not without risk.

Midline Cervical Cleft.—This uncommon anomaly (Fig. 189) may be mistaken for a thyroglossal fistula. The lesion is excised by Z-plasty.

TORTICOLLIS (Wry Neck)

This anomaly is due to developmental hypoplasia of the head, face and neck. As a result of damage to the short sternomastoid during delivery, a tender swelling may be noticed in the lower third of the muscle, three or four weeks after birth—the so-called *sternomastoid tumour*. Untreated the swelling disappears spontaneously within three months, but the parents must be warned that a wry neck may develop in later childhood. In about half the cases the degree of torticollis is slight or negligible and many patients with torticollis give no history of a previous sternomastoid tumour.

Clinical Features.—In a fully developed case of congenital torticollis (Fig. 190) the head is flexed to the affected side while the face is rotated to the opposite side. The head and neck appear to be displaced towards the unaffected side. There is hemiatrophy of the head and face on the affected side. The fibrosed sternomastoid stands out as a tight band and can be made more prominent by tilting the head away from the affected side. Not uncommonly the child corrects the tilting of the head by dropping the shoulder on the opposite side, thus enabling the head to be held upright. The patient may thus present with the complaint of drooping of the shoulder, and only when the shoulders are brought level can one see that the deformity is secondary to a torticollis.

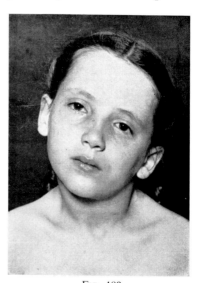

Fig. 190

Left-sided torticollis showing facial hemiatrophy.

The onset of the deformity is usually insidious and frequently first noticed by a neighbour or by a teacher when the child first goes to school. An infant has no real neck and the head sits almost directly on the shoulders. Only as the child grows and the neck forms about the age of 5 to 7 years does the short sternomastoid pull the head into the wry neck position (*vide* p. 4).

Differential Diagnosis.—In wry neck due to cervical hemi-vertebræ there is no definite tightness of the sternomastoid. " Rheumatic torticollis " may follow a seat in a draught; spasm of the sternomastoid from a tender underlying gland may cause a similar deformity. Compensatory cervical scoliosis may follow thoracic scoliosis or severe astigmatism. Spontaneous hyperæmic subluxation of the atlas (p. 342) presents as acute wry neck. Spasmodic wry neck (a variety of nervous tic) does not occur in childhood.

Treatment.—When a baby is found to have a sternomastoid " tumour " the mother is advised to carry the infant with the affected side towards her, and the cot is placed against a wall, so that to gaze around him the baby must stretch the short muscle. If torticollis does develop it is treated by open division of both heads of the sternomastoid through a small transverse incision just above the clavicle. Tight fascial bands are divided at the same time. In the female, preservation of the clavicular head may be justified to retain the proper outline of the neck. Following operation physiotherapy corrects the wry neck habit and helps to prevent recurrence. Neither subcutaneous tenotomy nor muscle slide of the sternomastoid off the mastoid process allows correction of the underlying tight bands of muscle and fascia.

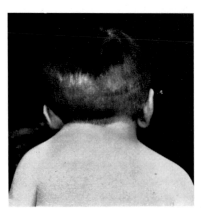

FIG. 191
Klippel-Feil deformity.

Klippel-Feil Syndrome.

This syndrome is characterised by fusion and partial absence of the upper cervical vertebræ giving an abnormally short neck and low hair line posteriorly (Fig. 191). Other developmental anomalies may be associated with the Klippel-Feil deformity : *webbing of the neck* (pterygium colli) can be improved by plastic surgery, but there is no satisfactory treatment of *congenital elevation of the scapula* (Sprengel's deformity).

CERVICAL LYMPHADENITIS

Inflammation of the lymph glands of the neck may be secondary to infection in the scalp, face, oral and nasal cavities or the external ear. In spite of systematic search the primary focus may not be found.

Acute Lymphadenitis.

The glands affected most commonly are in the anterior triangle or in the submandibular region (Fig. 17). The glands become fused together to form a firm tender mass. Discoloration of the skin and fluctuation are not apparent at once as the glands lie below the deep cervical fascia but suppuration is almost invariable in childhood. The offending organism is usually a penicillin-resistant staphylococcus. The constitutional upset varies greatly and is rarely affected by penicillin.

A kaolin poultice may be comforting while waiting for suppuration to become apparent. Pus is evacuated by inserting sinus forceps through a small skin incision.

Chronic Lymphadenitis.

Chronic non-tuberculous lymphadenitis may follow persistent low-grade infection in the catchment area. The affected glands vary in size from a pea to a grape and are only slightly tender on pressure. If the primary focus cannot be located and treated it may be difficult to eliminate the possibility of tuberculosis as a cause of the adenitis. The Mantoux reaction may be of help in the absence of prior B.C.G. vaccination.

Tuberculous Cervical Lymphadenitis.

The usual portal of entry is the tonsil, less commonly the adenoids. Extension upwards from lung infection and generalised tuberculous lymphadenopathy also occurs. The jugulo-digastric gland is usually involved but the infection also occurs in the glands of the posterior triangle, less commonly in the submental glands and occasionally in a gland in the suprasternal notch (Fig. 192). The affected glands show gradual, painless enlargement and at first remain discrete and rubbery. The infection may subside spontaneously at this point but the glands are more likely to undergo caseation and become adherent to the skin and subcutaneous tissue (Fig. 193).

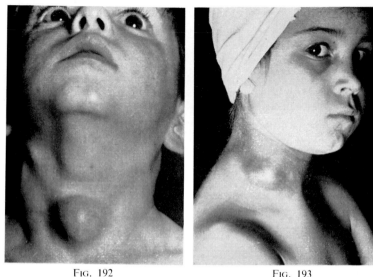

FIG. 192   FIG. 193

Fig. 192.—Tuberculous lymphadenitis (compare with Fig. 185).
Fig. 193.—Tuberculous lymphadenitis with involvement of skin.

Pain, sudden enlargement and reddening of the skin indicate secondary pyogenic infection. Caseating glands are now seldom allowed to rupture through the skin and the typical chronic sinus or depressed and adherent scar is rarely seen. The lesion may heal with calcification, which may be visible on X-ray.

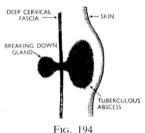

FIG. 194

Collar-stud abscess.

The diagnosis is usually easy, but chronic pyogenic lymphadenitis may simulate a tuberculous infection. A secondarily infected tuberculous adenitis may be mistaken for a simple acute cervical adenitis and incision and drainage may lead to a chronic discharging sinus. A collar-stud abscess may simulate a branchial cyst and the diagnosis is frequently confirmed only at operation. In the early stages lymphosarcoma, leukæmia and

Hodgkin's disease may enter into the differential diagnosis and a diagnostic biopsy may be called for.

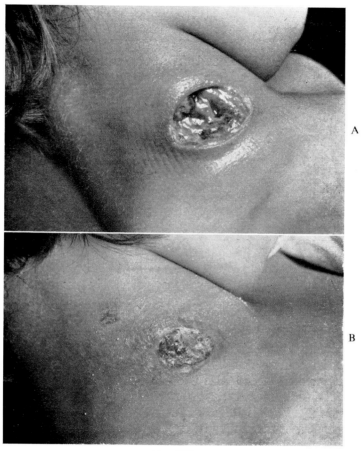

FIG. 195

A, Saucerisation of wound after removal of tuberculous gland which had involved skin (Fig. 193). B, Twelve days later. Soundly healed a month after operation.

Treatment.—Treatment is conservative in the early stages and removal of tonsils and adenoids should only be considered after the infection has subsided. If conservative treatment fails or if the glands caseate and infection penetrates the deep cervical fascia threatening the integrity of the skin, the affected glands should be expressed or excised. One must remember that the gland itself is below the deep cervical fascia and curettage of the superficial part of a collar-stud abscess will not eradicate the disease (Fig. 194). The opening in the fascia must be found and the gland removed. The skin wound is closed without drainage. If the skin is involved, the affected area of skin is excised and the wound closed without tension. If after removal of the diseased tissue primary suture is impossible, the wound should never be drained. All affected skin is cut away and the wound saucerised (Fig. 195, A). Healing will occur in a remarkably short time and with negligible scarring (Fig. 195, B).

When the wound is soundly healed the tonsils and adenoids are removed and sent for histological examination. If the tonsils are removed before excision of the cervical glands these may become infected from the raw tonsillar bed.

SPONTANEOUS HYPERÆMIC SUBLUXATION OF THE ATLAS

As this condition is almost invariably associated with inflammation in the neck, nasopharynx or near the base of the skull, it is convenient to consider it at this point. Our own cases have been associated with acute mastoiditis, pyogenic and tuberculous cervical adenitis and pyogenic infection of the cervical spine. Following inflammation in these areas the anterior arch of the atlas is decalcified, the attachment of the transverse ligament becomes insecure and the odontoid process is no longer held in close relationship to the arch of the atlas. Some slight trauma may be enough to avulse the ligament and the atlas is displaced forward. If the dislocation is complete sudden death will occur from pressure of the odontoid process on the cord. The excursion forward is, however, usually unilateral and spasm of the cervical muscles prevents the subluxation from becoming a complete dislocation. When the inflammatory process subsides recalcification takes place and spontaneous reduction may occur.

Clinical Features.—Shortly after such inflammatory lesions the child may present with the appearance of torticollis. There is an anxious expression on the patient's face. The head is held rigidly, slightly in front of the normal plane, tilted towards one shoulder and with the chin pointed to the opposite shoulder. There is no spasm of the sternomastoid muscle but any attempt at passive movement is resented. Radiography confirms the diagnosis.

Treatment.—The head and neck are immobilised between sand pillows or in a harness until the causal infection subsides. Spontaneous reduction may occur.

QUINSY (Peritonsillar Abscess)

Quinsy arises as a complication of acute tonsillitis. There is a unilateral boggy swelling bulging into the soft palate above the tonsil and displacing the uvula towards the opposite side. There is pyrexia, difficulty in swallowing, thick speech and pain radiating to the ear or down the neck.

Since the introduction of the sulphonamides quinsy has become a rare complication of acute tonsillitis. If an abscess forms, the child is placed with his neck fully extended and the head turned to the side so that pus cannot be inhaled and the abscess is evacuated with a guarded knife and sinus forceps.

RETROPHARYNGEAL ABSCESS

Acute suppuration may occur in the glands between the posterior pharyngeal wall and the prevertebral fascia, following tonsillitis or one of the fevers. There is high fever with dysphagia and dyspnœa. The swelling may be difficult to see in a young child, but it can always be palpated. If unrelieved the abscess may burst and flood the larynx and trachea. This condition also has become rare in recent years. When pus forms it is evacuated with the child lying on his side with the head down.

Chronic Retropharyngeal Abscess.—This condition may arise as a complication of tuberculosis of the cervical spine and the pus lies in front of the spine, but behind the prevertebral fascia. To avoid secondary pyogenic infection such an abscess should be opened through an incision behind the sternomastoid.

CHAPTER XXI

Spine and Pelvis

SPINA BIFIDA

THIS term is applied to a developmental gap in the vertebral column through which the contents of the spinal canal may protrude. Except in its simplest form (spina bifida occulta), it is usually a very grave anomaly and is commonly associated

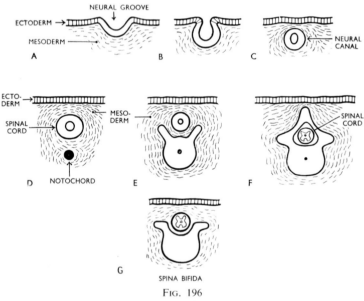

SPINA BIFIDA

FIG. 196

A to F, Development of vertebral column.

with anomalies of the spinal cord and paralysis of the lower limbs—both motor and sensory—with trophic and vasomotor changes in the skin and paralysis of the sphincters. There may be multiple developmental errors and many patients die at or soon after birth (Fig. 114).

The incidence in the general population is said to be 1 in

1,000 births. Having had one child with spina bifida, parents should be warned that the chance of the malformation appearing in any later child is approximately 1 in 40.

Embryology (Fig. 196).—Early in intra-uterine life the *neural groove* appears as a longitudinal furrow in the ectoderm on the

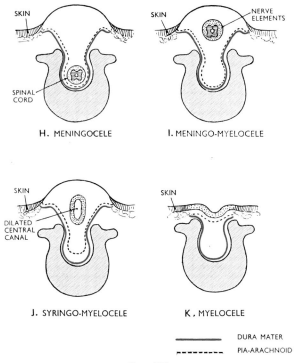

H. MENINGOCELE   I. MENINGO-MYELOCELE

J. SYRINGO-MYELOCELE   K. MYELOCELE

——————— DURA MATER
- - - - - - - - - PIA-ARACHNOID

FIG. 196
H to K, Types of spina bifida.

dorsal surface of the embryo. The edges of the furrow unite to form a tube from which the nervous system is developed. The tube becomes separated from the surface by mesoderm, and round the notochord the vertebral bodies develop. The developing vertebral arches fuse first in the thoracic region and fusion then extends up and down. Failure of fusion gives rise to spina bifida (Fig. 196, G) which is frequently associated with maldevelopment of the spinal cord and membranes (Fig. 196, H to K).

TYPES OF SPINA BIFIDA

1. **Spina Bifida Occulta.**—This is a common anomaly which is usually of no significance and is often discovered accidentally by radiography. Frequently only one vertebra (lumbar or sacral) is affected and there is no protrusion of cord or membranes. A local patch of hair, a nævus or a small depression on the lumbo-sacral region are suggestive of an underlying bone deficiency (Fig. 197). The condition rarely gives rise to symptoms in childhood. There is nothing to justify the belief that minor anomalies in spinal fusion have any causal relation to enuresis. In later childhood and adolescence neurological signs may appear, due to increasing tension produced at the site of the defect by disproportionate growth of vertebral column and spinal cord.

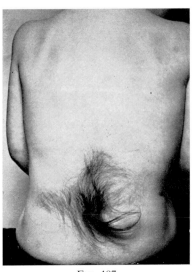

FIG. 197
Spina bifida occulta.

2. **Meningocele.**—There is a herniation of the meningeal coverings through a gap in the vertebral arches and this presents as a midline swelling in the back, most commonly in the lumbosacral region (Fig. 198) but occasionally in the cervical or thoracic region (Fig. 199). Rarely the defect presents to one or other side of the midline. The meningocele may be covered completely by normal skin or the skin may change to a thin and translucent covering which readily ulcerates and ruptures. No individual meningeal layers can be distinguished in this covering (Fig. 196, H). The swelling is elastic and may become more tense when the child cries. A meningocele may be transilluminated.

3. **Meningomyelocele** (Fig. 200).—To outward appearances the swelling may resemble the less common pure meningocele, but in this anomaly there are always nerve elements in the sac

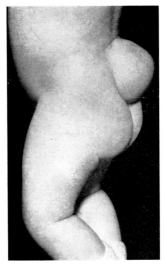

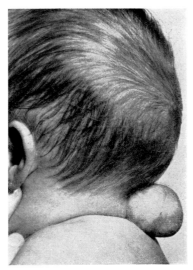

FIG. 198
Lumbar meningocele.

FIG. 199
Cervical meningocele.

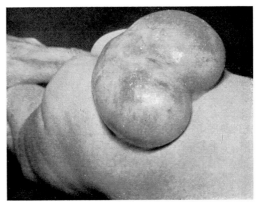

FIG. 200
Lumbar meningomyelocele.

(Fig. 196, I). These elements vary from normal or ectopic nerves, and ectopic spinal cord, to the cauda equina or the cord itself. The swelling may be entirely cystic or there may be solid elements. If cerebrospinal fluid is aspirated and replaced by air, a lateral radiograph may show the nerve elements coursing across the sac. Meningomyelocele is usually associated with motor and sensory paralysis of the legs, paralysis of the bladder

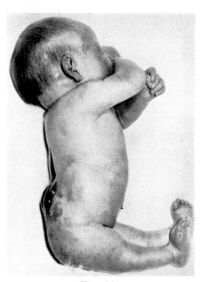

and bowel, and trophic ulcers develop readily. There may be associated club foot—usually talipes equino varus. Hydrocephalus may be present at birth or it may develop later. This form of hydrocephalus is commonly associated with the *Arnold-Chiari malformation*, in which a cone of medulla and cerebellum is prolonged downwards through the foramen magnum.

Fig. 201
Myelocele.

4. **Syringomyelocele** (Fig. 196, J).—In this rare anomaly the presenting features are similar to those of meningo-myelocele, but the central canal of the cord is greatly dilated. The condition is only of embryological interest.

5. **Myelocele.**—Arrest of development has occurred before closure of the neural groove (Fig. 196, K) and the infant presents with a raw elliptical area from which the open cord discharges cerebrospinal fluid (Fig. 201). This condition is rarely compatible with life. Many cases are stillborn; others die within a few days from infection of the cord and meninges.

DIFFERENTIAL DIAGNOSIS.—The only conditions which may give rise to difficulties in differential diagnosis are inclusion dermoid and sacrococcygeal teratoma.

TREATMENT.—No treatment benefits function, and any operative intervention is mainly for cosmetic purposes. If a thin-walled sac is ruptured, or is likely to rupture, early surgery is necessary to prevent infection of the cord or meninges. Provided that the sac is unlikely to rupture, surgery should not be attempted until the child is 3 months old. During this waiting period a thin-walled sac is protected by vaseline gauze and a suitable ring pad or a perforated hemisphere cut from an indiarubber ball. If there is paralysis of the limbs or sphincters or if hydrocephalus is present, these complications *cannot be benefited by surgical repair of the meningocele.* The parents must be given some idea of the future of their child and should be warned that the child may develop hydrocephalus (Chap. XVIII) or paralysis after operation.

When discussing the possibility of surgery one must consider *the size of the swelling, the coverings, the contents, the base or pedicle* and any *associated deformities.* If there is no clinical or radiographic evidence of nerve content, if the base of the sac will permit surgical closure and if there is no paralysis or hydrocephalus, the sac is excised, the membranes sutured and the gap in the vertebral arches closed with muscle or fascia. The operation is performed under antibiotic cover. Although a patient with meningomyelocele cannot be benefited by surgery it may be justifiable to excise the swelling or reduce its size to allow the child to be more readily nursed. Such deformities as club foot must be treated on orthopædic lines. Should a child with meningomyelocele survive without developing hydrocephalus, neurogenic bladder and difficulty in bowel control will present difficult problems for the rest of the patient's life. The common causes of death are urinary infection, meningitis or intercurrent infection.

There is no surgical treatment for myelocele or syringo-myelocele.

CONGENITAL SACRAL DERMAL SINUS

It is not uncommon to see a congenital sinus over the coccyx (Fig. 202). Some merely form a shallow depression (*sacro-coccygeal dimple*) and require no treatment. Others present a deeper, epithelium-lined tract which, although it may give rise to little trouble in early childhood, may lead to complications in adult life. Any time after puberty the combination of imperfect cleansing, collection of sebaceous material in the sinus and natural growth of hair in the sinus may lead to infection and abscess formation. The congenital dermal sinus is probably the same anomaly as the *pilonidal* sinus of adult life. Occasionally a dermal sinus over the sacrum or coccyx may be associated with a dermoid cyst; in the cervical, thoracic or

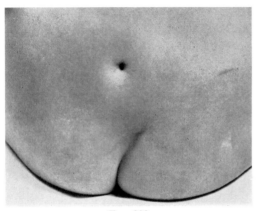

FIG. 202
Sacral dermal sinus.

lumbar region an enterogenous cyst may be found. Rarely a dermal sinus over the spine will communicate with the central nervous system and infection of the sinus may lead to meningitis.

Treatment.—A congenital dermal sinus in which the apex cannot be readily exposed should be excised before the child is old enough to be responsible for his own cleanliness.

DEFORMITIES OF THE SPINE

KYPHOSIS.—Localised kyphosis in childhood is almost invariably due to spinal tuberculosis (Fig. 206). Postural kyphosis is usually seen in the child with flat feet and protuberant abdomen, and before puberty this type of round back responds to appropriate exercises and adequate rest periods (Chap. I). Kyphosis due to osteochondritis of the spine (Scheuermann's disease) is rarely seen before puberty. Kyphosis may be a feature of generalised disease, *e.g.*, rickets and the muscular dystrophies.

LORDOSIS.—Lordosis is an increase in the anterior convexity of the lumbar spine. It is a common feature in flexion deformities of the hip and is most marked in bilateral congenital dislocation of the hip (Fig. 239). Treatment is directed to the hip lesions and these are considered in Chapter XXIII.

SCOLIOSIS.—This term is applied to lateral curvature of the spine. It occurs in many forms, differing in ætiology, clinical features, prognosis and treatment. A satisfactory classification is difficult but for the present purposes can be simplified without loss of accuracy into : *structural*, *postural* and *idiopathic*. In addition, scoliosis may occur as a secondary condition following pelvic tilt due to unequal limb length—developmental, post-traumatic, post-inflammatory or following increase in blood supply of one limb (*vide* limb lengthening, Chap. V). This *compensatory scoliosis* may also follow bronchiectasis, torticollis or poliomyelitis affecting the spinal muscles.

Structural Scoliosis.—This is the most common type of rotary lateral curvature in infancy and childhood. It is commonly due to hemivertebræ and the anomaly may occur in any part of the spinal column (Fig. 203). Treatment rarely presents a serious problem unless the deformity is severe. A supportive corset may be required from the time that the infant sits up, and later a corrective jacket and physiotherapy may be necessary. The deformity is usually mild and, although seldom progressive, paraplegia can occur in this type of scoliosis.

Postural Scoliosis.—This is usually a simple single curve within the normal physiological range. It is moderate in degree and, being essentially without structural change, is usually self-curing with a minimum of splinting and physiotherapy.

Many babies show a lateral curve of the spine in the first few months of life. This may persist until the erect posture is assumed, when it usually disappears spontaneously. In a few patients the lateral curve tends to increase and if untreated it is possible that the condition might progress to " idiopathic scoliosis " (*vide infra*). Although this condition may also be self-curing we prefer to treat the child in a Denis Browne splint (Fig. 204). This apparatus is worn (apart from removal for bathing and exercises) until the spine appears quite straight when the child is sitting up.

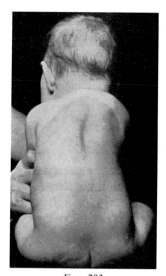

FIG. 203
Structural scoliosis due
to hemivertebræ.

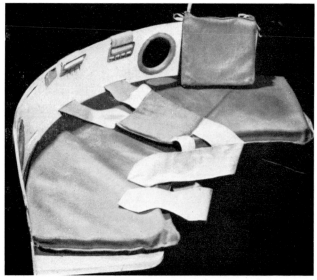

FIG. 204
Denis Browne scoliosis splint.

In school children or in adolescents there may be other evidence of muscular weakness such as rounded shoulders, protuberant abdomen and flat feet. The deformity is usually temporary and disappears when the patient's mode of life is properly organised, *i.e.*, suitable diet, avoidance of fatigue, adequate sleep and physiotherapy. In a few patients morphological changes develop and the condition undergoes transition into progressive scoliosis (*vide infra*).

Progressive Idiopathic Scoliosis.— This type of scoliosis may be indistinguishable from congenital postural scoliosis until after the age of 2 years and may be mistaken for simple postural scoliosis. The curve is usually in the dorsal spine, and both the curve and rotation increase in early life (Fig. 205). In spite of supports, exercises and even operation, this type of scoliosis is progressive and treatment taxes all the ingenuity of the orthopædic surgeon.

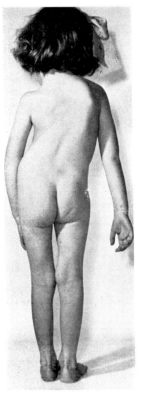

FIG. 205
Idiopathic scoliosis.

INJURIES OF THE SPINE

The spine of the child is normally much more flexible than that of the adult (except where the presence of congenital fusion of vertebræ may cause local limitation of movement) and fracture of the spine is uncommon. When it does occur the violence has usually been severe and has caused multiple associated injuries that prove fatal. Although actual fracture is rare, hæmorrhage is less uncommon and may cause pressure on the cord with resulting paralysis, temporary or permanent.

Street accidents account for most of the spinal injuries, but not infrequently children are buried while playing in a sand pit or quarry. The exact mechanism of the violence is thus often difficult to ascertain. The management of such spinal injuries in children follows that adopted in the adult, but a word of warning is perhaps justified for the lay person or even the first-aid worker called upon to attend the child. The normal adult is too heavy to be lifted by one individual, but there is a natural impulse to lift up an injured child in one's arms. Such action must almost inevitably result in flexion of the child's spine, with consequent risk of injury to the cord. As in the adult, the child should not be lifted from the scene of the accident until a stretcher is available for transport.

The diagnosis and treatment of injuries to the cord follow the same lines as those adopted in the adult. The prognosis in such injuries is no better than in the adult.

Cervical Spine.—Fractures and dislocations of the cervical spine are rare in childhood and seldom cause transection of the cord. Subluxation of the cervical spine occurs, but complete dislocation is rare. Head traction will relieve pain and spasm and allow facets to reset themselves within a few days.

Spontaneous hyperæmic subluxation of the atlas is considered in Chapter XX.

Dorsal Spine.—Compression fracture may occur in a fall from a height and in automobile accidents, but the fracture is rarely unstable. The compression is seldom great and it is unnecessary to reduce the deformity. To prevent further collapse the child may be nursed in hyperextension in a cast until the vertebral body becomes homogeneous. Even although there is slight wedging, there is no permanent disability.

Lumbar Spine.—Fractures below the first lumbar spine are almost unknown in children. Fractures of laminæ or pedicles are also rare, but may follow a torsion injury. They must be differentiated radiographically from ununited apophysis. No reduction is necessary and with rest, complete recovery is the rule.

HÆMATOGENOUS OSTEITIS OF THE SPINE

The spine is an uncommon site for acute osteitis, and when it occurs, accurate diagnosis is delayed owing to the depth of the lesion. In infancy the disease may affect the vertebral bodies and may develop insidiously in generalised osteitis of the newborn (Chap. IV). In older children the neural arches or transverse processes may be affected. The constitutional upset is severe and there may be neurological involvement before the site of the bone infection is obvious. The treatment of hæmatogenous osteitis is considered in Chapters IV and V.

TUBERCULOSIS OF THE SPINE

In recent years tuberculosis of the spine has become a relatively rare disease in childhood. The disease may occur in

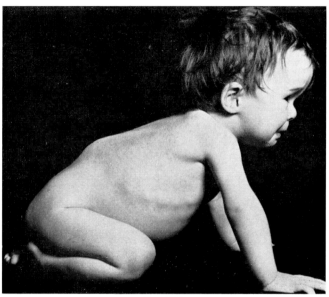

FIG. 206
Tuberculous kyphosis.

a child with a known primary pulmonary lesion, but more commonly it is seen in an apparently healthy child. It is a blood-borne infection and affects the cancellous bone of a vertebral body. The lower thoracic and upper lumbar vertebræ are most commonly affected.

Clinical Features.—In recent years the classical feature of the listless child complaining of pain in the back has been seen only rarely. Many children present with acute or chronic abdominal pain. Others are brought to the doctor because the mother has discovered a lump in the back following a fall or other injury (Fig. 206). In this second type of presentation clinical examination and radiography reveal a kyphotic deformity and disease which has been present for a fairly long period. Only a coincidental injury has brought the deformity

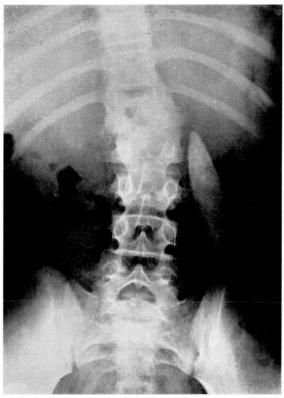

FIG. 207

Tuberculosis of first lumbar vertebra with
calcified psoas abscess.

to parental notice and usually nothing in the child's behaviour has suggested spinal disease.

On careful examination it is found that the child avoids jarring movements and has developed methods of keeping weight off the diseased vertebræ. Radiographic evidence of advanced disease may be present before the limitation of spinal movements has become evident.

Cold abscess is a common complication, but although it may be recognised on X-ray (Fig. 207) the disease is usually diagnosed before cold abscess is clinically recognisable. Paraplegia is rarely seen in childhood.

Treatment.—Treatment in a sanatorium is desirable. In the cervical region immobilisation is required for a year; in the dorso-lumbar region it may be two years before there is clinical and radiographic evidence of healing. Operation is rarely required in childhood, and antibiotics have improved the prognosis and shortened the duration of treatment.

TUMOURS

Sacrococcygeal Tumour (Fig. 208).—Tumours and cysts occur in this region of complex development. Most are

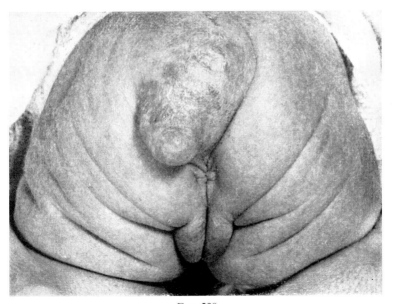

FIG. 208
Sacrococcygeal teratoma.

teratomatous and unless laboriously excised may undergo malignant change.

Chordoma (Fig. 209).—This uncommon tumour arises from remains of the notochord. It may occur in the sacrococcygeal region or at the base of the skull. In childhood it grows rapidly and total excision is usually impossible. The tumour may cause intestinal or urinary obstruction from pressure.

Spinal Cord Tumours.—Primary tumours of the spinal cord are uncommon in childhood and are rarely diagnosed during life. Primary glioma occurs and intracranial medullablastoma

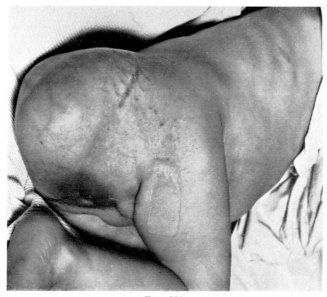

Fig. 209
Chordoma (scar over site of biopsy).

may metastasise to the cord. Extradural tumours involving the cord are sympathicoblastoma, neurofibroma and lipoma. Dermoid and enterogenous cysts within the spinal canal may give rise to pressure symptoms.

Signs and symptoms depend on the site of the lesion. After complete neurological examination, radiography following instillation of radio-opaque material into the canal will help to confirm the exact location of the tumour.

Pressure may be relieved by laminectomy, but radiotherapy may be the only method of treatment available.

PELVIS

Fractures of the pelvis due to crushing injuries or street accidents are not uncommon in children. The types of fracture follow closely those met with in adults, and reduction of the deformity is equally difficult. The functional recovery, even when reduction has not been effected, is much greater than in the adult. The capacity of the child's bones for restoration of normal structure is particularly striking in such cases.

The commonest sites of fracture are the rami of the pubis and ischium. In the absence of gross displacement no fixation is called for. Rest in bed for three to six weeks allows firm union and the normal architecture is soon restored. Where there is gross displacement, manipulation under general anæsthesia should be attempted.

The association of fractures of the rami with subluxation or even dislocation of the sacro-iliac synchondrosis follows the same pattern as in the adult. The subluxation or dislocation may occur either on the same side as the fracture or on the opposite side. This complication should always be suspected if the lateral fragments are both at a higher level than the medial. An attempt is made to reduce the sacro-iliac displacement by manipulation under general anæsthesia. If reduction is not complete there is no justification for resorting to open operation. A remarkable restoration of structure always occurs and normal function is almost invariable. When dealing with fracture of the pubic rami the possibility of rupture of the bladder or urethra must always be borne in mind. Should such a complication be found its treatment must always take precedence over treatment of the fracture. The child not accustomed to the hospital routine may attempt to micturate in bed, and the passing of a catheter is a routine precaution as a preliminary to examination and treatment of such cases. When dealing with the bladder or urethra the opportunity of correcting any bony displacement should not, however, be missed.

Ischio-pubic Osteochondrosis.—Before the ischio-pubic hiatus closes in children between 4 and 8 years, radiography frequently reveals exaggeration of the normal fusiform enlargement of the synchondrosis (Fig. 210). This may be mistaken for callus or infection. The lesion may cause limp and limitation of abduction of the hip joint, but the radiographic appearances

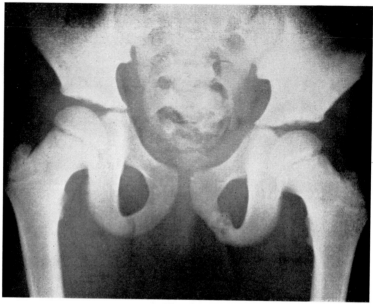

FIG. 210
Ischio-pubic osteochondrosis.

may occur in the absence of symptoms. The limp and limited abduction of the affected hip are relieved with a few days' rest in bed and the fusiform enlargement eventually disappears.

CHAPTER XXII

Upper Limb

DEVELOPMENTAL ANOMALIES

Syndactyly.

Development of the Hand.—About the sixth week of intra-uterine life there is a flapper-like broadening of the distal end of the upper limb bud. Four vertical grooves appear and these deepen until the flapper becomes separated into five parts. The thumb is the first to separate and the fingers separate at their distal ends first. Failure of separation may take place between two or more adjacent fingers and this failure may be partial or complete.

Clinical Features.—Webbing of the fingers is a common anomaly (Fig. 211) and may be associated with *microdactyly* or *ring stricture* (Fig. 212). Two or more fingers may be involved and the anomaly may be bilateral. If the webbing is partial the two fingers are joined by a skin web at their base ; if complete the digits are united in their entire length. The interphalangeal joints may be imperfectly developed with gross limitation of flexion. In the few cases in which the thumb is involved the fusion is never extensive.

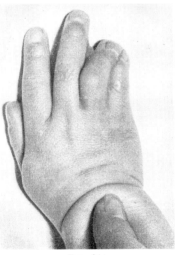

FIG. 211
Syndactyly.

Treatment.—Operation should be postponed until the age of 2 or 3 years. The web is constructed from dorsal and palmar triangular skin flaps with their bases hinged at the

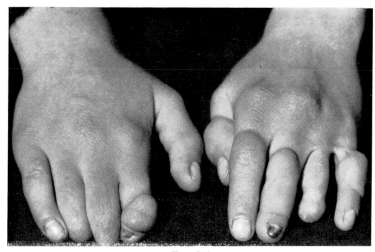

FIG. 212

Ring stricture and " intra-uterine amputation."

level of adjoining metacarpal heads. When fusion is complete the fingers are separated, using Z-incisions, and the raw surfaces are covered with split-skin or free full-thickness grafts.

Polydactyly.

Supernumerary digits are common and usually take a rudimentary form, although the nail may be well formed

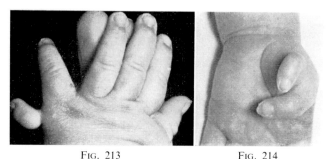

FIG. 213   FIG. 214

Fig. 213.—Common form of polydactyly rudimentary digit.
Fig. 214.—Bifid thumb.

(Fig. 213). Rudimentary digits may be attached to either radial or ulnar side of the hand. They are easily removed shortly after birth. Less commonly the digit may be fully formed with a separate metacarpal. A bifid thumb may arise from the thumb metacarpal (Fig. 214). Removal of supernumerary fingers rarely presents any problem, but when the thumb is double it may be wise to wait for some years to see which is the more useful

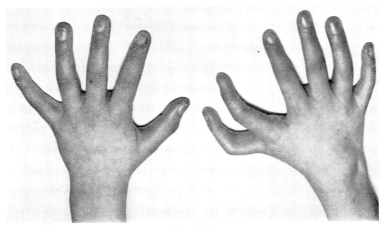

FIG. 215

Polydactyly : all fingers (triphalangeal thumb).

digit. A child may be born with five (or even six) fingers instead of four fingers and a thumb (Fig. 215). A complex plastic procedure is required to turn this triphalangeal finger into an æsthetically pleasing and functioning thumb. Congenital absence of the thumb is usually associated with absence of all or part of the radius and constitutes a serious disability (Fig. 216).

Local Gigantism (Macrodactyly).

One or more digits may be of almost adult size at birth (Fig. 217). The disproportion may become less marked with increasing age, but if growth cannot be restrained by radiotherapy amputation may be required to allow proper use of the hand. The results of plastic procedures are disappointing.

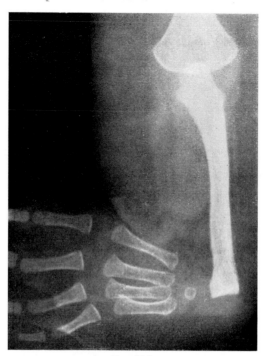

FIG. 216
Absence of thumb and radius.

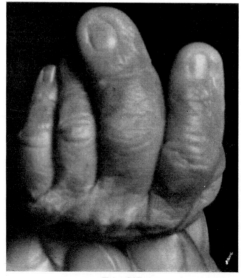

FIG. 217
Gigantism of fingers.

364

Radio-ulnar Synostosis.

The upper ends of the radius and ulna are fused (Fig. 218), the forearm is fixed in pronation and the palm cannot be turned upwards. The results of surgery are disappointing owing to associated neuromuscular defects.

Absence of Radius.

The anomaly causes club hand (Fig. 216). The defect may be partial or complete and the thumb may be absent. Despite the deformity the limb may have surprisingly good function. At an early age the soft tissue deformity is corrected as far as possible by manipulation, plaster casts and splints. Passive daily stretching is carried out by the parents until the child is old enough to co-operate with the physiotherapist. Some improvement in the deformity can be gained by osteotomy of the curved ulna, and after displacing the carpus over the distal end of the ulna a fibular bone graft is inserted to replace the distal end of the absent radius.

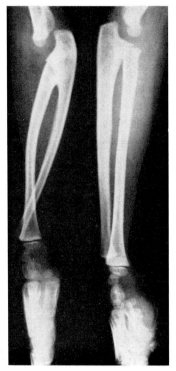

FIG. 218

Radio-ulnar synostosis
(right arm).

Hemihypertrophy.

Hemihypertrophy may affect the whole of one side of the body. Occasionally an arm may show hypertrophy associated with extensive hæmangioma formation or arteriovenous fistulæ.

Trigger Thumb.

There is a congenital constriction in the sheath of the flexor pollicis longus tendon and a flexion deformity of the interphalangeal joint of the thumb. The thumb cannot be actively

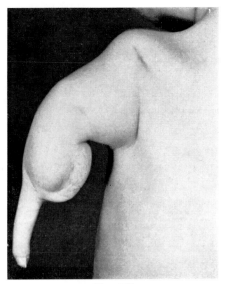

Fig. 219
Gross anomaly of left arm.

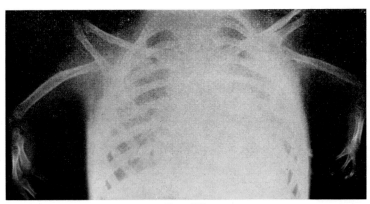

Fig. 220
Phocomelia (seal limb).

extended. (In the adult a similar deformity may arise from repeated trauma.) The deformity may be bilateral and is usually noticed at birth. A firm nodule can be felt in front of the metacarpo-phalangeal joint. Occasionally other fingers are affected by *stenosing tendovaginitis*.
Treatment is simple and effective. A longitudinal incision is made along the tendon sheath, either by subcutaneous tenotomy or after direct exposure of the swelling through a transverse incision in the skin crease.

Miscellaneous Anomalies.

Gross developmental anomalies are shown in Figures 219 to 221. These deformities are treated by fitting a suitable prosthesis when the child is old enough to appreciate its use.

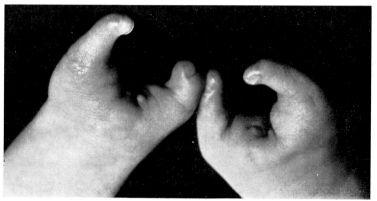

FIG. 221
Lobster-claw deformity of hands. Mother had similar deformity.

FRACTURES AND DISLOCATIONS

Clavicle.

The clavicle forms the only bony connection between the shoulder girdle and trunk, and it is hardly surprising that it is one of the most commonly fractured bones in the body. The clavicle is liable to break when force is applied to the out-stretched hand, the elbow or the shoulder.

Birth fracture of the clavicle is considered in Chapter III.

In infancy fracture of the clavicle presents with pseudoparalysis and pain when the arm is moved. It must be differentiated from osteitis of the clavicle, scapula or upper humerus. The symptoms may be relieved by the application of a flannelette figure-of-eight bandage for ten days. The mother can be reassured that any swelling (due to massive callus) will disappear entirely in a few months. In children, reduction of a fractured clavicle is rarely necessary under the age of 6 years. A padded figure-of-eight bandage is applied and tightened every morning by the parent. It is retained for three weeks. From 6 to 12 years greenstick fractures are treated with a padded figure-of-eight bandage for four weeks. If there is marked displacement this is reduced before immobilisation.

Scapula.

Most fractures of the scapula are due to direct violence. Even if there is marked displacement treatment is conservative. Unless the fracture is combined with other injuries requiring rest in bed, a simple sling is the only treatment necessary.

Injuries at the Shoulder Joint.

Dislocation and epiphyseal injuries are rare in childhood.

Fractures of the surgical neck and upper third of the humerus are not uncommon. Anterior, posterior and rotational displacement may accompany both adduction and abduction types of injury, and lateral as well as anteroposterior X-ray films are required. Impaction is common and 10 to 20 degrees of angulation is permissible. Although the initial appearance may look unsatisfactory moulding takes place in six months to a year. If the fracture is not impacted it may be aligned by a hanging plaster cast as in the adult. Following severe trauma bed rest with lateral traction is desirable. Reduction by open operation should be avoided, especially if the patient is a girl in whom the presence of an unsightly scar might be resented in later life.

Pulled Shoulder.

One of the commonest shoulder injuries is caused by the solicitous but ignorant parent, nursemaid or older brother or sister. The toddler is helped up a stair or on to a high pavement by a vigorous jerk on the arm. If there is not full co-operation from the child the shoulder may be over-stretched, causing an acute sprain. The same mechanism operates when the child is kept from falling by jerking on the arm. There is a pseudo-paralysis, and if no history is available the condition may be mistaken for poliomyelitis. There is power in the arm below the shoulder, pain on attempted movement of the shoulder and a negative X-ray. The condition is relieved by rest in a sling. When the force of the jerk is transmitted in a different way a *pulled elbow* may result (p. 375).

Middle Third of Shaft of Humerus.

The common oblique fracture of the middle third of the humerus is easily controlled by two plaster of Paris slabs extending from the shoulder to the wrist, the elbow being flexed to a right angle. The arm is supported in a sling. A transverse fracture may require traction and manipulation to correct deformity.

INJURIES ABOUT THE ELBOW

The elbow joint is a particularly vulnerable region in the child and there is wide range in the variety and degree of displacement of fractures. The following are the more common types of bone injury in order of frequency :—

1. Supracondylar fractures :
   (*a*) extension type.
   (*b*) flexion type.
2. Separation of lateral condyle.
3. Separation of medial condyle.
4. Separation of medial epicondyle.
5. T-shaped fracture.

1. Supracondylar Fractures.

(*a*) *Extension Type* (99 per cent.).—This injury is caused by a fall on the outstretched arm. The line of fracture runs transversely across the shaft immediately above the condyles and from below upwards and backwards. The deformity is threefold, the

22

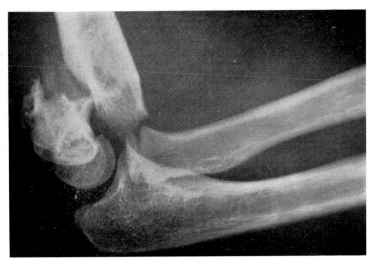

FIG. 222
Extension type of supracondylar fracture of humerus.

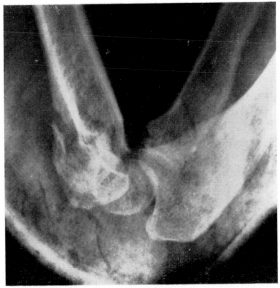

FIG. 223
Fracture in Fig. 222, after reduction of deformity.

lower fragment being displaced backwards, tilted to the medial or lateral side and rotated relatively to the long axis of the humerus (Fig. 222). The fracture should be regarded as an emergency and treated as soon as possible after the injury. Reduction should be carried out only by an experienced surgeon. While the traction is applied the forearm is carried forward to flex the elbow and reduction is maintained by an assistant controlling the arm and continuing traction on the flexed elbow. Correction of the lateral or medial and of the rotational displacement is then carried out. Swelling may make it impossible to palpate the bony points and difficult to determine if reduction has been satisfactory (Fig. 223). Injection of hyaluronidase into the hæmatoma may help to disperse the swelling. Confirmation by immediate X-ray examination is essential. If reduction is satisfactory a plaster slab is applied from the deltoid to the wrist. The application of a circular cast is an invitation to Volkmann's paralysis. The amount of flexion of the elbow is determined by the radial pulse and capillary circulation of the fingers. An ample margin of safety should be allowed, bearing in mind that further hæmorrhage and swelling will result from the manipulation. The arm is supported by a collar-and-cuff sling. The circulation must be watched carefully for the twenty-four hours following manipulation, and any signs of interference dealt with promptly as described in Chapter V. The child is encouraged to exercise the wrist and fingers and after three weeks the collar-and-cuff sling and the plaster are replaced by a triangular sling. Movements of the elbow are then encouraged and the sling discarded after a further two weeks. On no account should massage or passive movements be permitted. Exuberant callus and myositis ossificans will disappear if left unmolested. Reversal of the carrying angle may be due to uncorrected medial displacement but may occur later due to accelerated growth of the lateral condyle.

Examples of this fracture do occur which defy correction of the deformity by manipulation. It is justifiable in such cases, where the deformity is gross, to resort to open operation in preference to repeated manipulation.

(b) *Flexion type* (1 per cent.) (Fig. 224).—A fall upon the flexed forearm or upon the elbow is the usual cause of this type of fracture. The fracture is reduced and immobilised in sufficient

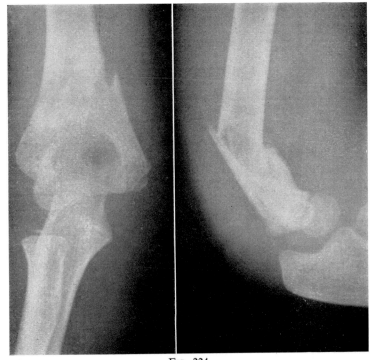

FIG. 224
Flexion type of supracondylar fracture.

extension to prevent a recurrence of the anterior displacement of the lower fragment.

2. Fracture of the Lateral Condyle.

This type of fracture varies from the incomplete or flake fracture to a complete separation of the condyle including the capitellum and part of the trochlea.

The flake fracture occurs when the radial collateral ligament tears away its insertion ; the X-ray film shows a thin flake of bone only slightly separated. Displacement is usually minimal and no treatment is called for other than the use of an arm sling with the elbow flexed at right angles. The child is encouraged to move the elbow within the sling for a week or ten days. Thereafter the sling is removed and ordinary use in dressing and feeding encouraged.

In the complete fracture the fragment may be markedly

displaced or rotated through 90 degrees or more (Fig. 225), and frequently there is also partial subluxation of the joint. Correction of the displacement by manipulation is rarely successful and it is well to be prepared for open operation. Even with the site of fracture exposed it is curiously difficult to replace the fragment which is often firmly engaged within the joint. By traction and rotation the fragment can be disengaged and accurately replaced and fixed by suture of the aponeurosis or by a metal pin. Immobilisation by plaster is not necessary. The use of an arm sling is all that is required and voluntary movements are encouraged immediately after operation. Failure of union with displacement of the fragment distally may be followed by a most unsightly deformity, but excellent function may be attained despite the deformity.

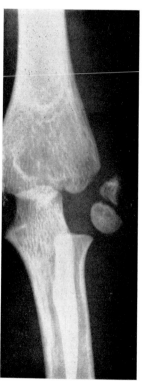

Fig. 225
Fracture of lateral condyle of humerus.

3. Fracture of Medial Condyle.

This type of injury corresponds to the T-shaped fracture in the adult caused by a fall on the point of the elbow in which the ulna is driven upwards as a wedge separating the two humeral condyles. This T-shaped fracture is rare in children, but the medial condyle may be sheared off by similar violence, the line of fracture passing through the trochlea. Correction of the displacement by manipulation is more easily attained than is that of the lateral condyle. A posterior slab is applied with the elbow as fully flexed as the circulation permits.

4. Fracture of the Medial Epicondyle.

This injury varies from a slight partial avulsion with negligible displacement to complete separation with displacement into the joint. The slight form is treated by the use of an arm sling with the elbow flexed for three weeks. Earlier freedom with consequent pulling of the flexor muscles may result in fibrous union and prolonged tenderness. In the more severe form the medial collateral ligament is torn and the fragment is displaced into the joint. The absence of the epicondylar prominence on clinical examination is confirmed by the X-ray films. Reduction by manipulation is occasionally successful. If attempt at reduction fails, open operation is carried out and the fragment extracted from the joint by a hook and fixed with sutures through the aponeurosis. The arm is supported in a sling with the elbow flexed for three weeks. The sequel of ulnar neuritis is extremely rare in children.

5. T-shaped Fracture.

The severe T-shaped fractures of the lower end of the humerus are extremely rare in children. Satisfactory correction of the displacement is difficult and there should be no hesitation in resorting to open operation in such cases. The ulnar nerve is displayed and protected and the fragments pinned in position. The pins are removed at the end of six weeks. The joint is immobilised with plaster slabs for two or three weeks only. Thereafter active movements are encouraged.

Fracture of Olecranon.

Fracture of the olecranon is relatively uncommon. It usually results from a direct blow on the tip of the elbow, but it may be associated with fracture of the radial neck or a forward dislocation of the elbow joint. In examining the X-ray film of a suspected fracture the possibility of twin centres of ossification should be borne in mind. When the fragment is small and displacement slight the arm need only be rested in a sling for two weeks. If the fracture is through the base with considerable separation of the fragments the arm is fixed in full extension with a posterior plaster slab for at least six weeks.

Neck of Radius.

There are two common forms of injury to the head and neck of the radius. One is essentially a separation of the upper radial epiphysis. The head is forced against the capitellum and tilted to the lateral side with crushing of the adjacent metaphysis, but it remains within the orbicular ligament. The impaction makes correction of the deformity almost impossible, but in most cases the architecture of the bone is restored with the normal use of the arm. The other form of this injury is a greenstick fracture of the neck of the radius with similar tilting of the head to the lateral side and angling of the neck inwards. Correction of this deformity may be difficult. No splinting is called for, but the arm is rested in a sling and pronation and supination movements are encouraged.

Normal function may not be attained for many months, but the temptation to resort to open operation should be resisted as the results are never satisfactory.

Dislocation of the Elbow Joint.

Posterior dislocation of the forearm bones upon the humerus is a common injury of childhood and is usually the result of a fall upon the outstretched hand. The loss of mobility and derangement of the normal relations of the olecranon and condyles enable the injury to be distinguished from the supracondylar fracture. Reduction by traction is usually easy, but in children a general anæsthetic is helpful and kindly. The elbow is flexed as far as is comfortable and the arm supported in a triangular sling. Early voluntary movements are encouraged, but on no account should massage or passive movements be applied. Complications such as nerve injury are rare and normal function should be restored in three or four weeks.

Pulled Elbow.

Subluxation of the radial head from the annular ligament is common in children from two to six years. In this age group the radial head is no greater in diameter than the shaft. The injury is produced by a jerk on the child's upraised arm (see " pulled shoulder," p. 368). It may also occur when the arm is caught between the bars of a crib. The injury is very painful and the arm is held stiffly in moderate flexion and mid-pronation. The child screams and resists all attempts to examine the arm.

After warning the child a quick manipulation into supination produces an audible and palpable click. Movements then become normal and pain disappears. The elbow is immobilised in a collar-and-cuff sling for a week to prevent recurrence which is not uncommon.

INJURIES TO FOREARM, WRIST AND HAND

Fractures of the forearm occur in the following order of frequency; *distal third* (75 per cent.), *middle third* (20 per cent.), *proximal third* (5 per cent.). At the distal end they are commonly produced by indirect violence from a fall on the outstretched hand—the same force that produces a Colles' fracture in the adult.

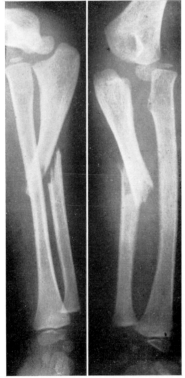

Upper Third of Ulna.

Fracture of the upper third of the ulna is not very common in children and when it does occur differs somewhat from that met with in the adult. According to the direction of the violence the fragments may be angled forwards or backwards. Theoretically this angulation cannot occur without dislocation of the head of the radius as occurs in the Monteggia fracture in the adult (Fig. 226). Correction of the deformity is often difficult, but every effort should be made to achieve it as even a small amount of angulation interferes with pronation and supination. After correction, anterior and posterior plaster slabs are applied controlling both elbow and wrist joints.

Fig. 226
Monteggia type of fracture of ulna.

Fractures of the Middle Third of both Bones.

Though the violence is usually indirect the bones frequently break at the same or nearly the same level (Fig. 227). The line of fracture, however, is not transverse but oblique or irregular. Commonly the fracture is of the greenstick type, either of both bones or of one only, the other being complete. The lower fragments are bent towards the radial side and frequently pronated. Reduction of the displacement without rendering the fracture complete is not easy, and the deformity will usually recur within the cast. There must be no hesitation in rendering the fracture complete. Plaster slabs are applied with the forearm in mid position between pronation and supination. They must immobilise both the elbow and wrist joints, extending to just short of the metacarpo-phalangeal joints, with a plaster strap across the palm. The thumb and fingers are left free and movements encouraged.

When the fractures are complete overriding of the fragments is usually present as well as angling. Reduction may be effected by strong traction on the forearm, the elbow being flexed to

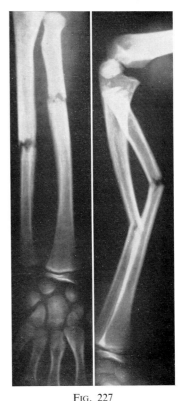

Fig. 227

Fracture of radius and ulna, to show importance of two views.

90 degrees and the arm firmly held by an assistant. It is curiously difficult sometimes to disengage the fragments, and considerable manipulation with traction may be necessary before complete reduction is obtained. When the radius is broken above the insertion of the pronator radii teres the forearm is held in full supination while the plaster is applied. The forearm

should never be completely encircled with plaster lest the swelling consequent upon the manipulation cause obstruction of the venous return. The closest watch must be kept upon the fingers and any sign of pressure dealt with at once as described in Chapter V. Immobilisation is continued for four to six weeks.

Fractures in the Lower Third.

There are three common fractures in this situation.

1. *Incomplete Compression Fracture of the Lower Third of the Radius.*—Local tenderness is the only sign of injury to the bone and the X-ray shows the transverse line of compressed

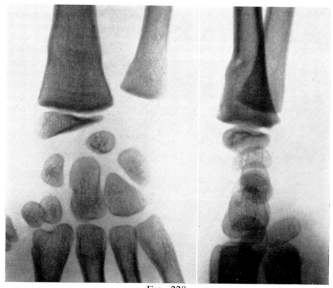

FIG. 228
Compression fracture of cortex of radius.

cortex (Fig. 228). No treatment is necessary save the use of an arm sling for seven to ten days.

2. *Separation of the Lower Radial Epiphysis.*—A true separation of this epiphysis does occur, but in the majority of the injuries so described the epiphysis carries with it a wedge of the dorsum of the metaphysis and the injury is more accurately described as a fracture (Fig. 229). The clinical picture resembles

that of the Colles' fracture, which is much less common in children. The typical " dinner fork " deformity is present, the epiphysis being displaced and rotated dorsally. A varying degree of displacement to the radial side is usually but not invariably present. In the more severe degrees of radial displacement, fracture of the styloid process of the ulna is constantly present. The appearances in the X-ray film are characteristic, but in the less severe injuries the anteroposterior view may show surprisingly little evidence of the bone injury.

Correction of the deformity is usually obtained without difficulty, but it may be necessary to disimpact the fragments before the displacement can be reduced. The method of reduction is similar to that employed in the treatment of a Colles' fracture. There is, however, a greater risk in children of the epiphysis slipping back a little when the swelling has subsided and the plaster fits less firmly. For this reason it is wiser to place the wrist in a position of slight flexion before applying the plaster. The increased tension of the extensor tendons assists in maintaining

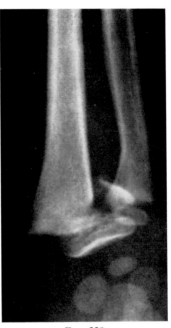

FIG. 229

Fracture-separation of lower radial epiphysis.

correction of the deformity without impairing free use of the fingers and thumb. There is no risk of any subsequent limitation of dorsiflexion in children. The use of an arm sling is advisable for a week or ten days, but the child is encouraged to make use of the arm and hand for feeding and dressing. The plaster is removed in three weeks.

3. *Fractures of both Bones about one to two inches above the Epiphysis.*—The fracture may be complete or incomplete and the usual deformity is a simple backward displacement of the

lower fragments. Reduction is usually easy and the plaster slabs must fix the elbow joint as well as the wrist. It is wise to maintain immobilisation for four to six weeks as union seems slower at this site. Movement of the fingers and thumb must be encouraged. Rarely it may be found impossible to overcome the shortening of the fragments, and in such cases it is justifiable to resort to open operation.

WRIST AND HAND

Sprained wrist and fracture or dislocation of one of the carpal bones are extremely rare in young children, but *from the age of* 10 *or* 12 *years fracture of the scaphoid is not infrequent.* Any boy of this age who is said to have " sprained his wrist " should be subjected to a most careful X-ray examination. As in the adult the line of fracture is easily missed unless oblique views of the wrist with the hand in radial deviation are taken. Fracture of the scaphoid tubercle is the more usual type, but fracture of the waist may occur. The former unites quickly with rest in an arm sling but the latter requires prolonged immobilisation as in the adult. There is not, however, in children the same risk of permanent disturbance of function or of arthritis should the fracture fail to unite. The wrist soon adapts its mechanics to the " extra " bone and normal function is restored. There is no justification for operative measures to promote union or for excision of the bone.

Ligamentous injuries of the carpus require two weeks of complete immobilisation.

Fractures of the metacarpals and phalanges follow the same pattern as in the adult. Flexion fracture of the neck of the metacarpal bone of the index or of the little finger is not un-common. Correction of the deformity can be effected by direct pressure on the head through the flexed proximal phalanx. Correction is usually stable and a light plaster is then applied to control the wrist and the proximal phalanges. In the common oblique fracture of the shaft of the metacarpal there is rarely any displacement and the application of a plaster cast for three weeks is all that is necessary.

Fractures of the phalanges present rather a problem in treatment as the fingers are small and local splinting difficult to apply. It is quite justifiable in children to include an adjacent finger when applying a small plaster strip as a splint with the finger flexed at both joints. The most satisfactory results in fractures of the metacarpals and of the metatarsals follow early resumption of function.

Open Injuries of the Hand.

Wounds may involve damage to skin by burning or avulsion, laceration of nerves and tendons and open injuries of bones and joints. First-aid treatment is aimed at avoidance of infection and future disability. A sterile dressing is applied and the hand splinted in the position of function, that is, the wrist in 30 degrees dorsiflexion, metacarpo-phalangeal and distal interphalangeal joints in 45 degrees of flexion and the middle interphalangeal joints in almost 90 degrees flexion. Even hæmorrhage from a divided radial artery can be controlled by gentle pressure. With the dressing in position tests of function are carried out without exposing the wound. If the child cannot flex the distal joint of a finger against resistance the profundus tendon is cut. If he cannot perceive light touch to the finger the digital nerve has been severed or severely contused. If he cannot extend the last two joints of his fingers and spread the fingers apart and bring them together the motor ulnar nerve has been damaged. If the median motor nerve is damaged he cannot extend the thumb as in reaching for a glass.

If the patient reaches hospital within six hours of the injury most wounds will heal without infection. Contaminated wounds not adequately cleansed in an operating theatre until after six hours will usually develop infection. Antibiotics are given prophylactically and tetanus antitoxin or a booster dose of toxoid is administered. During operation joint dislocations and bone fragments are reduced. Tendons are seldom repaired when fractures are present in the same area but are sutured with fine silk or stainless-steel wire four or five weeks later. An attempt is always made to unite severed nerves.

Crushed Finger Tip.

If the finger tip is crushed but the bone is not denuded the wound is gently but thoroughly cleansed. Damaged tissue is approximated by the longitudinal application of narrow strips of gauze moistened in collodion or Nobecutane and a gentle pressure dressing is applied.   Fractures of the distal phalanx require no further treatment.   If the nail is partially avulsed it should be trimmed off proximally leaving the distal part as a splint.   If the tip of the finger is partially amputated it should be stitched back on as the regenerative powers of the tissues of the child are remarkable.   If the amputation is complete further bone should not be removed but the stump covered with a free split-skin graft.

When the terminal phalanx is contused but the skin is intact, relief from pain and early disappearance of swelling may be obtained by inunction of the part with hydrocortisone ointment. We have used a bland ointment containing hydrocortisone acetate which is gently rubbed into the injured digit for two or three minutes.   This procedure is repeated at hourly intervals and relief is usually obtained within a few hours.

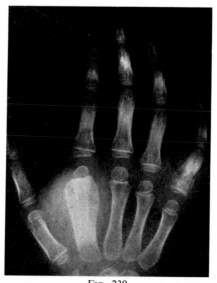

FIG. 230
Tuberculous lesions of second metacarpal
and proximal phalanx of fifth finger.

Tuberculous Dactylitis.

Tuberculosis may occasionally affect a metacarpal or phalanx in the first five years of life (Spina ventosa).   The interior of the bone is converted into tuberculous granulation tissue and a spindle-shaped swelling develops. The radiographic appearance may resemble that of a central enchondroma. With antibiotic therapy and adequate immobilisation in plaster of Paris the disease slowly heals. In miliary tuberculosis there may be multiple lesions of the metacarpals and phalanges (Fig. 230).

Ganglion.

As in the adult a smooth ovoid painless swelling arises on the dorsum of the wrist close to the tendon of the extensor carpi radialis. A few ganglia in children subside following injection of hyaluronidase, but most require the insertion of a *seton*. A heavy silk suture is passed through the ganglion on a cutting needle and left *in situ* for four or five days. Excision is rarely justifiable in children.

CHAPTER XXIII

Lower Limb

DEVELOPMENTAL ANOMALIES

SYNDACTYLY, polydactyly and *local gigantism* affect the foot. Syndactyly causes little disability and no treatment is required. In polydactyly (Fig. 231) amputation of the extra digit or digits is required to allow the fitting of normal footwear. Polydactyly and syndactyly may both occur in the same patient (Fig. 232). Local giantism, as illustrated in Figure 233, is treated by amputation of the large digit. When the entire leg is hypertrophied (Fig. 234) there may be tilting of the pelvis to the opposite side and scoliosis owing to the unequal length of the legs.

Overlapping Fifth Toes.—The fifth toe may overlap the fourth and there is a tight skin fold and shortening of the extensor tendons. The condition may be familial and is often bilateral. Mild degrees of the deformity may be cured by prolonged strapping with adhesive tape. Most require operative treatment which consists of Z-plasty of the skin web, extensor tendon lengthening and capsulotomy of the metatarsophalangeal joint.

— CLUB FOOT (Talipes)

Talipes equino-varus.

This deformity is usually the result of a developmental anomaly, though in some cases it may be due to malposition *in utero*. There is inversion of the forefoot combined with adduction. The heel is smaller than normal and lies to the inner side of the midline of the ankle. There is usually plantar flexion (equinus). The medial border of the foot is concave, the lateral convex. The plantar aspect of the foot faces medially or is even upturned (Fig. 235). In bilateral cases the deformity is always unequal, one foot being more deformed than the other. If the deformity is unilateral the affected foot is smaller than normal.

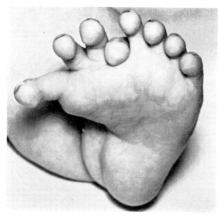

FIG. 231
Polydactyly.

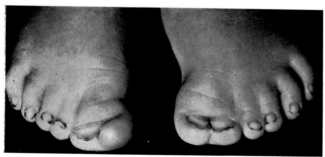

FIG. 232
Syndactyly and polydactyly.

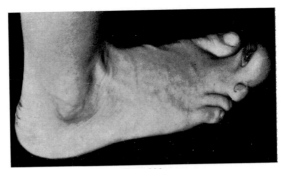

FIG. 233
Giantism of a digit.

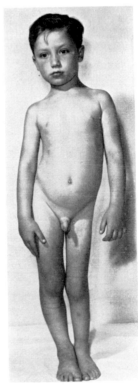

FIG. 234
Hypertrophy of right leg
with pelvic tilt to left and
compensatory scoliosis.

Treatment.—There is a persistent tendency to recurrence after apparent complete correction. At the outset parents are warned that a permanent cure of a severe talipes equino-varus cannot be expected under five years. Treatment should start within a week of birth and supervision should be maintained for five to fifteen years. The foot is manipulated forcibly into the calcaneo-valgus position (*vide infra*) and at the first manipulation an attempt is made to force the foot round until the little toe

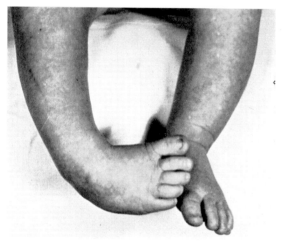

FIG. 235
Right talipes equino-varus.

touches the outer aspect of the leg. Over-correction is maintained by Denis Browne splints. The over-correction into valgus is increased in successive manipulations at intervals of two weeks and it is maintained by packing up the outer side of the sole plate of the splint with adhesive felt (Fig. 236). After three to five months correction should be complete and the Denis Browne splint is then replaced by a removable splint which can be applied by the mother (Fig. 237). This calcaneus splint is worn when the child is asleep. Walking is encouraged as soon as possible and during the day the child is urged to run about.

In relapsed or late untreated cases the feet present a rigid deformity. Such cases are treated by wedged plasters or by

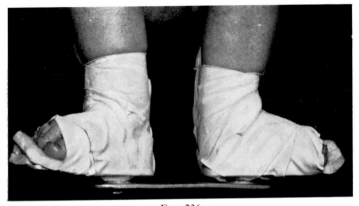

FIG. 236

Talipes equino-varus partially corrected; correction maintained in Denis Browne splint.

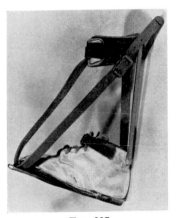

FIG. 237

Removable splint used to maintain correction in talipes equino-varus.

forcible manipulation.   Posterior capsulotomy and lengthening of the tendo Achillis may be required.   Wedge tarsectomy and arthrodesis should rarely be performed in childhood.

Talipes calcaneo-valgus.

This is the most common form of talipes seen by the family doctor.   It is usually a mere exaggeration of the normal calcaneus position of a newborn baby's foot. There is excessive dorsiflexion at the ankle and valgus displacement (pronation) of the foot. If there has been a marked increase in intra-uterine mechanical pressure the deformity is associated with weak muscles or with congenital dislocation of the hip. These children tend to walk late and often develop knock-knee.

Treatment.—In most cases the deformity can be readily corrected and the mother can be reassured that with home manipulation the anomaly will disappear. If there is any doubt that the deformity may be more than an exaggeration of the normal calcaneus position the foot is splinted in the varus position until it can be held naturally inverted.

Although talipes is usually a developmental anomaly similar deformities occur in association with spina bifida (Chap. XXI), or as a secondary deformity in spastic or flaccid paralysis (Chap. XXIV). In such cases the permanent use of corrective footwear with lateral steels is necessary.

Metatarsus varus.

Like equino-varus this form of talipes may be due to malposition *in utero.* There is adduction of the forefoot and when the child starts to walk he tends to trip over his own feet. The footwear quickly becomes misshapen.

Treatment.—The foot is manipulated into an over-corrected position of forefoot abduction which is maintained by a splint. Properly treated, the deformity should be corrected within a few months.

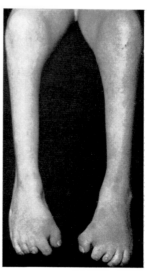

Fig. 238

Arthrogryposis multiplex congenita.

Arthrogryposis multiplex congenita.

As a result of gross intra-uterine pressure combined with malposition there may be weakness of muscles and stiffness in all four limbs (Fig. 238). The knees are usually fixed in extension but there are flexion deformities of the other joints. The lack of results from treatment is depressing.

CONGENITAL GENU RECURVATUM

When a baby is born with the knees hyperextended the deformity is very striking. The anomaly is probably a result of malposition *in utero* and there is usually a breech presentation. The hips are flexed and not infrequently they are actually dislocated. The tibia is hyperextended on the femur and the skin is wrinkled over the knee and tightly stretched over the popliteal fossa.

Despite the apparent severity of the deformity, the prognosis is good. Splints or corrective plaster casts are applied and usually within a few days the knees can be brought back to the neutral position and thereafter they are slowly flexed. It may be wise to hold the knees in flexion for a few months, using a removable splint to allow the physiotherapist to exercise the muscles. Rarely there is a tendency to recurrence and splints and exercises are continued until walking is well established.

CONGENITAL DISLOCATION OF THE HIP

This deformity may be unilateral or bilateral. It is much more common in girls than in boys (8 to 1). The ætiology is obscure but the deformity is probably due to defective development of the acetabulum plus a mechanical thrust from the uterine wall which drives the femoral head downwards and backwards. When the infant extends its legs after birth the powerful longitudinal muscles move the femoral head upwards. The upward movement is increased on walking by the pressure of body weight.

Surgical Anatomy.—The upper rim of the acetabulum fails to develop, the head of the femur is small and the neck shortened and sometimes anteverted. The joint capsule may become stretched and assume an hour-glass shape. The pelvi-femoral muscles become shortened (adductors, hamstrings, sartorius, gracilis, tensor fascia femoris and rectus femoris); the pelvi-trochanteric muscles are stretched (obturators, quadratus femoris, glutei and gemelli).

Clinical Features.—If newborn babies were thoroughly examined dislocations of the hip would be detected early in life.

Usually the diagnosis is not made until the child attempts to walk. She may be slow in walking and a limp (in unilateral dislocation) or characteristic waddling gait (in bilateral dislocation) then draws attention to the defect. Compensatory

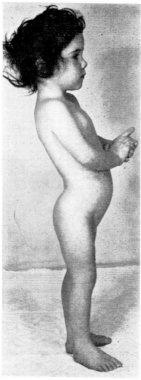

FIG. 239

Lumbar lordosis and protuberant abdomen in congenital dislocation of hips.

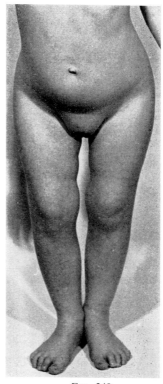

FIG. 240

Pelvic tilt in congenital dislocation of right hip.

lordosis develops early (Fig. 239) and the pelvis is tilted downwards on the affected side (Fig. 240). In *unilateral cases* there is shortening of the affected leg. The great trochanter is unduly prominent and lies above Nelaton's line. If the hip is flexed and fully abducted there is limitation of abduction and external rotation. If the normal hip is then flexed and abducted and the two sides compared it will be seen that on the affected side the angle between the thigh and the trunk is obtuse instead of acute and the normally smooth curve of the buttock and thigh is broken (Fig. 241). Due to displacement of the femoral head the femoral artery loses its support and femoral pulsation is difficult to feel. The femoral head can be felt posteriorly in its abnormal position. " Telescoping " may be felt when the femur is moved up and down in its long axis. *Trendelenburg's Test—* When the child stands on the normal limb and raises the affected limb from the ground the contracted abductor muscles of the hip on the normal side raise the pelvis on the affected side, the upward rotation taking place at the fulcrum formed by a stable

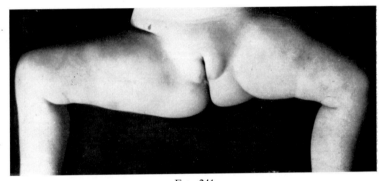

Fig. 241
Congenital dislocation of left hip.

hip joint. Consequently when viewed from behind the buttock on the affected side is seen to rise with this movement. When the child stands on the affected leg with the sound limb off the ground the pelvis drops downwards on the " sound side " and therefore when viewed from behind the buttock on the sound side is seen to drop and remain at a lower level. This occurs because the fulcrum at the hip joint is unstable and in consequence the hip abductors cannot support the pelvis and the body weight. Trendelenburg's test is also positive in gluteal palsy following anterior poliomyelitis.

In *bilateral cases* the legs appear too short for the body, the perineum is broadened and the trochanters are unduly prominent. There is a waddling gait and an increase in lumbar lordosis. Both femoral pulses are difficult to feel, abduction and external rotation are limited, the femoral heads are displaced and telescoping may be elicited on both sides.

Radiographic Appearances.—The femoral capital epiphyses are smaller than normal and in unilateral cases the epiphysis may not be seen on the affected side. The femoral heads may be obviously dislocated on to the dorsum ilii and the femoral neck foreshortened due to anteversion. *Shenton's line* (the arc formed by the under surface of the neck of the femur and the obturator foramen) is broken (Fig. 242). If the radiographic

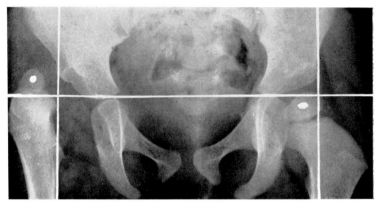

FIG. 242

Radiographic appearances in congenital dislocation of right hip.

diagnosis is in doubt a horizontal line is drawn on the X-ray film through the translucent triradiate cartilages and a vertical line through the outermost part of the acetabular roof. If the lesion is unilateral the vertical line is drawn on the sound side, and on the other side a parallel is drawn at an equal distance from the midline. Normally the femoral capital epiphyses lie below the horizontal and medial to the vertical line. If the femoral head lies lateral to the vertical line or above the horizontal line the hip will dislocate or has dislocated (Fig. 242). The cartilaginous limbus which forms the rim of the acetabulum may be a bar to reduction. Its position can be visualised in an arthrogram following injection of a contrast medium into the hip joint.

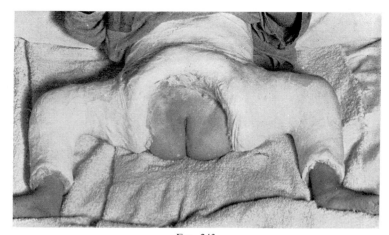

FIG. 243

Congenital dislocation of hip, immobilised in " frog " position in plaster of Paris after reduction.

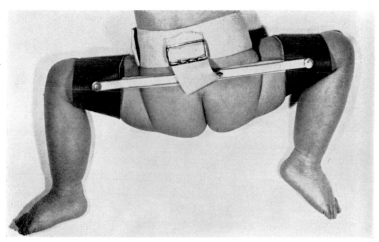

FIG. 244

Denis Browne type of apparatus on patient with reduced bilateral congenital dislocation of hip.

Treatment.—Treatment consists in bringing the head of the femur within the acetabulum and maintaining it in position with plaster of Paris or splints. Reduction can be carried out by manipulation under general anæsthesia and the hips are then immobilised in plaster of Paris with the thighs flexed and widely abducted (the so-called " frog " position) for six to eight weeks (Fig. 243). Most surgeons now prefer to obtain reduction by gradual abduction with skin traction in a frame. Reduction is maintained in plaster of Paris for about two months. Immobilisation thereafter is only partial and restricted mobility is controlled by the Denis Browne apparatus for a further nine months (Fig. 244). The child is left free to get about in any way she likes—crawling, walking on all fours or in a position like a Cossack dancer with knees bent and buttocks close to the floor. An alternative method is to continue the use of a plaster of Paris spica for from six to nine months. During this period the plaster is changed three or four times, or oftener if there is frequent soiling. The degree of abduction is lessened each time. After removal of the plaster a period of physiotherapy precedes weight-bearing.

Until the age of 2 years reduction is usually attained without difficulty and the prognosis is good unless the degree of aplasia is extreme. In older children who have been walking for some time contractures may make reduction impossible even after a period of traction and abduction, and operation is necessary.

In some children though reduction can be attained by manipulation the joint remains unstable. In such cases operation is again necessary and it is usual to reconstruct the acetabulum by making a bony shelf above the acetabular margin.

After the age of 8 or 10 years reduction may be impossible but some improvement in function may be obtained by anterior transposition of the femoral head or by subtrochanteric osteotomy.

Some gross developmental anomalies are illustrated in Figures 245 to 247. Although the deformity in Figure 247 would appear to be hopeless the boy is now ambulant in artificial limbs which have been slowly built up over a period of years (Fig. 248, A, B and C).

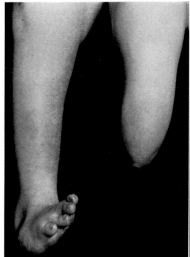

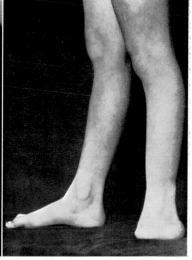

FIG. 245
" Congenital amputation "
of leg.

FIG. 246
" Congenital amputation "
of forefoot.

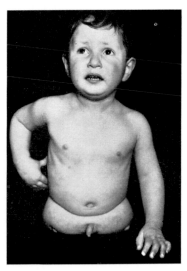

FIG. 247
Bilateral " congenital amputation "
through hips.

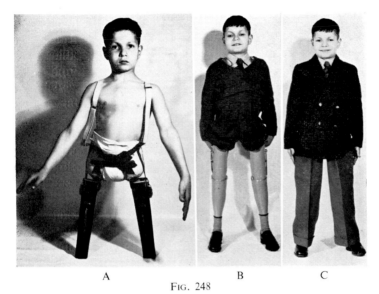

A   B   C

FIG. 248

Patient shown in Fig. 247 wearing intermediate prosthesis. A, Aged 6 years.
B and C, Prosthesis at 9 years.

COMMON POSTURAL DEFECTS

Intelligent observation of the posture of normal children
will refute the suggestion that the legs should be straight.
During the first two years of life there is some degree of genu
varum with an inward twist of the lower end of the leg. When
napkins are finally discarded and the child is fully ambulant
the knees may develop a valgus " deformity " which is maximal
between 4 and 5 years, the malleoli being 2 in. apart. The
normal infant's foot has little arch and even this is often
concealed by a pad of fat ; the heels are usually everted.

Flat Foot.

The child is brought to the doctor because the parents
have noticed the flat or pronated feet, because of a pigeon-toed
gait or because the child complains of pain in the foot or leg.
The clinician looks not for a flat foot but for a foot which is
functioning in a position that throws strain on the ligaments
and muscles. The longitudinal and anterior arches are examined

in recumbency and on weight-bearing. The position of the os calcis in relation to the weight-bearing line is noted. Any eversion of the heel is best seen from behind with the foot at eye level.

" Valgus ankles " are probably normal when a child begins to walk and in most cases the deformity disappears spontaneously. If the eversion of the heels persists or is marked in a young child, an $\frac{1}{8}$-in. wedge is applied to the medial aspect of the heels of the shoes and longer rest periods are advised. In the older child the parents usually complain not of the feet but of the shoes. Treatment can often be based on the way the shoes are worn down. When the shoes are worn down on the inside valgus wedges are applied to the heels and a medial prolongation to the heel may be added. If the uppers are broken down on the inside valgus stiffening is added to the valgus wedging of the heels. The child is instructed in suitable exercises. A third type of shoe deformity is encountered in which the shoe is trodden down on the outer side. The child has no disability, but the economic problem of distortion of footwear can be partially met by fitting crepe-rubber soles and heels. Walking exercises are prescribed.

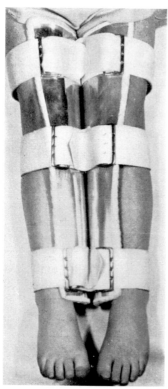

FIG. 249
" Mermaid " splint

Knock Knees (Genu valgum).

Nowadays knock knee and bow leg are seldom due to rickets. When a child of 2 or 3 years stands with his knees touching and the malleoli are no more than $1\frac{1}{2}$ in. to 2 in. apart, the mother can be assured that the condition will be cured before the age of 5. Adequate rest periods are advised particularly in heavy children. If the knock knee is associated with everted heels $\frac{1}{8}$-in. valgus wedging of the heels is prescribed. Although this is unlikely to affect the growth of the femoral condyles it certainly helps to correct the knee deformity. When the malleoli are more than $2\frac{1}{2}$ in. apart or where valgus wedges alone fail to correct the deformity "Mermaid" splints (Fig. 249) are made to fit the patient and are worn in bed at night.

Bow Legs (Genu varum).

These children are usually well developed and the deformity is self-curing, the cure starting soon after the napkins (which force the thighs apart) are discarded. If the legs are still bowed after the age of 2 a modified "Mermaid" splint can be worn at night. Osteochondrosis of the medial tibial condyle (Blount's disease) (Fig. 250) may lead to genu varum and this condition should be excluded by X-ray. Severe deformity from resistant rickets may occasionally require osteoclasis or osteotomy.

THE LIMPING CHILD

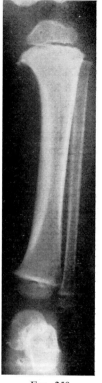

FIG. 250

Osteochondrosis of medial tibial condyle : Blount's disease.

The causes of a limp are many and varied and it is sometimes difficult to determine the site of the causal lesion in a young child. From the history, from observation of the gait and from clinical examination, however, it is usually possible to decide whether the cause is to be found in the bones, the joints or the muscles and ligaments. Not uncommonly no lesion can be discovered and it is well to bear in mind that children will sometimes limp to draw attention to themselves or even in imitation of a limping adult. Moreover, children may firmly deny the history of an injury if it has been sustained during some forbidden activity. Even in the course of ordinary play they may subject their joints and muscles to strain beyond the normal range without any marked pain at the time, and when pain arises later they may quite honestly deny any injury or hurt.

If the limp has been present since the child started to walk the most likely causes are congenital dislocation of the hip joint, spastic hemiplegia, congenital anomalies of the limb or pelvis, undiagnosed neonatal osteitis with damage to the femoral head or undiagnosed poliomyelitis.

In an older child a limp of recent onset is commonly due to minor injuries to the bones or joints often unnoticed by the child. Such lesions are self-curing and the child soon ceases to limp, usually in a matter of days or a few weeks. In some cases the limp will persist long after the pain has ceased.

The causal lesion may be in the foot, the leg, the knee or hip joint. In the foot painful heel, osteochondritis of the tarsal scaphoid and *march fracture* of a metatarsal are all met with in children. In the region of the knee osteochondritis of the tibial apophysis (Osgood-Schlatter's disease) is uncommon before puberty but traction injuries to the apophysis are common in younger children. A less common cause of local pain in the inner side of the knee is an osteochondrosis of the medial tibial condyle (Blount's disease) (Fig. 250). This is associated with a differential growth rate and bowing of the leg.

The greatest difficulties arise when the lesion seems to be in the region of the hip joint. The pain may be slight and inter-mittent and referred by the child vaguely to the buttock, the groin or even the knee. It may be felt only on movement or may be more severe at night in bed. Physical signs may be slight or equivocal. Limitation of passive movement may affect only one range of movement or it may involve all the movements of which the joint is capable; it may be found throughout the whole range of a movement or may be elicited only at the extremes of movement. The limitation may be extra-articular in origin, due, for example, to spasm of the psoas muscle associated with an intra-abdominal lesion such as deep iliac adenitis or a pelvic abscess, or with a psoas abscess arising in a tuberculous lesion of the spine.

There are however three conditions common in childhood, originating in the hip joint but differing widely in cause and prognosis, that call for comment in some detail. These are *synovitis of the hip joint*, traumatic or infective ; *osteochondritis of the femoral capital epiphysis* (Perthes' disease) ; and *tuberculous disease* of the hip joint.

SYNOVITIS OF THE HIP

This is the most common cause of pain and spasm in the hip. The synovitis is usually traumatic in origin although a history of injury may be difficult to obtain. Passive movement is painful and limitation is present throughout the range of all movements. There is no constitutional disturbance and the child is usually comfortable in bed. The erythrocyte sedimentation rate is normal.

A subacute infective synovitis is also common—probably following trauma in a child with bacteræmia. In such patients the temperature is elevated, there is acute pain and limitation of all hip joint movements. It may be difficult to exclude osteitis of the upper femur or pyogenic arthritis.

Treatment.—Both types of synovitis subside with a few days' rest in bed, but in the infective type skin traction and four-hourly aspirin may be required to give relief from pain. If the child is toxic blood is taken for culture and an antibiotic is administered until one is certain that there is no serious pyogenic infection in bone or joint. The heart is examined and if an apical systolic murmur is present juvenile rheumatism must be considered. Rheumatism may start with pain in the hip and the pain does not always move to another joint.

OSTEOCHONDRITIS OF THE FEMORAL CAPITAL EPIPHYSIS (PERTHES' DISEASE)

This is a deforming condition of the femoral head caused by interference with its blood supply. It is most common in boys between the ages of 2 and 10 years, affecting usually only one limb but sometimes both. The most constant early sign is a limp which is intermittent and most marked after exercise and when the child is tired. Although pain is not complained of spontaneously the child will sometimes admit that he limps because his leg is sore. The general health is good although the boy tires more readily than his fellows. The only physical sign

24

found in the early stages is remarkably constant and consists of limitation of the range of abduction and of internal rotation of the hip joint. Flexion, extension and adduction are normal and there is no muscle atrophy or shortening of the limb.

The radiographic appearances are usually well marked and in sharp contrast to the comparatively mild clinical changes.

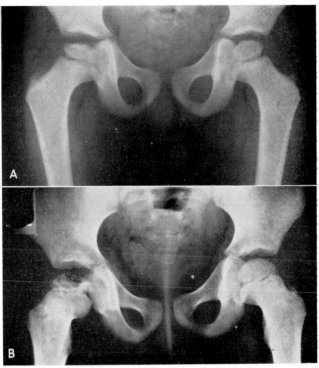

FIG. 251
Perthes' disease. A, Aged 4 years. B, Aged 5 years.

The earliest change noticeable in cases of recent origin is slight increase in the density of the epiphyseal shadow. This is followed very soon by flattening of the normal curvature as though some degree of compression had occurred (Fig. 251, A). Then areas of rarefaction appear, producing the appearance of fragmentation of the femoral head (Fig. 251, B). The areas of irregular density are gradually replaced by areas of decalcification. At the same time the flattening becomes more marked with spreading at the periphery, producing a mushroom-like appearance (Fig. 251, c). After a period varying from one to four years the bony structure is restored as recalcification proceeds, until the appearance is almost normal (Fig. 251, d). In most cases some degree of flattening persists despite clinical cure. In a minority of cases the femoral neck and even the

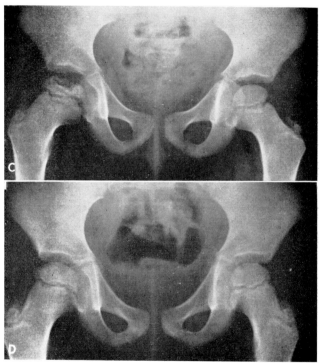

Fig. 251
Perthes' disease. C, Aged 6 years. D, Aged 8 years.

acetabulum become involved in the process and gross deformity of the head and neck follows with considerable limitation of abduction and rotation (Fig. 252).

Prognosis.—Osteochondritis is a self-limiting disease with ultimate spontaneous recovery. If weight-bearing is allowed during the active phase of the disease there is likely to be permanent flattening and deformity of the femoral head. In

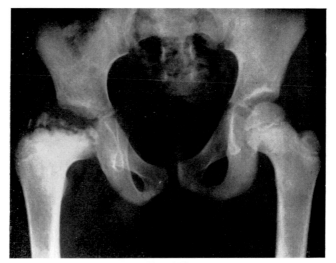

FIG. 252

Severe osteochondritis of head and neck of femur.

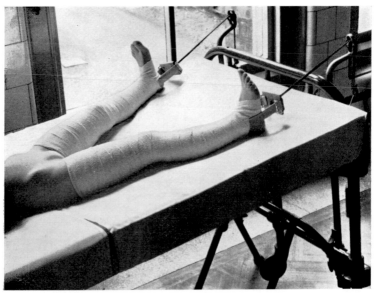

FIG. 253

Skin traction used for fracture of femur and Perthes' disease.

spite of the deformity there is little evidence that osteochondritis leads to osteo-arthritis of the hip in later life.

Treatment.—Weight-bearing is forbidden until there is radio-graphic evidence of satisfactory reformation of the femoral head. Bed rest may last for one to three years. (In some patients with osteochondritis involving the femoral neck as long as eight years may elapse before there is satisfactory consolidation of the bone.) It is impossible to keep an otherwise healthy child at rest in bed for such lengthy periods without some form of restraint. This restraint is best maintained with skin traction with weights and pulleys (Fig. 253). Before school age this treatment can be carried out at home, but after the age of 5 years treatment is maintained in an institution which can provide education of a standard accepted by the local Education Authority. When radiographic consolidation is well advanced early ambulation is sometimes allowed, using a Thomas walking caliper to restrain the patient's wilder activities.

TUBERCULOSIS OF THE HIP JOINT

Tuberculosis commonly affects the hip joint before the age of 10 years. The blood-borne infection usually attacks the synovial membrane; less frequently the disease starts in Babcock's triangle on the under surface of the neck of the femur or in the acetabulum. The hip lesion is usually secondary to a focus in the lung and is due to a human strain of the tubercle bacillus in most cases.

Clinical Features.—A limp is usually the first sign, but pain may be an early feature and this may be referred to the knee. On examination there is wasting of the thigh and buttock and this may be present very early. There is limitation of joint movement in all directions in contrast to the limitation only of abduction and internal rotation in osteochondritis. There may be apparent lengthening of the leg when effusion into the joint leads to abduction of the hip; later the thigh is adducted from muscle spasm and there is apparent shortening of the leg. Night-starting pains indicate erosion of articular cartilage. True shortening occurs when the bone is eroded or the femoral head dislocated (Fig. 254).

Diagnosis.—Limp, limitation of *all* movements and muscle

atrophy should make one suspect tuberculosis *even when the general health is good and there is no radiographic evidence of joint disease.* A Mantoux test is done, the lung fields are X-rayed, the erythrocyte sedimentation rate measured and a white blood cell count performed. During these investigations the hip is immobilised by the application of skin traction. Should radiography reveal bone atrophy a biopsy of the deep inguinal glands is performed. If no bacilli are revealed and the diagnosis is still in doubt a synovial biopsy is carried out.

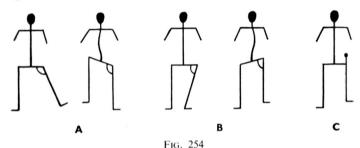

A   B   C

FIG. 254

Tuberculosis of left hip. A, Effusion leading to abduction. When legs are parallel, pelvis tilts with apparent lengthening of left leg. B, Adduction of hip. When legs are parallel, the left leg shows apparent shortening. C, Erosion or dislocation causes actual shortening.

Treatment.—Tuberculosis of the hip is a manifestation of a general disease so that a sanatorium regime is imperative. Treatment is by prolonged immobilisation, first by traction to correct deformity and then in the optimum position in a frame or in a plaster of Paris case. Streptomycin, para-aminosalicylic acid and isoniazid have greatly shortened the period of treatment, have reduced the incidence of complications and allow a direct surgical attack on the joint without the risk of sinus formation or dissemination of the disease.

COXA VARA

The normal angle formed by the femoral neck with the shaft of the femur is 135 degrees, and any decrease in the neck-shaft angle is known as *coxa vara.* It is a feature of many different conditions—congenital dislocation of the hip, Perthes' disease, various forms of arthritis, slipped epiphysis (*vide infra* Fractures), rickets, achondroplasia, hypothyroidism, etc. In addition, many writers have described the condition of *idiopathic coxa vara*, said to be due to " a failure of mineralisation of the femoral neck." Although once common, this condition is no longer seen in the Royal Hospital for Sick Children. When the patient is fully investigated, an underlying cause can almost always be found. " Idiopathic " coxa vara has vanished with the disappearance of severe rickets ! Nevertheless, coxa vara is occasionally seen in young children and the clinical features merit a brief description.

Clinical Features.—The child, who is usually over the age of 3, is brought to the doctor because of a limp or, if the lesion is bilateral, with a waddling gait. Abduction of the hip is limited, there is a positive Trendelenburg test (see Congenital Dislocation of the Hip), the perineum may be widened and the trochanters prominent. The condition may be confused with congenital dislocation of the hip, but the diagnosis is made clear by radiography. The femoral neck forms a right angle with the shaft and the translucent area occupied by the epiphyseal line is unusually wide. There is usually premature closure of the epiphyseal line and the deformity rarely progresses after the age of 12.

Treatment.—Bed rest and skin traction do not affect the deformity. Subtrochanteric osteotomy may be required at puberty.

COXA VALGA

In children who have never walked because of developmental defects or severe paralysis, the angle between the femoral neck and shaft remains greater than 140 degrees—a condition referred to as *coxa valga*. The deformity is usually present in children with paralytic dislocation of the hip. The clinical features are those of the associated disease and treatment of the coxa valga is rarely required.

PARALYTIC DISLOCATION OF HIP

Posterior dislocation of the hips may occur in the flail lower limbs of poliomyelitis and myelomeningocele ; less commonly, it occurs in spastic paralysis. Fixation of the hips in an abducted position helps to prevent dislocation and aids in maintaining reduction once this has been achieved.

THE KNEE

Acute Prepatellar Bursitis.—In childhood prepatellar bursitis is commonly secondary to a superficial septic focus in the region. The swelling tends to be more diffuse than in the adult and when there is a sympathetic effusion into the knee joint the lesion may resemble closely a septic arthritis of the knee. The condition may subside following administration of parenteral penicillin or it may be necessary to evacuate pus.

Chronic prepatellar bursitis is not seen in childhood.

Semimembranosus Bursa.—A swelling appears between the tendon of the semimembranosus and the medial head of the gastrocnemius. It is rendered tense and more apparent when the knee joint is fully extended. The swelling may disappear spontaneously in a few weeks and excision is rarely necessary. Many cases have been cured rapidly following aspiration and instillation of hyaluronidase.

Congenital Discoid Meniscus.—The fœtal meniscus consists of a complete disc and sometimes normal resorption of the central portion does not take place. The anomaly usually occurs in the lateral meniscus. The child's knee clicks in flexion and extension and there may be effusion into the joint. An older child may complain that the knee gives way.

The condition is treated by excision of the disc. It is difficult to persuade a child to move the painful leg properly after operation so that it is advisable to teach him quadriceps exercises *before* operation.

Recurrent Dislocation of the Patella.—The patella may be dislocated at birth or dislocation may be due to trauma. Recurrent dislocation however is a result of an abnormal direction of pull of the quadriceps muscle. It is more common in the female and tends to be familial.

Clinical Features.—The child is usually over 6 years and the condition is most commonly seen in the rapidly growing young adolescent. There is a history of recurring pain or swelling in the knee and the incidents usually occur when the child has been sitting for a prolonged period. The dislocation is rarely seen by the doctor but there is usually fluid in the joint for forty-eight hours after each incident. There may be atrophy of the thigh. With the knee extended and the quadriceps relaxed the patella can be pushed over the lateral condyle of the femur.

Treatment.—During the growing period the knee is supported by a crepe bandage or an elastic knee cap and the physiotherapist arranges quadriceps drill. After the age of 15 it may be necessary to transfer medially the insertion of the patellar tendon. If operation is carried out too early there may be damage to the growing apophysis with interference with growth.

Osteochondritis Dissecans.—Although more common in adult life, this disease also occurs in children. The medial femoral condyle is the most common site, but it can affect the ankle, hip or elbow. It is more common in males and may be bilateral. There is aseptic necrosis of subchondral bone and the fragment, which may separate, includes subchondral bone and cartilage.

There is recurrent pain in the knee, intermittent swelling and a history of clicking and weakness in the joint. There may be atrophy of the thigh. Radiography shows a radiolucent line separating a small dense fragment of bone or the fragment may be seen free in the joint.

The lesion may heal with conservative treatment in a non-weight-bearing splint for four to six months. If the fragment has become detached, it is removed.

Monarticular Arthritis.—In this condition, chronic synovial thickening and increase in joint fluid simulates rheumatoid arthritis limited to one joint. It is fairly common in the ankle and it may affect the hip or elbow but is characteristically seen in the knee. It occurs most commonly between the ages of 3 and 10 years.

The patient presents with chronic swelling of the knee of weeks' or months' duration. Pain is slight but a limp is common. There is synovial thickening and aspiration of joint fluid reveals cellular or chemical changes similar to those found in rheumatoid arthritis. A Mantoux test is performed and the knee joint and lung fields are X-rayed. If the test is positive and tuberculosis cannot be eliminated from the differential diagnosis, joint biopsy is performed.

The knee may be flexed and traction may be necessary to secure full extension. Thereafter absolute rest to the knee is achieved by a plaster of Paris case or a specially made splint. Gradual resumption of weight-bearing is allowed after three or four months. The erythrocyte sedimentation rate is checked at regular intervals. A complete cure is effected in most cases but a few develop rheumatoid arthritis.

The Foreign-body Knee.—Foreign bodies such as needles, glass, wood or clothing may penetrate the knee joint and give rise to a clinical picture similar to monarticular arthritis. There is chronic swelling of the knee and X-ray may reveal the foreign body. The aspirated joint fluid usually contains a large quantity of fibrin clot.

The joint is opened and the fibrin clot and any accessible foreign body removed.

Septic Arthritis.—Blood-borne septic arthritis is rare but the knee may be infected from osteitis of the lower femur or upper tibia. Direct infection may follow a puncture wound of the knee.

The knee is swollen and acutely painful and tender and there are signs of toxæmia. The differential diagnosis is from *popliteal adenitis* and *acute prepatellar bursitis*. In septic arthritis the swelling is most apparent in the region of the suprapatellar pouch.

Penicillin is administered and the leg is immobilised by skin traction. The causal organism is grown from a blood culture or from the aspirated joint fluid. The treatment of septic arthritis is more fully considered in Chapter V.

Tuberculosis.—There is relatively painless chronic swelling of the knee with synovial thickening, and early atrophy of the thigh. The Mantoux test is positive, the erythrocyte sedimentation rate is raised and aspiration of joint fluid reveals 1,000 to 2,000 white cells per cubic millimetre—mainly polymorphonuclear. Radiography shows fluid in the joint and decalcification of bone; rarely there may be bone destruction in the epiphysis. The diagnosis is confirmed by synovial biopsy.

As in bone and joint tuberculosis elsewhere, sanatorium treatment is desirable. Streptomycin, P.A.S. and isoniazid are administered and the knee is immobilised in a bivalved, unilateral hip spica. Since the introduction of effective antibiotic therapy, it is justifiable to try to preserve movement in the joint by removing the leg from the spica for daily exercises.

PAINFUL HEEL

This is a common complaint in childhood. Apart from definite injuries and low-grade osteitis of the calcaneus, the painful heel may be due to the following conditions.

Strain of the Tendo Achillis.—This is usually the result of the vigorous activities of childhood. There may be fullness and tenderness over the tendon. The condition is relieved by strapping and rest. If the strain persists, a half-inch cork elevator is fitted inside the heel of the shoe and heat and gentle massage prescribed.

Calcaneal Bursitis.—The pain arises in an adventitious bursa over the tendo Achillis caused by the pressure of ill-fitting shoes. A cork elevator is fitted and suitable footwear obtained.

Calcaneal Apophysitis (Osteochondritis: Sever's disease).—This form of osteochondritis rarely occurs in childhood. There is pain and tenderness in the back of the heel and radiography shows patchy sclerosis of the apophysis. A heel elevator is fitted to the shoe and acute pain is relieved by strapping. The condition is self-curing.

PAINFUL FOOT

Foot Strain.—Over-activity and insufficient rest often cause ligamentous strains of the inner side of the foot and ankle. The child limps and often stands on the outer border of the foot with the toes curled under. The feet are more comfortable without shoes.

The symptoms are relieved by the application of adhesive strapping to the feet with the heels inverted.

Osteochondritis of the Tarsal Scaphoid (Köhler's disease).—This condition occurs between the ages of 3 and 6 years and there is pain and swelling on the dorsum of the foot. The pain is aggravated by walking and the child usually bears weight on the outer border of the foot. Radiography reveals sclerosis and flattening of the scaphoid (Fig. 255) and there may be some fragmentation. The condition can be simulated by tuberculosis of the scaphoid and the prognosis should be guarded until the radiographic changes are typical. Pain is usually relieved by strapping and when the possibility of tuberculosis has been ruled

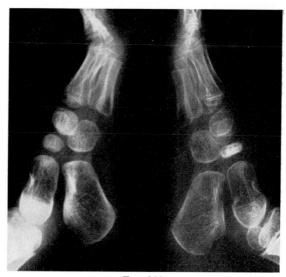

FIG. 255
Osteochondritis of right tarsal scaphoid
(Köhler's disease).

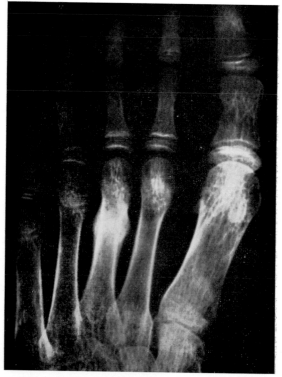

FIG. 256
Stress fracture of third metatarsal.

out the parents can be reassured that osteochondritis is a self-curing condition.

March Fracture (Pied forcé).—This form of stress fracture affecting the second, third or fourth metatarsal is seen occasionally in childhood. The patient complains of pain in the foot and there is pain and tenderness over the affected metatarsal. The radiographic appearances are the same as in the young adult (Fig. 256). Acute pain is relieved by strapping and firm footwear and dancing and strenuous games should be avoided for a few weeks.

CAVUS FOOT

A high-arched foot with forefoot equinus and claw toes can produce severe disability. The deformity is rarely seen before the age of 3 years. Various neurological conditions may be responsible for the deformity—spina bifida or other lesions of the spinal cord such as Friedreich's ataxia and infantile paralysis. In many patients there is no history or definite evidence of any predisposing disease, but slight atrophy of the limb suggests a mild and undiagnosed attack of poliomyelitis some time in the past.

The child is clumsy in walking and falls frequently. Later there is pain on walking and callosities develop under the heads of the metatarsals. Corns may develop on the prominences of the hammer toes.

Mild degrees of the deformity respond to manipulation. More severe cases are treated by plantar fasciotomy and wrenching or by a modified Steindler operation in which the short muscles and ligaments are elevated off the calcaneus; the long extensor tendons are transplanted to the metatarsal heads.

IDIOPATHIC GANGRENE IN THE NEWBORN

On three occasions we have treated infants with gangrene of the forefoot occurring in the neonatal period (Fig. 257). In none was there evidence of syphilis or other vascular disease nor was there evidence of birth trauma. In one instance the baby was resuscitated by injection of a stimulant into the umbilical

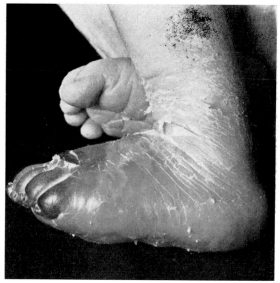

FIG. 257

Idiopathic gangrene of the forefoot in a baby aged 2 weeks.

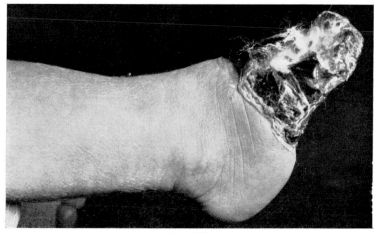

FIG. 258

Spontaneous separation taking place in neonatal gangrene of foot.

" vein." Even if the injection had been given into the umbilical artery by accident one must postulate some anomalous connection between the umbilical and the common or external iliac arteries before such a catastrophe could occur.

The gangrene is dry and spontaneous separation takes place (Fig. 258). The stump is covered by a skin graft (Fig. 259).

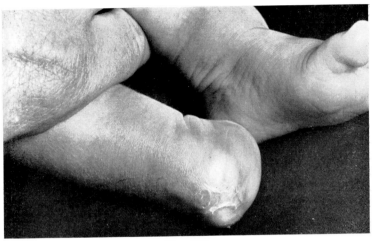

FIG. 259
Grafted stump of foot following neonatal gangrene.

Suitably blocked footwear is provided when the child starts to walk.

Gangrene of the foot has been reported as a complication of intravenous therapy via the saphenous vein at the medial malleolus. We have not experienced this tragic complication of intravenous therapy in infancy or childhood.

PSEUDOHYPERTROPHIC MUSCULAR DYSTROPHY

Many patients with this primary myopathy first report with flat feet or a stumbling gait, and although the loss of muscle function affects more than the legs, it is convenient to consider the disease in this section. The myopathy is frequently familial and is more common among male than female siblings. The diagnosis is usually obvious before the age of 6 years. The muscle weakness is symmetrical, progressive and characterised by enlargement of muscle groups, most typically seen in the calf muscles. Atrophy of the shoulder girdle muscles may be present from the onset or may follow later.

The child has difficulty in climbing stairs, is easily fatigued and the gait is characterised by stumbling and frequent falls. The calves are enlarged (like a professional footballer) and feel doughy on palpation. When the patient is placed on the floor he rolls over and rises to his feet by " climbing up his thighs " —that is, he aids extension of the knees by supporting the quadriceps with his hands. Many of the children become obese due to inactivity. The condition is slowly progressive and the patient is finally bedridden. Many succumb to respiratory or other infection during late childhood or adolescence.

No treatment affects the progress of the disease. The child is kept ambulant as long as possible, at first with the encouragement of a physiotherapist and, later, supported by calipers and a suitable brace. Stretching exercises may delay the onset of contractures. When the child is no longer able to walk, treatment of contractures must not be too enthusiastic. The patient has not many years to live and must be able to sit up in bed or in a chair. It is quite unjustifiable to keep the legs and spine straight by keeping the child flat on his back.

FRACTURES

FEMUR

Fracture of the neck of the femur is rare in childhood but it may occur in association with severe multiple injuries which may prove fatal.

Slipped Femoral Epiphysis.

Although this condition is more common after puberty it may occur earlier. The patients are often fat and flabby and they complain of pain in the hip or knee and walk with a limp. All movements of the hip are limited and radiography shows slipping of the epiphysis, usually associated with coxa vara. Treatment is by bed rest with skin traction. Reduction usually takes place in a few weeks but traction should be maintained for two months. With minimal trauma or none at all, the capital epiphysis may separate completely off the neck in either the early or late stage of the disease. If seen promptly in the early stage, gentle closed reduction is performed followed by nailing. Reduction by open operation should be avoided because of the risk of avascular necrosis of the femoral head. Subtrochanteric osteotomy should not be performed in this condition until the epiphysis has fused.

Subtrochanteric and Upper Third Fractures.

The upper fragment in this type of fracture is flexed, abducted and externally rotated. Effective control of the fragment is impossible and accordingly the lower fragment must be brought into alignment with it. Under general anæsthesia traction is applied to the limb followed by flexion, abduction and external rotation. A complete plaster spica is applied as far as the lower tibia, the knee joint being flexed to 45 degrees. The plaster is kept on for a minimum period of eight weeks.

Fracture of the Middle Third.

In this, the commonest type of fracture of the femur in childhood, the method of treatment depends upon the age of the child.

1. *Birth Fractures.*—Treatment is described on page 22. Very rarely these fractures are complicated by damage to the lumbo-sacral plexus. The flaccid paralysis of the leg which follows this nerve injury may also occur without bone damage.

2. *From Infancy to Four Years of Age.*—The method of choice for this age group is vertical traction. Adhesive strapping is applied to *both* legs and the cords from the stirrups are tied to a cross bar fixed to the sides of the cot so that the buttocks are just free of the mattress. The position seems to be comfortable and nursing is greatly facilitated (Fig. 260). Firm union occurs in about four weeks.

3. *From Four Years Onwards.*—The most popular method of treatment is the application of a plaster spica. In the common oblique or spiral fracture there is usually little displacement and but little shortening (Fig. 261). The maintenance of the normal slight anterior bowing is particularly important and the spica is applied to include the pelvis and the foot. Union is complete in four to six weeks after which a period of a week in bed is desirable to allow restoration of normal muscle tone and movements before weight-bearing is permitted.

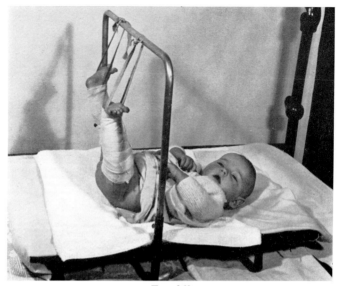

Fig. 260
Fracture of femur in infant, immobilised in gallows splint.

In the transverse type of fracture, angling, lateral displacement and considerable shortening may be present (Fig. 262). Firm traction and careful manipulation are called for to correct these deformities before the spica is applied.

For the oblique or spiral fracture an alternative method of treatment has been used in the Royal Hospital for Sick Children, Glasgow, for many years with satisfactory results. The method consists of free horizontal traction by weight and pulley with the end of the bed raised to increase the counter traction of the child's weight. No attempt is made to immobilise the fracture and the child is free to move about in bed or even turn round or sit up. Traction is constant and normal alignment maintained (Fig. 253). Within a day or two the child seems comfortable and nursing presents no difficulties. Firm union with a large mass of callus occurs in three weeks, after which the child is allowed freedom in bed for a further week before attempting to bear weight on the limb. The children are comfortable and enjoy the freedom of moving about and sitting up in bed.

In older children the additional use of a Thomas knee splint for the first ten days or so is perhaps desirable. The

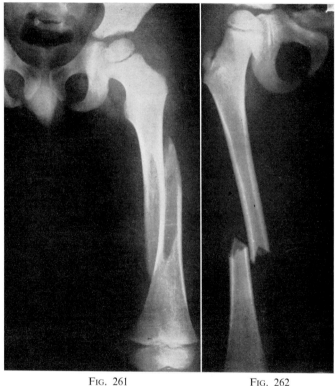

FIG. 261   FIG. 262

Fig. 261.—Oblique fracture of femur.
Fig. 262.—Transverse fracture of femur.

slings require constant supervision and adjustment. When firm callus is palpable the splint may be discarded and free traction maintained for the remaining period.

Fracture of the Lower Third.

This fracture is usually transverse with backward tilting of the lower fragment and overriding of the fragments. The displacement is corrected by manipulation under anæsthesia with the knee flexed to 90 degrees. The position is maintained until a plaster spica is applied from the groin to the toes. A careful watch must be kept on the circulation of the limb. The spica is kept on for six weeks and the usual period of freedom in bed allowed before weight-bearing is permitted.

The most common supracondylar fracture in children is the incomplete compression fracture without gross displacement. A simple straight walking plaster is applied from the groin to the toes and weight-bearing allowed. The plaster can be removed in six weeks' time.

PATELLA

This is an uncommon fracture in children and the types of lesion are similar to those in adults. If there is little separation of the fragments a crepe bandage is applied and weight-bearing allowed. This is removed in two weeks and movements of the knee joint and power of the quadriceps are soon normal. Where wide separation of the fragments occurs open operation and suture of the aponeurosis is advisable before application of the plaster cast. There is no justification for excision of the patella as full function is invariably attained by the treatment described above.

TIBIA AND FIBULA

Stress Injury to the Tibial Tubercle.

This type of injury is common in children before fusion of the epiphysis. In active and vigorous children the quadriceps attachment to the tubercle is subjected to frequent strain. The lateral expansions of the tendon prevent a complete separation of the epiphysis but partial separation may result in pain and tenderness localised to the tubercle and often called Osgood-Schlatter's disease. (Analogous lesions are found at the base of the fifth metatarsal and the posterior facet of the os calcis to which is attached the tendo Achillis.) The condition in most cases is self-curing if the more vigorous games are prohibited.

Fractures of the Tibial Tuberosities.

The more severe forms of this fracture with separation and depression of the fragments are rare in children. Complete correction of the displacement is essential in such cases and there should be no hesitation in resorting to open operation and pinning of the fragment accurately in place. Even so there is a risk that the growth area may be damaged with consequent persistent inequality of growth. Should this occur the employment of stapling in an attempt to delay the growth on the sound side is justifiable. Unfortunately the result is uncertain.

The less severe forms in which slight depression only is present are best treated by immobilisation of the joint in its normal position for at least two months. Thereafter a further period of at least six months' weight-bearing in a walking caliper should be enforced.

Fractures of the Middle Third.

The commonest type of fracture of the tibia in a child is the oblique or spiral fracture of the middle third of the bone. It

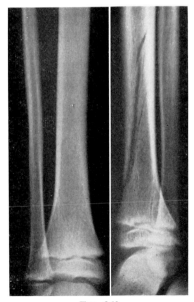

FIG. 263
Fracture of the tibia, apparent only
in the lateral view.

is frequently greenstick in character without displacement or abnormal mobility and only the lateral X-ray film reveals the thin crack as the cause of the local tenderness (Fig. 263). The fracture may be complete but if the fibula remains intact displacement is usually slight. Not infrequently the torsional strain fractures the fibula as well but at a different level, usually the upper end. Such fractures are treated by the application of a walking plaster case from mid-thigh to the toes for three to six weeks. The child is encouraged to walk as soon as the pain and discomfort cease and when the cast is removed normal gait is soon established.

Fracture of the Lower Third.

Fracture of the lower third of the tibia is commonly due to direct violence and the fibula is broken at or about the same level. Deformity may be marked and correction difficult. Under general anæsthesia traction is applied with the knee flexed over the end of the table. The fragments are then moulded into correct alignment, particular care being taken to restore the normal anterior bowing, and the plaster case is then applied from mid-thigh to the toes. A careful watch is kept on the circulation. This plaster is kept on for four weeks and is then replaced by a below-knee walking plaster for a further three weeks. Should difficulty be experienced in bringing the foot to a right angle without causing backward bowing of the fragments there need be no hesitation in applying the plaster with the foot in slight plantar flexion. Full range of ankle joint movement is always attained subsequently.

Fracture Separation of the Lower Tibial Epiphysis.

This type of injury is analogous to the fracture separation of the lower radial epiphysis and usually a small wedge of the metaphysis is detached from the postero-lateral area and accompanies the displaced epiphysis, the fibula being fractured $1\frac{1}{2}$ to 2 in. above its tip. The greatest care must be taken to correct the displacement fully and a plaster case is applied with the heel well inverted for a period of four weeks. Thereafter it is replaced by a walking cast for a further three weeks.

Fractures of the Malleoli.

Minor fractures of the malleoli without displacement are not uncommon and are treated by the application of a below-knee walking plaster.

Frequently the medial malleolus is fractured at its base accompanied by a fracture of the lower end of the fibula about $1\frac{1}{2}$ in. above the tip. Some degree of lateral displacement may accompany this injury and in applying the plaster cast the heel should be well inverted. At the end of three weeks this case is replaced by a walking plaster for a further three weeks.

FRACTURES OF THE BONES OF THE FOOT

Os Calcis.—The more severe types of fracture of the os calcis are rare but incomplete fractures in the form of cracks are not uncommon. The diagnosis may be made only from the X-ray film as displacement is rare. A below-knee walking plaster cast is applied to the base of the phalanges and weight-bearing allowed. The plaster is removed after three weeks.

Talus.—Fracture of the talus, though uncommon, may occur in association with severe crushing injuries, the bone being driven upwards between the tibia and fibula. Should the bone be dislocated and its blood supply cut off avascular necrosis will develop. Regeneration in such cases is slow and prolonged freedom from weight-bearing essential until the X-ray film shows satisfactory recalcification.

Fracture of the other small bones of the foot is uncommon. Union occurs readily if the foot is immobilised in a plaster cast for four weeks.

Fracture of the Metatarsal Bones and Phalanges.—Fracture of the base of the fifth metatarsal is not uncommon and requires no treatment beyond rest in bed for two weeks. Alternatively a light walking plaster may be applied for the same period. Care must be taken not to mistake the common presence of an accessory bone—the os vesalanium—for a fracture.

A badly crushed foot is moulded back to its normal contours, held in a padded plaster cast and elevated on pillows. When the swelling subsides an unpadded plaster is applied. The meta-tarsals eventually remould themselves and the function is excellent.

Broken phalanges are splinted or bound to an adjacent toe.

CHAPTER XXIV

Paralysis in Childhood

OBSTETRICAL PARALYSIS

FORCIBLE manipulation or traction on the arm during delivery may damage the brachial plexus (Chap. III. Birth Trauma). In *Erb-Duchenne paralysis* the fifth and sixth cervical nerves or their roots are damaged, causing paralysis of the abductors and lateral rotators of the shoulder and flexors of the elbow. The arm hangs at the side in an attitude of internal

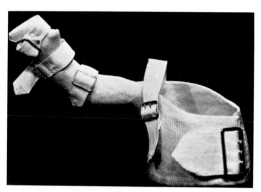

Fig. 264
Modified Fairbank splint (made from Glassona) for right Erb's palsy.

rotation with the forearm pronated and with flexed fingers and wrist. The differential diagnosis is from fracture of the clavicle or humerus and from neonatal osteitis. During the first ten days of life the sleeve should be pinned to the pillow to keep the shoulder abducted and the elbow flexed (Fig. 8); most cases recover within this time. If the arm cannot be fully abducted by the end of the second week it is immobilised in a modified Fairbank's splint made to fit the patient (Fig. 264). The splint is worn night and day and removed only for bathing and for massage and passive exercises. Recovery is usually complete within three months if there is no permanent damage to the plexus. A complication of this injury is subluxation of the head of the radius (Fig. 265); this leads to limitation of flexion and external rotation.

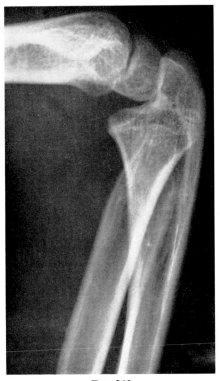

FIG. 265
Subluxation of head of radius complicating
Erb's palsy. (Child now 6 years old.)

If the injury is severe there may be paralysis of the whole arm. Treatment is carried out on similar lines but complete recovery is unlikely.

Very rarely, the lumbo-sacral plexus is damaged, but obviously this lesion is more difficult to produce than a similar lesion in the brachial plexus. There is flaccid paralysis of the leg. In the few cases we have seen recovery has never been complete.

LESIONS OF PERIPHERAL NERVES

Median Nerve.—Damage to the median nerve may follow wounds of the forearm—usually from glass. Median nerve palsy may also be associated with Volkmann's paralysis. A lesion above the elbow involves the flexor muscles of the wrist, the fingers and thumb, pronator teres and pronator quadratus as well as the oppenens pollicis, flexor pollicis brevis and the superficial head of the abductor pollicis.

Clinical Features.—There is atrophy of the thenar eminence and sensory loss in the thumb, index and middle fingers and half of the ring finger. There may be trophic disturbances and wasting of the terminal phalanx of the index finger, the finger being thin, pointed and conical.

Treatment.—The ideal treatment of a divided nerve is immediate end-to-end suture and this can usually be carried out safely within the first ten or twelve hours after injury. If the wound is grossly contaminated or if there is delay in treatment secondary suture is performed as soon as the wound is soundly healed. If this is not possible *in situ* the nerve is transposed in front of the pronator teres and suture performed. If end-to-end suture is impossible the sensory branch of the radial nerve is anastomosed to the median at the wrist to give a return of sensation.

Ulnar Nerve.—Ulnar palsy may follow cuts at the wrist (the median nerve may be damaged at the same time). The ulnar nerve supplies the intrinsic muscles of the hand; there is anæsthesia of the palmar aspect of the fifth and the ulnar side of the ring finger. Ulnar palsy may be a complication of supracondylar fracture of the humerus. It may be an immediate complication or may occur later due to increasing deformity of the elbow. The results following suture at the wrist are only fair. No splint is used and early movements are encouraged. In delayed ulnar palsy following supracondylar fracture anterior transplantation of the nerve is carried out.

Radial Nerve.—Radial palsy may follow contusion of the upper arm. There is drop-wrist. Following suitable splintage the results are good.

SPASTIC PARALYSIS

The term *cerebral palsy* covers a large group of patients with lesions of mixed ætiology. Intracranial birth injury is the most important single cause and almost half the patients present with spastic paralysis. Following loss of cerebral inhibition muscle tone is increased, reflexes are exaggerated and there is a state of hypertonus. There is weakness, stiffness and loss of control of the affected limb rather than definite paralysis. Later there may be atrophy, contraction and deformity; athetoid movements may be seen. The paralysis may take the form of a monoplegia, paraplegia, hemiplegia or quadriplegia (diplegia) (Fig. 266). The pædiatric surgeon tends to classify the patient according to the most predominant handicap. Although it is desirable to give parents some idea of the future prospects for their child, it is exceedingly difficult to give an accurate prognosis in the young child.

The cerebral damage may be *antenatal*, due to cerebral agenesis, Rhesus incompatibility or kernicterus; *natal*, due to asphyxia or birth injury; *post-natal*, following meningitis, encephalitis or trauma.

Clinical Features.—If the damage has been severe death occurs early. In mild cases of spastic paralysis it is difficult to make a diagnosis in the early months of life and the final assessment may be very difficult during the first two years. The child is slow in sitting up, slow in standing, walking and talking. The affected limb or limbs may be smaller than normal. There is no reaction of degeneration. There is inco-ordination of movements rather than paralysis. Speech, sight and hearing may be involved and there may be convulsions. Disturbances of sensation are rare. There are varying degrees of mental deficiency, but at the best the child is usually emotionally unstable. Thirteen per cent. are idiots and 50 per cent. are feeble-minded. The mental condition improves when the child becomes ambulant following physiotherapy, appropriate splintage or operation, and the improvement may be dramatic once the child is capable of mixing with other children. Deformities occur as the result of spasm or from the pull of stronger muscle groups.

Treatment.—Treatment consists essentially of training the

child to overcome the effects of the spasm and inco-ordination of the muscles. The results depend largely upon the degree of mental impairment present and the extent of co-operation from the child and from the parents. The physiotherapist aims at relaxation of spasm, encouragement of co-ordination and

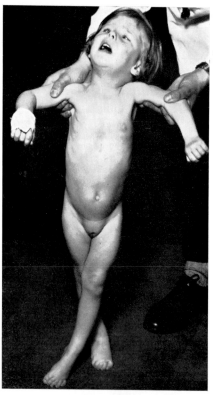

Fig. 266
Spastic diplegia.

prevention of contractures, and for this a sound knowledge of child psychology is essential. Where speech is affected the services of a speech therapist are enlisted to allow the child to benefit from the ordinary school education.

Night splints may be required to aid in the prevention of contractures and ambulatory splints and appliances to encourage walking. Operative treatment may be required in older children from 5 years onwards. This may take the form of relief of severe spasm by cutting part or all of the nerve supply—most commonly section of the obturator nerve in severe adduction spasm. Where contractures have been allowed to occur the contracted muscles may be cut or the tendons lengthened. Surgery may help to secure the erect posture when the knees are flexed. Adductor tenotomy however is rarely satisfactory, and lengthening of the tendo Achillis usually does more harm than good. In persistent equinus, passive stretching exercises, wedged plaster casts or suitable splints or footwear help to improve function of the anterior tibial muscles. Operative treatment is usually only a preliminary step to allow the physiotherapist to carry out essential treatment more effectively.

ACUTE ANTERIOR POLIOMYELITIS

This is an acute infective fever which is usually sporadic but may be epidemic. The disease is due to a filterable virus reaching the central nervous system through the nasopharynx or gut. There is fever, muscle tenderness and paralysis which at first may be widespread due to inflammatory œdema of the cells in the anterior horn of the cord. As the inflammatory products are absorbed there is partial recovery. Any residual paralysis is related to the areas of the cord which are irreparably damaged. Muscles which are still completely paralysed six months after the onset of the disease are permanently paralysed. Almost all recovery in a muscle takes place by the twelfth month and recovery in an individual muscle is complete after twenty-four months. Paralysis most commonly affects the leg, arm and trunk in that order.

Treatment.—The patient is isolated in a fever hospital and is initially given complete functional rest. To relax all paralysed muscles thorough and continuous splintage is applied early in the disease. Joints are immobilised in the neutral position and splints are adjusted as groups of muscles recover. If paralysis is extensive a complete plaster shell may be necessary. A respirator will be required for bulbar palsy. The stage of recovery lasts from six months to two years and presents many orthopædic problems. At first the child is given non-weight-bearing exercises and then comes re-education and suitable splintage, *e.g.*, an abduction or aeroplane splint for paralysis of the shoulder girdle, a cock-up splint for a drop-wrist, a walking caliper for leg palsies, a back brace to support spinal muscles combined with a corset if the abdominal muscles are affected. Drop-foot splints, lateral irons and T-straps are fitted as required. Massage and graduated exercises are given. Operative treatment is not considered until two years after the onset of the disease, and few operations are performed before puberty. Operations take the form of tendon transplantations, stabilising of flail joints, lengthening of a short limb or operations devised to overcome contractures.

Recent advances in immunology have led to the introduction of poliomyelitis vaccine and vaccination programmes are in progress in most civilised countries. Within a few years this dreaded crippling disease may be reduced in incidence and severity, and in the lifetime of some of our readers poliomyelitis may become a rare disease.

Index

* When Conrad Ramstedt first described his procedure, he spelt his name Rammstedt.

Printed in Great Britain at THE DARIEN PRESS LTD., Edinburgh